T0251490

100 Notable Names
from General Practice

100 Notable Names from General Practice

Edited by

Neil Metcalfe
General Practitioner
York, UK

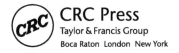

CRC Press
Taylor & Francis Group
Boca Raton London New York

CRC Press is an imprint of the
Taylor & Francis Group, an **informa** business

CRC Press
Taylor & Francis Group
6000 Broken Sound Parkway NW, Suite 300
Boca Raton, FL 33487-2742

© 2019 by Taylor & Francis Group, LLC
CRC Press is an imprint of Taylor & Francis Group, an Informa business

No claim to original U.S. Government works
Printed on acid-free paper

International Standard Book Number-13: 978-1-138-09950-0 (Hardback)
International Standard Book Number-13: 978-1-498-75198-8 (Paperback)

This book contains information obtained from authentic and highly regarded sources. While all reasonable efforts have been made to publish reliable data and information, neither the author[s] nor the publisher can accept any legal responsibility or liability for any errors or omissions that may be made. The publishers wish to make clear that any views or opinions expressed in this book by individual editors, authors or contributors are personal to them and do not necessarily reflect the views/opinions of the publishers. The information or guidance contained in this book is intended for use by medical, scientific or health-care professionals and is provided strictly as a supplement to the medical or other professional's own judgement, their knowledge of the patient's medical history, relevant manufacturer's instructions and the appropriate best practice guidelines. Because of the rapid advances in medical science, any information or advice on dosages, procedures or diagnoses should be independently verified. The reader is strongly urged to consult the relevant national drug formulary and the drug companies' and device or material manufacturers' printed instructions, and their websites, before administering or utilizing any of the drugs, devices or materials mentioned in this book. This book does not indicate whether a particular treatment is appropriate or suitable for a particular individual. Ultimately it is the sole responsibility of the medical professional to make his or her own professional judgements, so as to advise and treat patients appropriately. The authors and publishers have also attempted to trace the copyright holders of all material reproduced in this publication and apologize to copyright holders if permission to publish in this form has not been obtained. If any copyright material has not been acknowledged please write and let us know so we may rectify in any future reprint.

Except as permitted under U.S. Copyright Law, no part of this book may be reprinted, reproduced, transmitted, or utilized in any form by any electronic, mechanical, or other means, now known or hereafter invented, including photocopying, microfilming, and recording, or in any information storage or retrieval system, without written permission from the publishers.

For permission to photocopy or use material electronically from this work, please access www.copyright.com (http://www.copyright.com/) or contact the Copyright Clearance Center, Inc. (CCC), 222 Rosewood Drive, Danvers, MA 01923, 978-750-8400. CCC is a not-for-profit organization that provides licenses and registration for a variety of users. For organizations that have been granted a photocopy license by the CCC, a separate system of payment has been arranged.

Trademark Notice: Product or corporate names may be trademarks or registered trademarks, and are used only for identification and explanation without intent to infringe.

Visit the Taylor & Francis Web site at
http://www.taylorandfrancis.com

and the CRC Press Web site at
http://www.crcpress.com

To Wilfie, Toby and Beatrice.

CONTENTS

PART 1: General Practitioners Pre-Twentieth Century

PART 2: General Practitioners from the First Half of the Twentieth Century

PART 3: Contributions from General Practitioners 1950–1967

PART 4: Featured General Practitioners from the Last 50 Years (1967–2017)

LIST OF ABBREVIATIONS

BChir	Bachelor of Surgery
BMA	British Medical Association
BMJ	*British Medical Journal*
CBE	Commander of the Order of the British Empire
DBE	Dame Commander of the Order of the British Empire
DSc	Doctor of Science
EBMA	European Board of Medical Assessors
FRCGP	Fellowship of the Royal College of General Practitioners
FRCP	Fellow of the Royal College of Physicians
FRCS	Fellow of the Royal College of Surgeons
GMC	General Medical Council
GMSC	General Medical Services Committee (of the BMA), post 1998 the GPC
GP	General Practitioner
GPC	General Practitioners Committee (of the BMA), post 1998 the GMSC
HIMS	Highlands and Islands Medical Service
JCPTGP	Joint Committee on Postgraduate Training for General Practice
LLD	Doctor of Laws
LRCM	Licentiate of the Royal Conservatory of Music (Canada)
LRCP	Licentiate of the Royal College of Physicians
LRCS	Licentiate of the Royal College of Surgeons
LSA	Licentiate of the Society of Apothecaries
MB	Bachelor of Medicine
MBBChir	Bachelor of Medicine, Bachelor of Surgery
MBBS	Bachelor of Medicine, Bachelor of Surgery
MBChB	Bachelor of Medicine, Bachelor of Surgery
MBE	Member of the Order of the British Empire
MD	Doctor of Medicine (United Kingdom)
MDDUS	Medical and Dental Defence Union of Scotland
MOH	Medical Officer of Health
MP	Member of Parliament
MPhils	Master of Philosophy
MRC	Medical Research Council
MRCGP	Membership of the Royal College of General Practitioners
MRCP	Member of the Royal College of Physicians
MRCS	Member of the Royal College of Surgeons
MSc	Master of Science
NHI	National Health Insurance
NHS	National Health Service
NIA	National Insurance Act
OBE	Officer of the Order of the British Empire
Oxford DNB	Oxford Dictionary of National Biography
PhD	Doctor of Philosophy
RAF	Royal Air Force
RAMC	Royal Army Medical Corps
RCGP	Royal College of General Practitioners (pre-1967 The College of General Practitioners)
RCP	Royal College of Physicians
RCS	Royal College of Surgeons
RMO	Resident Medical Officer
RNVR	Royal Naval Volunteer Reserve
The College	The College of General Practitioners [from 1967 Royal College of General Practitioners (RCGP)]

UWCM	University of Wales College of Medicine
VTWP	Vocational Training Working Party
WHO	World Health Organization
WONCA	World Health Organization of National Colleges, Academies, and Academic Associations of General Practitioners/Family Physicians (after 1992 World Organization of Family Doctors)

ACKNOWLEDGEMENTS

I would like to express my gratitude to the many people who helped see me complete this book. I am very appreciative to Dr Jo Koster at Taylor & Francis who kindly, at the start of the project, was both supportive and enthusiastic in my going forward with the idea of this book; her support and advice throughout have been invaluable. Her colleagues, Julia Molloy and Ben O'Hara, have also been extremely helpful at various times of the project, together with those who have further helped in the editing, proofreading and design of the manuscript.

Once the project got started, I needed skilled and interested authors and co-authors and so wish to thank all who have contributed written material for the 100 main chapters. I may never have again so many emails to be involved with in a project as this one, so thank you for their understanding and communication which has led to their ability to keep to the required style and content for the chapters.

In order to assist my own research as well as that of other authors of this book, I am thankful to several archives and libraries. In particular, Dr Sharon Messenger at the Royal College of General Practitioners (RCGP) archive has been enthusiastic throughout in her support but has also helped provide written content suggestions as well as access to many of the images used in the book. She has been most obliging in granting me and a number of the authors access to her interesting and easy-to-use archive. Fiona Watson, librarian at the RCGP, has helped with numerous literature searches and a number of requests; I am grateful for the consistency of her timely and courteous manner throughout. At the British Medical Association (BMA) Records and Archives, Lee Sands and Ben Davis have also been extremely helpful for providing both accurate information on when any featured general practitioners had roles at the BMA as well as a number of images.

I am very grateful to all those who facilitated the progress of this book. Each devolved council of the RCGP helped make useful suggestions, provided contacts as well as information to help. There were many colleagues and family members of the featured general practitioners in this book who provided anecdotes, images, papers and personal facts which helped the manuscripts become more accurate and better reflected their family, personal and working lives. Furthermore, I am especially beholden to colleagues who read some of the chapters. Professor Jonathan Reinarz gave me expert advice on the introduction to the book; Professor Sir Denis Pereira Gray shared his knowledge on the introductions to the four separate parts of the book as well as the chapters on Richard McConaghey and John Burdon, whilst Dr Chris Timmins made perceptive points on John Fry. In addition, I am indebted for all those who have kindly granted permission to reproduce the figures included in the book.

Above all I would like to thank my family. Without the loving sacrifices and devotion provided throughout my childhood and beyond by my parents, Colin and Leonie, my ambition to be a general practitioner and have a career with various interests that it has brought me would very possibly never have materialised. This is something that I will forever be grateful for. Lastly, and not least, I thank my lovely wife, Harriet, for putting up with constant papers and jottings spread throughout our house, as well as my wonderful children who always make me smile and who have all attempted at one time or another to make interesting additions to this book's manuscript.

EDITOR

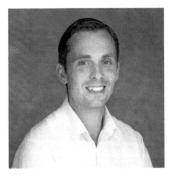

Dr Neil Metcalfe, BMedSc (Hons) MBChB DRCOG DCH PGCME FRCGP, is a general practitioner in York, England. He earned both of his undergraduate degrees from the University of Birmingham, where his medical degree in 2004 followed an earlier intercalated honours degree in the History of Medicine. Whilst a medical student, he was awarded prizes in anaesthetics, general practice, tropical medicine and writing. He qualified as a general practitioner in 2008, achieving MRCGP with distinction. He has published over 100 papers in English and French journals on subjects including dermatology, general practice, medical education and the history of medicine. He has presented at international meetings and delivered a keynote speech on the history of military medicine at the Association of Anaesthetists of Great Britain and Ireland. He is an honorary senior clinical tutor at Hull York Medical School and has created and delivers several undergraduate modules at a number of medical schools in England, including in the history of medicine. In 2013, he was awarded the first-ever RCGP First 5 GP Enterprise Award before being voted the overall winner of the RCGP Enterprise Award. He was elected FRCGP in 2016.

CONTRIBUTORS

Anizatul Ahmad
3rd year medical student
University of Leeds

Rizwan Akhtar
5th year medical student
University of Leeds

Mariam Altheyab
4th year medical student
University of Leeds

Phoebe Anderson
5th year medical student
University of Manchester

Philippa Banks
3rd year medical student
University of Leeds

Matthew Betts
4th year medical student
University of Manchester

Duncan Blues
Foundation doctor
Edinburgh

Tadhg J.G. Blunt
5th year medical student
University of Manchester

Fraser McMillan Brooks
5th year medical student
University of Manchester

Sophie Joyce Brotherton
Locum SpR Fellow (Registrar) in Acute Medicine
Wirral University Teaching Hospital NHS
    Foundation Trust

Emily Brown
Locum junior doctor
North Bristol Trust

Matt Butler
Foundation doctor
North Middlesex University Hospital

Charmaine Carter
General practitioner specialist trainee
North West Deanery

Caroline Cartlidge
4th year medical student
University of Leeds

James Clark
General practitioner specialist trainee
Salford Royal
NHS Foundation Trust

Fiona Cowie
5th year medical student
University of Aberdeen

Anna-Marie Dale
4th year medical student
University of Leeds

Adam Davies
4th year medical student
University of Leeds

John Anthony Doherty
5th year medical student (with European Studies)
University of Manchester

Freya Doswell
4th year medical student
Hull York Medical School

Jessica Dunphy
Foundation doctor
Doncaster Royal Infirmary

Rebecca Dunphy
General practitioner specialist trainee
North West Deanery

Camille Gajria
General practitioner
London

Abigail Gittens
5th year medical student
University of Leeds

Christopher Goode
Foundation doctor
Hull and East Yorkshire Hospitals

Alan Gopal
Academic junior doctor
Hull and East Yorkshire Hospitals

Chanu Gunasekara
Foundation doctor
Leeds

Katherine Halford
Foundation doctor
Hull Royal Infirmary

Alaina Halim
5th year medical student
University of Manchester

Lucy Hamer
4th year medical student
University of Leeds

Geraldine M. Hayes
5th year medical student (with European studies)
University of Manchester

Rebecca Jane Helliwell
4th year medical student
University of Leeds

George Higginbotham
3rd year medical student
University of Leeds

Julia Humphreys
General practitioner and senior clinical lecturer
Manchester Medical School
University of Manchester

Sohail A. Iftakhar
Foundation doctor
Oldham

Armaan Iqbal
Intercalating medical student
University of Leeds

Ayesha Islam
4th year medical student
University of Leeds

Adam J. Jakes
Obstetrics & Gynaecology academic clinical fellow
Guy's & St Thomas' Hospital

Daniel James
General practitioner
Bury St. Edmunds

Ivan Jobling
Foundation doctor
West Yorkshire

Emma-Jane Jones
4th year medical student
University of Leeds

Kayleigh Jones
Foundation doctor
York

Krishma Kataria
5th year medical student
University of Aberdeen

Mohammedabbas Khaki
General practitioner
North West London

Atia Khan
Foundation doctor
Halifax

Hiba Khan
5th year medical student
Hull York Medical School

Saadiyah Khan
4th year medical student
University of Leeds

Rebecca Kingston
Foundation doctor
Great Western Hospital

Aidan Lee
Anaesthesiology resident
University of Toronto

Joanna Legg
Intercalating psychology student
Kings College London

Jeannine D. Lemon
3rd year medical student
University of Leeds

Alexandra Macnamara
Clinical teaching fellow
Hull York Medical School

Olivia Macnamara
5th year medical student
University of Nottingham

Mehreen Mahfooz
Foundation doctor
York

Jean-Claude Massey
5th year medical student
University of Manchester

Sayyada Mawji
General practitioner specialist trainee
North West London Deanery

Clare McGenity
Foundation doctor
Mid Yorkshire Hospitals Trust

Mason McGlynn
4th year medical student
University of Leeds

Sharon Messenger
Archivist
Royal College of General Practitioners

Harriet Metcalfe
Student recruitment manager
York St. John University

Neil Metcalfe
General practitioner
York

Imogen Monks
Foundation doctor
Watford

Katherine Moor
5th year medical student
University of Leeds

Sophie Moriarty
4th year medical student
University of Leeds

Eleanor Morris
3rd year medical student
Hull York Medical School

Martha Kate Nicholson
5th year medical student
Hull York Medical School

Rhea Nicholson
4th year medical student
University of Leeds

Amy L. Northall
3rd year medical student
University of Sheffield

Odon Nsungu
2nd year medical student
University of Grenada

Olivia Owen
Foundation doctor
University of Hospitals Leicester Trust

James Parry-Reece
4th year medical student
Hull York Medical School

Georgie Patrick
5th year medical student
University of Manchester

Stuart Pinder
5th year medical student
University of Leeds

Zahra Ramzan
2nd year medical student
University of Leeds

Rohin Reddy
3rd year medical student
Hull York Medical School

Hannah Louise Regan
Foundation doctor
Liverpool

Nathan Samuel
3rd year medical student
Hull York Medical School

Sabrina Samuels
Foundation doctor
United Lincolnshire Hospitals

Priyana Sen
Foundation doctor
Leicester

Priya J. Shah
4th year intercalating medical student
University of Leeds

Saumil Shah
4th year medical student
Hull York Medical School

Umair Shahid
5th year medical student
University of Leeds

Zoe Shipley
Foundation doctor
Derby

Olivia Sjökvist
Foundation doctor
Winchester

Isabel Slark
4th year medical student
University of Leeds

David M. Smith
Academic junior doctor
Yorkshire Hospitals

Collette Isabel Stadler
General practitioner specialist trainee
Cambridge

Lukas Kurt Josef Stadler
Research scientist
University of Cambridge

William Mark Stevens
3rd year medical student
University of Leeds

Neena Suchdev
Foundation Doctor
Newcastle

Sarah K. Taylor
5th year medical student
Hull York Medical School

Paula Tebay
Trainer with The Art Room
Oxford

Emma L. Vinton
Medical writer and community psychiatric nurse
Newcastle Upon Tyne

Daniel Ward
General practitioner
Essex

Fiona Watson
Librarian
Royal College of General Practitioners

Patricia Wilkie
Honorary President and Chairman
National Association for Patient Participation

Bernadette Wolff
4th year medical student
University of Nottingham

Samuel Wood
Foundation doctor
York

Rebecca N. Woollin
Foundation doctor
Sunderland

Rashi Yadav
4th year medical student
University of Leeds

INTRODUCTION

Learning from medical history is crucial and established. Hippocrates wrote in the fourth century BC that 'the physician should know what the physician before him has known if he does not want to deprive himself and others'.[1] This pattern of knowledge and experience accumulation was supported in more recent times by the eminent physician Sir William Osler (1849–1919) who said 'History maketh a young man to be old, without either wrinkles or grey hairs; privileging him with the experience of age, without either the infirmities or inconveniences thereof'.[2] Guidance from the General Medical Council's (GMC's) *Tomorrow's Doctors*,[3] which was first published in 1993, did much indirectly to try and establish medical history within medical schools. New curricula was introduced when suggestions to move from courses that aimed to merely gain knowledge to those that permitted a learning process were taken on board by medical schools.[3] This is because many saw medical history as a subject that helps students to develop critical and analytical skills, enhance writing skills and allow them to broaden their educational horizons.[4] This can be as a result of exposing the reader to worlds and histories beyond the classroom, lecture theatres, laboratories or hospital wards.[4] The same skills set can be obtained whether approaching the subject from a medical, scientific or humanities background. It has now become an academic discipline in its own right.

One facet of medical history is medical biography. Originally, the main method for medical history research and teaching was through the biographies of past great medics and surgeons. Just two such examples from the nineteenth century include John Glaister's (1856–1932) *Dr William Smellie and his Contemporaries: A Contribution to the History of Midwifery in the Eighteenth Century*[5] as well as Joseph Adams' (1756–1818) *Memoirs of the Life and Doctrines of the Late John Hunter* (1818).[6] Medical biography details the lives and careers of these individuals.

Particularly in the second half of the twentieth century, biography as a research tool was maligned by some historians.[7] Vita Fortunati, Professor of English Literature at the University of Bologna, wrote using the comparative example of the biography of literature that it was not felt important in the 1960s to know the lives of the authors when reviewing literary works; however, this ceased in the late 1980s when it was realised instead to be a useful instrument in the interpretation of the literary texts.[7] She reported that scientific biography took longer to be accepted and that is was a paradox because the history of science had been regularly popular with the public and useful in popularising science, nevertheless that there had been a lack of recognition, on the part of the historians of science, of the usefulness of such a tool.[7] Several of the reasons for the mistrust in biography by some historians was written in a review by Mark Jackson (1959–).[8] The former physician and now professor and also Director of the Welcome Centre for Cultures and Environments of Health at the University of Exeter mentioned that some historians had considered biographies to be too narrow a method of study; focusing on an individual was at the expense of learning about the bigger picture of how society functioned through economical, political and cultural influences.[8] He went on to mention some had an issue with most medical biographies in that they used to feature only the great names, often those with eponyms.[8] Some examples include the eponyms for medical diseases named after Sir Percival Pott (1714–1788) and Sir James Paget (1814–1899), or eponyms for clinical signs named after Sir Jonathan Hutchinson (1828–1913), such as Hutchinson's pupil, freckle, teeth and triad. Focusing on such names meant that the sample size of people written about was too small; not enough medical biographies of the ordinary man or woman, such as laboratory workers, nurses or patients were written to allow generalisations of a particular branch or type of medical practitioner to be made. Furthermore, there can be difficulties, as also discussed by Thomas Söderqvist,[9] emeritus professor of Medical Museion at the University of Copenhagen, related to the disadvantages of being drawn into the lives of their subjects, as if having known them, and perhaps becoming too subjective and uncritical.[8]

The study of medical biography, however, was summarised by both Fortunati and Ann Jackson to being more accepted today than previously and that it can offer a useful research method of medical history.[7,8] This was particularly felt to be those biographies which include both the low and high points of their subjects lives and accomplishments. One argument supporting this is that if studying a social, cultural or political influence on a medical history subject then answers can only be obtained if the people being mentioned are known about.[8] Secondly, observing the highs and lows in life stories, whether personal or career related, can, as Osler frequently argued, be illuminating, inspiring and educational.[10] This is also echoed in the book on western medicine written by Professor Jacalyn Duffin (1950–), who, like Osler, is a Canadian physician, historian and educator. In her *History of Medicine: A Scandalously Short Introduction* (1999) she describes a pedagogical tool to stimulate the interest of even the most tunnel-visioned medical students: a game of heroes and villains.[11] In the game, students choose a figure from a list of names from the history of medicine. Then, by using primary and secondary sources, the students decide whether the figures were villains or heroes. The winner of the game is the student who first recognises that whether a person is a villain or hero depends on how you look at their life. If the student or reader can identify with some parts of the history and events described then they can be inspired by them, as well as learn something for their own edification. This potentially wider public appeal of medical biography in itself can also promote the medical historians who have researched and published about it to a broader audience, helping them become valid and important contributors to medical history.[12]

Attempts to include medical biographies in the medical history literature have been met with mixed results. Medical history has countless books, journals, museums and archives devoted to it, but what about medical biography? Of course, there are numerous biographies and autobiographies of individual medical practitioners, such as the biographies written by Duffin of René Laennec (1781–1826)[13] and James Langstaff (1825–1889),[14] as well as Professor Michael Bliss' studies of Harvey Cushing (1869–1939)[15] and Osler[16] being excellent modern examples. In terms of collections of biographies, by far the largest is the *Oxford Dictionary of National Biography* (*Oxford DNB*),[17] which is the successor to the 22-volume *Dictionary of National Biography* published between 1894 and 1902 and updated with decennial supplements. At the time of writing, amongst the 72 million words from 60,061 entries that the *Oxford DNB* has produced on British nationals who have died, 3278 medical biographies are present, some of which have been revised and rewritten over time. More internationally diverse and specific to health professionals is the *Dictionary of Medical Biography* (2006), edited by husband-and-wife medical historians Professor William and Helen Bynum.[18] Amongst its five volumes are 1140 entries which include coverage across medical systems, time periods and cultures. Anne Digby, Emeritus Professor of history at Oxford Brookes University, in her review of it mentioned 'it is an impressive addition to the existing number of dictionaries of medical or scientific biography which, given the potential of the subject, is still surprisingly limited in scope'.[19] This is similar with journals, as medical biography does feature regularly in medical history, general medical or medical speciality journals. There is, however, just one journal specific to medical biography. Since 1993, the *Journal of Medical Biography* has been published quarterly, and, by the end of 2016, has published 1608 medical biographies in total.[20] However, not all of these entries are of people as they can include entries regarding museums, statues and blue plaques amongst others.

Attention now turns to medical biographies about general practitioners. In terms of books, Sir Zachary Cope (1881–1974) wrote *Some Famous General Practitioners and Other Medical Historical Essays* (1961) which had one chapter of the whole book containing 11 biographies about general practitioners from around the world.[21] When using the *Oxford DNB* and specifically searching by statement of occupation featuring physician, surgeon or general practitioner there are 1428, 578 and 26 entries respectively, which means that general practitioners feature in 1.28 per cent of the total biographies from that group of occupations. This is slightly higher than the results produced, using the same search, within the titles of the articles in the *Journal of Medical Biography* where the eight papers on general practitioners account for 0.50 per cent of the total biographies. In the *Dictionary of Medical Biography* there were 17 (1.49 per cent) entries dedicated to general practice within the history of medicine across the world.[20] It must be mentioned that there are limitations in obtaining these numbers because previous biographers, editors and the medical professionals themselves have varied in their nomenclature of work categories. Terms such as apothecary, apothecary-surgeon, consultant, medic, medical practitioner, military surgeon, quack and specialist are just some of the phrases, which according to the resource can be included or excluded in the broader categories of physician, surgeon or general practitioner.

Does the low percentage of general practitioner biographies represent the actual percentage of doctors who work as general practitioners? The answer is that it does not. In November 2016, there were 67,758 general practitioners registered with the GMC in the United Kingdom, which was 43.3 per cent of the total workforce who had completed training.[22] From a study of the Organisation for Economic Co-operation and Development in 2013, an average of 30 per cent of all medical doctors working from 33 countries were general practitioners.[23] The same study revealed that the percentage of general practitioners in the workforce had, on average, lowered over the decades.[23] This information, therefore, suggests that there is a significant discrepancy between the percentage of general practitioners being written about and that of hospital specialists. Considering that the history of general practice also seems limited to the studies and works of Irvine Loudon's (1924–2015) *Medical Care and the General Practitioner 1750–1850* (1986)[24] Digby's *The Evolution of British General Practice 1850–1949* (1999),[25] and the edited *General Practice under the National Health Service 1948–1997* (1998),[26] one could generally conclude to an absence of histories of general practice, particularly when compared to the dozens of histories available on hospitals and hospital specialities. This book aims to help fill some of that gap by providing a collection of short biographies of general practitioners.

In structuring and organising this book, initial parameters had to be determined. Due to a combination of my being a general practitioner having trained and worked in the National Health Service (NHS), having an active interest in British medical history and having experienced the lengths of time occasionally required to obtain primary historical sources, where survival of general practitioner records seems to be lower than those of hospital records and specialists records and a possible cause for their histories being absent, it was deemed appropriate to focus the book on British general practice. All general practitioners to be included had to have worked in the British Isles as a general practitioner even if born, trained or ultimately celebrated for work elsewhere. A time frame for the book had to be determined. The wish was to include as wide a range of time periods from British general practice as possible, and to include broadly similar numbers of general practitioners from each period. Since the William Rose (1640–1711) cases of 1703 and 1704 have been considered by many to establish the legal foundations for general practice in England, all general practitioners included worked as such after 1703. This includes some that are alive and practising today.

Making decisions regarding which general practitioners to include required careful thought. In order to allow each biography to feature sufficiently detailed information, be a respectable mode of academic reference and permit at the same time the book to feature as many general practitioners as possible, within tight overall word count pressures, a total number of 100 biographies, each similar in length, was set. A general practitioner with a notable career may have had an influence on one or more areas such as medical education, medical politics, the organisational structure of general practice, research and all of these of course either at local or national levels. There is a recognised need in medical history since the 1980s to reflect regional variation and so it has been important to reflect provincial practice in a number of cases.[27] As biographies also feature lives away from work, general practitioners who have influenced the arts, national politics and welfare, non-medical academia and sport have also been included. Finally, considering the difficulties women suffered from, given the prejudices male scientists historically held against them, it has been proposed by Fortunati that biographies of female scientists could provide an important pedagogical function in the education of girls and young women in order to help introduce them to the world of science and research.[7] Therefore, on applying this to medical science, biographies of perhaps historically lesser-known female general practitioners have been included, taking into account the discrepancy in the ratio of male to female general practitioners which has existed for centuries until only recently. Eleven chapters are on biographies of female general practitioners. All of this helps to hopefully ensure a breadth of general practitioner biographies.

Despite these reasons, some readers may be surprised by some names having been included or excluded. Further reasoning takes into account, to a degree, the list put together in 2010 by a panel of leading general practitioners to mark the 50th anniversary of *Pulse* entitled *50 GPs Who Shaped (or Will Shape) General Practice*.[28] General practitioners chosen with focus on their general practice careers have had careers that reflect the changes in practice over this three-century period. Consequently, many general practitioners could unfortunately not be included, even if having held certain high-ranking positions with national or international organisations. From the BMA and RCGP only those appointed to the most influential role at the BMA, the Chairman of Council and the general practitioners whose careers are already acknowledged to be exemplary when being appointed to President of the RCGP, which is the constitutional head and most prestigious position at that organisation, could be fitted in. Similarly, not all general practitioners who have represented their country in sport could be included. Just taking the England Rugby Football Union team as an example, there have been to date 65 medical doctors to have represented the team. Not all of their careers are known about, but 17 of them are known to have been general practitioners working in Great Britain.[29] Ultimately, those selected from the sporting world included WG Grace (1848–1915), for being the first international sports star, as well as those who obtained the pinnacle of many sports, an Olympic gold medal.

There are two names included that I believe are worth specifically explaining to some readers. Firstly, Joseph Collings (1918–1971) was an Australian general practitioner who spent time in British general practice. His time may not have been necessarily spent consulting patients but he did observe 104 general practitioners from 55 practices across the United Kingdom in the late 1940s and his report, *The Collings Report*, has been cited as 'the single most effective factor in mobilising opinion in favour of constructive change, and as a catalysing contribution to the formation of the RCGP'.[30] The other name is Harold Shipman (1946–2004). He has been included as his murders led to significant changes to British general practice. It was felt this was more than Bodkin Adams (1899–1983) who was a convicted fraudster and, although a suspected serial killer, was never convicted of murder. The case exemplifies what Jonathan Reinarz and Rebecca Wynter, respectively professor and post-doctoral researcher at the History of Medicine Unit at the University of Birmingham, discussed in *Complaints, Controversies and Grievances in Medicine* (2015).[31] They concluded that controversy and complaints can be powerful, have important ways which can inform wide historical and contemporary discussions and be used as a positive agent of health care development. The same *Pulse*[28] article, mentioned above, also placed Shipman as the 5th most influential general practitioner from the past on British general practice which, rather like Duffin's aforementioned 'Heroes and Villains' exercise, shows that different views can be created on the same piece of history. To omit such a name as Shipman would be to ignore the impact, however deadly and hopefully never repeatable, he had on the history of general practice.

From the outset a variety of skilled and interested writers were sought. This has been obtained by using contributions from people with backgrounds ranging from archivists to general practitioners, medical writers to lecturers. Medical history still has some way to go to be included in the curriculum of all medical schools in the United Kingdom[32] but since there is interest in the subject within the student population, and as a means to help their learning as per the reasons already detailed, interested medical students were recruited. Interestingly, some of the authors since undertaking their writing for this book have revealed their new interest in, whilst others reconfirmed their career wish to, becoming general practitioners.

Each biography has been written in a similar style due to both a list of criteria as well as editing. Whenever possible, dates of the lives of closely associated names to the biographies have been given in the main chapters, particularly any medical doctors, to allow the reader further information that may help if ever wishing to undertake further study of associated individuals. All chapters have a 'further reading' section to provide those searching for more information with some of the main sources, since the biographies, although containing major positive and negative careers aspects, are necessarily concise.

The book has been split into several parts. A generally chronological approach has been employed so that general practitioners have been collated according to the time period in which they were most notable. The first part includes general practitioners from before the twentieth century and the second part discusses those who practised during the first half of the twentieth century. The third part concerns the early years of the second half of the twentieth century, particularly focusing on the names involved in the creation or early years of, the RCGP. The final section concerns those names from the last 50 years up to the time of writing.

As a result the book offers options on how it can be used. It could be read from start to finish, as each part has an introduction that mentions some of the main changes and activities of that period, and thus presents names in a generally chronological order. Alternatively, the reader can take a more thematic approach, looking at themes such as medical education, medical politics, research, societal involvement and look for particular general practitioners from across the centuries involved in those themes. Some general practitioners do feature in other people's biographies so the lives of those linked together can be followed from one biography to the next by cross-referencing. Furthermore, there are chapters which offer an insight into British general practice and to society as a whole so can be dipped into for personal interest. It should be reiterated that this book is not a specific history of British general practice text, for which readers are referred to the three main volumes already mentioned.[24-26] If wishing to read historical aspects to the RCGP, there are several writings available specifically related to that organisation.[33-35] However, it does offer a fresh approach by using biographies to describe some of the major parts of the history of general practice, reveal the hitherto largest number and range of contributions of general practitioners in medical and social history, as well as introduce the reader to some unfamiliar names rather than be devoted to classical general practitioners of distinction.

There is a proverb 'Footprints in the sand hills of life are not made by sitting down'. What features in many of these lives is the energies and dedication that many of these people have displayed. This has helped benefit many today, either directly or indirectly, in one form or another. There is no doubt that many other careers and lives are being conducted currently that are affecting us similarly today and in the future about whom people will be interested in writing about and reading. I hope you enjoy reading about the footprints already made.

Neil Metcalfe (January 2017)

References

1. Hunter D. History as a dimension of medicine. *Middlesex Hospital Journal* 1968;68:20–26.

2. Osler W. A note on the teaching of the history of the history of medicine. *British Medical Journal* 1902;2:93.

3. GMC. *Tomorrow's Doctors*. London: GMC, 1993.

4. Metcalfe NH, Stuart E. A short history of providing medical history within the British medical education curriculum. *Medical Humanities* 2014;40:31–37.

5. Glaister J. *Dr. William Smellie and his Contemporaries: A Contribution to the History of Midwifery in the Eighteenth Century.* Glasgow: James Maclehose & Sons; 1894.

6. Adams J. *Memoirs of the Life and Doctrines of the Late John Hunter*. London: J. Callow & J. Hunter; 1818.

7. Fortunati V. Mirror shards: Conflicting images between Marie Curie's autobiography and her biographies. In: Franceschi ZA, Govoni P (eds.). *Writing About Lives in Science: (Auto)Biography, Gender, and Genre*. Göttingen: V&R Unipress; 2014.

8. Jackson M. Biography as history. *Journal of Medical Biography* 2004;12:63–65.

9. Söderqvist T. How to write the recent history of immunology – Is the time really ripe for a narrative synthesis? *Immunology Today* 1993;14:565–68.

10. Osler W. *An Alabama Student and Other Biographical Essays*. Oxford: Clarendon Press; 1908.

11. Duffin J. *History of Medicine: A Scandalously Short Introduction*. Toronto: University of Toronto Press; 1999.

12. Nye MJ. Scientific biography: History of science by another means? *Isis* 2006;97:322–29.

13. Duffin J. *To See with a Better Eye: A Life of R. T. H. Laennec*. Princeton, NJ: Princeton University Press; 1998.

14. Duffin J. Langstaff: *A Nineteenth-century Medical Life*. Toronto: University of Toronto Press; 1993.

15. Bliss M. Harvey Cushing: *A Life in Surgery*. Oxford: Oxford University Press; 2007.

16. Bliss M. William Osler: *A Life in Medicine*. Oxford: Oxford University Press; 2007.

17. *Oxford Dictionary of National Biography*. Oxford: Oxford University Press; 2004–16.

18. Bynum WF, Bynum H (eds.). *Dictionary of Medical Biography*. London: Greenwood Press; 2006.

19. Digby A. Dictionary of medical biography. *Medical History* 2008;52(2):280–81.

20. Personal correspondence with Dr. Andrew Larner, Editor of the *Journal of Medical Biography*.

21. Cope Z. *Some Famous General Practitioners and Other Medical Historical Essays*. London: Pitman Medical Publishing Co. Ltd; 1961.

22. Personal correspondence with Mrs. Tista Chakravarty-Gannon, Principle Regional Liaison Adviser, General Medical Council.

23. OECG. *Health at a Glance 2015: OECD Indicators*. Paris: OECD Publishing; 2015.

24. Loudon I. *Medical Care and the General Practitioner 1750–1850*. Oxford: Clarendon Press; 1986.

25. Digby A. The *Evolution of British General Practice 1850–1949*. Oxford: Oxford University Press; 1999.

26. Loudon I, Horder J, Webster J (eds.). *Practice under the National Health Service 1948–1997*. Oxford: Clarendon Press; 1998.

27. Personal correspondence with Professor Jonathan Reinarz, Director of The History of Medicine Unit and Professor of the History of Medicine, University of Birmingham.

28. Anon. 50 general practitioners who shaped (or will shape) General Practice. *Pulse* 2010;17 March:18–21.

29. Personal correspondence with Mr. Richard Steele, Rugby Historian and a Committee Member and Researcher at World Rugby Museum, Twickenham, London.

30. Hunt JH. The foundation of a College. The conception, birth, and early days of the College of General Practitioners. *The Journal of the Royal College of General Practitioners* 1973;23(126):5–20.

31. Reinarz J. Wynter R. *Complaints, Controversies and Grievances in Medicine*. Oxford: Routledge; 2015.

32. Metcalfe NH, Brown AK. History of medicine student selected components at UK medical schools: A questionnaire based study. *Journal of the Royal Society of Medicine Short Reports* 2011;2(10):77.

33. Fry J, Hunt Lord of Fawley, Pinsent RJF (eds.). *A History of the Royal College of General Practitioners: The First 25 Years*. Lancaster: MTP Press; 1983.

34. Pereira Gray DJ (ed.). *Forty Years On: The Story of the First Forty Years of the Royal College of General Practitioners*. London: Atalink; 1992.

35. Johnston DJ (ed.). *Sixty Years of Knowledge and Compassion: The RCGP in Ireland 1952–2012*. Belfast: RCGP; 2012.

PART 1: GENERAL PRACTITIONERS PRE-TWENTIETH CENTURY

Featured General Practitioners Who Made Their Main Contributions before the Twentieth Century

The first part of this book will focus on general practitioners whose main contributions occurred before the twentieth century. This time period includes the emergence of general practice as we know it today. Therefore, some of the main names featured in the associations, journals and medical politics that helped lead to a number of acts are mentioned. Attention will then move on to those whose academic and research pursuits helped general practice and medicine, before also including those who were notable for their contributions to society.

Medical Politics and Medical Education Pre-Twentieth Century

Prior to the nineteenth century there was a rigid hierarchical and tripartite structure within the medical profession.[1] Physicians (FRCP) were seen to be the elite of the profession following having attended universities. This was usually at University of Oxford or University of Cambridge and they would normally also be Fellows of the Royal College of Physicians (RCP) which had been founded in 1518 during the reign of King Henry VIII.[2] Those having attended other universities usually practised under the licentiateship of this college. The physicians were able to practise in London and within seven miles of the City. They were the only ones permissible to prescribe 'physic' or medicine. The surgeons and barbers of London came together under the Medical Act of 1540 to form a company and were generally thought of as craftsman. Advances in surgery as well as the flourishing of hospitals during the eighteenth century meant the two separated in 1745 when the Company of Surgeons was established before the Royal College of Surgeons (RCS) of London was created in 1800. The third branch of the structure was the apothecaries. They were tradesmen who dispensed medicines and belonged to the Worshipful Company of Grocers that had been established in 1345. A separate Section of Apothecaries was created in 1607 and King James I granted a Royal Charter in 1617 to create the Worshipful Society of Apothecaries.

There has long been conflict between the physicians and the apothecaries. Much of this was initially to do with who had the right to prescribe. The plague in 1666 had seen the physicians flee the City leaving the Apothecaries to provide much of the care, particularly to the poor.[3] This had led to many apothecaries to dispense as well as to prescribe to the lower classes.[1] The Royal College of Physicians (RCP) had always claimed that the Physicians alone had the right to prescribe and that apothecaries should only dispense medications. This conflict came to a head in 1703 when William Rose an Apothecary, was prosecuted by the RCP for prescribing.[1,4] He initially lost and was fined but the case was reheard at the House of Lords on 15 March 1704 when Rose and the Worshipful Society of Apothecaries were found in favour to be permitted to prescribe and dispense drugs.[1,2,4] This did much to legally permit a combining of roles and a new term, 'general practitioner' was first seen in the literature a decade later in 1714,[5] though 'surgeon-apothecary' was much more frequently used during the following 100 years[1–4] and so interchangeable use of the terms will be used subject to the time period being described.

In the early nineteenth century there was new unrest in the medical profession. Medical and scientific breakthroughs were aiding many physicians and surgeons not only with actual successful treatments but also with their own prestige. This esteem was thought by some to be tainted by the blurring of roles that had happened and had seen the surgeon-apothecary combine both roles and also various types of practitioners to see themselves as a family doctor.[1] Pressure on the apothecaries themselves also came from the surgeons that had been discharged from the Army Services being able to work as surgeon-apothecaries without any actual formal training in pharmacy due to the Medical Acts of 1749 and 1763 exempting all officers from any form of apprenticeship.[6] Considering that a study in Lincolnshire by Edward Harrison (1766–1838), in 1806, showed that there were nine untrained practitioners or 'quacks' to every one doctor belonging to a recognised body,[7] those working solely as an apothecary had much competition.[1] As they were still bound to being permitted to be paid only for the dispensing of medicines and any medical advice to be given for free, temptation to overprescribe was a reality for many.

Formed from this unrest was the Apothecaries Act of 1815. There were a lot of contributors to this but the contributions of George Man Burrows and Robert Kerrison were especially important. Burrows had been disillusioned with the unrest within the apothecary and surgeon-apothecary fields such that he helped form the London Association of Apothecaries in 1812, ultimately becoming the Associated Apothecaries and Surgeon-Apothecaries due to an increase in provincial membership. He was its first chairman, something he later wrote that he would have declined if he had known the work that it would entail such as the 130 committee meetings and answering of over 1500 letters. In the three years to 1815, his work revolved aiming to improve medical education and increase the respectability of the profession.[8] Kerrison joined later that year and wrote various pieces on medical reform and his campaigning against much opposition from the medical colleges ultimately led to the passing of the Apothecaries Act on 1 August 1815. This Act was the first to introduce the need for all apothecaries to be licensed, be at least 21 years of age and to pass an examination. The Licentiate of the Society of Apothecaries (LSA) was the main, though not sole, licence and was not just for those within the confines of the City and for the seven miles around it but now a national requirement, something that drastically increased the regulatory and administrative needs of the Worshipful Society of Apothecaries. The standard for the licence gradually increased and, in 1827, midwifery and diseases of women and children were added; by 1834, apprentices had to pass an examination at the end of their training and submit a formal testimonial, and, in 1839, a medical paper was introduced.[1] A written exam in Latin from 1849, and then in 1851, one including Greek and maths, was necessary to be passed.[1]

Following on from both the work before and following the Apothecaries Act, various medical education activities occurred. The *London Medical Repository* was the voice of the Association of Apothecaries and Surgeon-Apothecaries and saw Anthony Todd Thomson join Burrows and William Royston as joint editors in 1814, a year after its first volume. Another general practitioner, Thomas Wakley, founded *The Lancet* on 5 October 1823 with the aim to spread medical knowledge amongst the medical profession but also to combat nepotism that he saw affecting hospital post appointments. There were a number of private medical schools that were created but were replaced by medical schools attached to hospitals. London University, now University College London, was the first to cater to new aspirants to general practice in 1826, and following the Report of the Select Committee on Medical Education in 1834, nine provincial medical schools were running in 1858.[1] There were also many medical associations that were formed. For example, The Metropolitan Society of General Practitioners was founded in 1831 and The National Association of General Practitioners was founded and presided by Robert Pennington in 1843. The latter had the aim of inaugurating a College of General Practitioners, Surgery and Midwifery. Opposition again came for the Royal Colleges, particularly that of the RCS, and negotiations ultimately broke down. More successful in its longevity was the Provincial Medical and Surgical Association founded in Worcester in 1832, which ultimately became the BMA in 1856.

In the second half of the nineteenth century the hierarchical system still continued and initial optimism amongst general practitioners to advance and improve this branch of medicine faded away.[4] The Medical Act of 1858 revealed all legally qualified practitioners to be equal before the law, whether or not they had qualified through obtaining one or more of the Membership of the Royal College of Surgeons (MRCS), the diploma of Licentiate of the Royal College of Physicians (LRCP), LSA or medical degrees. The Worshipful Society of Apothecaries was recognised and given a seat on the newly formed GMC. Regrettably for some there was again disagreement on a conjoint qualification with the RCP refusing to oversee training and examination of general practitioners.[1] The Medical Act of 1886 defined a qualifying examination as one in medicine, surgery and midwifery though both the RCP and RCS refused to admit the Worshipful Society of Apothecaries. Instead, the Colleges set up a joint examination, the MRCS LRCP, between themselves. This left the Worshipful Society of Apothecaries to have an ever-reducing influence. However, the Worshipful Society of Apothecaries can be said to have helped with the development of training, examining and setting standards, all especially in the first half of the nineteenth century, which proved important in establishing the general practitioner within the medical system.

Research by General Practitioners Pre-Twentieth Century

The eighteenth century was not totally bereft of surgeon-apothecaries highly respected for their work. A view of this time for many is that there were large gaps in performance between the leading names of the London physicians and surgeons and with those practising as country doctors. It was deemed that the knowledge of physic and pharmacy was primitive in the provinces and surgical skills lacking. However, from this group efforts were being made to advance medicine by surgeon-apothecaries and their lives deserve recording. John Huxham from Plymouth conducted annual series of recordings between 1724 and 1748 into the prevalence of epidemic disease. He was possibly the first to classify influenza and his work was associated with the discovery of scurvy. Similarly, Edward Jenner was the discoverer of vaccination. He first inoculated an eight-year-old boy named James Phipps in 1796 with pus taken from the cowpox blister from a local milkmaid, called Sarah Nelmes, and later inoculated Phipps with a smallpox blister, who subsequently did not go on to get smallpox. The possibility of purchasing a degree from a university, in his case from St Andrews, despite never having set foot in Scotland, merely requiring the references of two others, meant he had by then transferred to being a physician but at least 20 of his initial years as a doctor were as a surgeon-apothecary in Gloucestershire and his case load had led him to such discoveries.

Specific research on neurological structures and conditions was aided by several general practitioners in the early and mid-nineteenth century. *An Essay on the Shaking Palsy*[9] in 1817 by James Parkinson was the first to describe the condition with which he is now synonymous. Eleven years later John Abercrombie published the first textbook in neuropathology entitled *Pathological and Practical Researches on Diseases of the Brain and Spinal Cord* (1828).[10]

This subject was itself first defined by Abercrombie who, from an initial general practitioner career, went onto publish different subjects as well to become physician in Scotland to King George IV in Scotland. Particularly around the mid-nineteenth century Jacob Clarke undertook much histological research when time permitted. His work led him be the first to establish the location of the dorsal or 'Clarke's' nucleus of the spinal cord and describing the posterior vesicular column. Pioneering discoveries in other neurological conditions such as amyotrophic lateral sclerosis were also undertaken later.

Thomas Hunt enjoyed a productive career. He did much to advance epidemiology when, in 1846, he pioneered a new plan for the advancement of medical sciences submitted to the South Eastern Branch of the Provincial Medical and Surgical Association. He undertook a questionnaire of members that led to a new method of collective data collection. He also did much in dermatology that included working at the Western Dispensary for Diseases of the Skin as well and undertaking research on the potential benefits of arsenic.

Around the mid-nineteenth century, several pioneers of infectious disease work are noted. William Budd, initially from Devon, had tried unsuccessfully, in 1939, to convince contemporaries that typhoid fever was spread through close contact of infected individuals. Later, when working in Bristol in 1847, he was able to be more successful in his work when showing that contaminated water was the cause of a typhoid fever epidemic. He linked this to cholera as well but was beaten to publication and notoriety with the condition, and epidemiology and public health as a whole, by John Snow. It was Snow who, again following a number of years looking into water causation theory, was able, in 1854, to demonstrate the source of a local cholera outbreak in Soho when priming the Broad Street Pump. His relatively short life also saw him being an early user, advocate and researcher in anaesthesia, using anaesthesia during two births by Queen Victoria and receiving her approval of it; one of several reasons for its use being accepted into society.[11]

The latter half of the nineteenth century witnessed several general practitioners who ultimately become the 'fathers' of different medical and surgical branches. Charles Blackley, whilst working as a general practitioner in Lancashire, undertook multiple experiments regarding hay fever. Ideas from his experiments were discussed regularly with Charles Darwin and he is a leading historical name in the discovery of the pathogenesis of this condition. Hugh Owen Thomas had come from a family of 'bone setters' and although there were opponents to his work whilst alive, due to his work being continued and promoted by his nephew including during the First World War (1914–1918) he is posthumously seen as 'the father of British orthopaedics'. Similarly Charles MacMunn did much in his lifetime with the spectroscope that was not widely accepted contemporaneously. However, with developments after his death ultimately showing how accurate he had been, his research has been seen as important in the understanding of intracellular biochemistry. As general practice workload meant a range of patients were seen, general practice encompassed work at asylums, friendly societies, mines, railway companies and other industries. Whilst initially a medical officer with the customs service in Amoy, now Xiamen in South East China, Patrick Manson undertook research on the *Filia* parasite. His interest and successful discoveries ultimately led to a career devoted to tropical diseases, which sees him now recognised as 'the father of tropical medicine'.

The final name to include, however, is one that should feature in any historical description of general practice. James Mackenzie was born in Scotland in 1853 and much of the general practice part of his career took place in the nineteenth century. This was in Burnley, Lancashire, where he felt that university had not prepared him for the work he was doing and that much information on the early signs and symptoms of illness that might present to a general practitioner were missing. This led him to actively record many patient consultations and cardiology was the speciality that particularly benefitted from this. He wrote numerous papers and using his own polygraph, the forerunner to the electrocardiogram, he described different arrhythmias. In 1902, he published *The Study of the Pulse*,[12] which documented 28 years of personal research in Burnley. He later became a specialist in charge of the cardiology department at the London Hospital. In 1919, he founded the St Andrews Institute of Clinical Research, again aiming to find out more about early presentation of disease to general practitioners.

General Practitioners Helping Pre-Twentieth-Century Society

English literature and some non-medical literature genres benefited from several general practitioners at this time. Francis Adams was a classical scholar whose passion for Greek led him to translate many texts into English, to the benefit of many students and readers. The writings of Arthur Conan Doyle created various novels including those featuring the detective Sherlock Holmes, a character still popular today. In natural history, much research and literature was provided by Jonathan Couch and Gideon Mantell. Couch contributed much to the field of ichthyology (the zoological study of fish) including commendable work on the pilchard and his four volume illustrated *History of the Fishes of the British Islands* (1862–1865).[13] Mantell had an interest in palaeopathology that led him to discover the dinosaur Igunadon in 1822.

The work of the police has possibly benefited from the career of Henry Faulds. He was involved in a medical mission to Japan with the United Presbyterian Church of Scotland from 1873. He became very involved in the Japanese culture and was interested in the fingerprint impressions that had remained on shards of ancient Japanese pottery. He concluded that fingerprints had to be unique to each individual and could, therefore, be used for identification. He used this knowledge successfully in two legal cases in Japan and he attempted to showcase its use in forensics to the metropolitan police. The practice has become vital evidence in criminal investigations although contemporaneous society and history were not kind to Faulds, crediting the discovery to others, leading to him being known as 'the forgotten Scot'.

More successfully acknowledged was John Rhodes who did much with regard to being a poor-law reformer. As a member of the Chorlton Board of Guardians he spent a lot of time in the Chorlton Workhouse, later the Withington Hospital in South Manchester. There he deplored the dietary provisions and his criticisms led to changes in the calculations of the calorific needs of patients. In the workhouses he also instigated the employment of nurses as well as the employment of patients suffering from severe epilepsy. He did much epidemiological data collection on the poor and their medical requirements, which were then used in his campaigning, unofficially, for better provisions and for which he is positively remembered historically.

The final two general practitioners included in this time period differ in their recognisability. Representing the more locally known general practitioners who showed enterprise and provided a variety of contributions was William Close. He invented an array of equipment to help society. For miners, he devised a new technique for sand-tamping explosive charges, and for the Isle of Walney where he was based in Cumbria, he designed a hydraulic pump. For musicians he patented the drainage spittle-cock to help prevent moisture accumulating in brass instruments as well as developing a new type of trumpet. He also helped create new inks as well as provide much on local history though his deeds were not well known from his short life, perhaps due to performing them relatively remotely. A different general practitioner however, was infinitely better known during that period to the extent that his initials were instantly recognisable then and still are by many now. 'WG' Grace was the first international sports star due to his cricketing feats, though in later years he was perhaps better known in society for his rather non-athletic figure. Considering cricketing tours to Australia and other Commonwealth countries were then done by ship and so were many months long, it may surprise some that he was able to keep his general practice in Gloucestershire, albeit with the assistance of frequent and long-term locums.

References

1. Bloor DU. The rise of the general practitioner in the nineteenth century. *Journal of the Royal College of General Practitioners* 1978;28:288–91.

2. McConaghey RMS. Proposals to found a Royal College of General Practitioners in the nineteenth century. *Journal of the Royal College of General Practitioners* 1972;22:775–88.

3. Copeman WSC. *A History of the Worshipful Company of Apothecaries of London*. London: Pergamon; 1968.

4. Loudon ISL. The origin of the general practitioner. *Journal of the Royal College of General Practitioners* 1983;33:13–18.

5. Bellers J. *An Essay Towards the Improvement of Physic*. London: J. Sowle; 1714.

6. Hamilton B. The medical professions in the eighteenth century. *The Economic History Review* 1951;4(2):141–69.

7. Harrison E. *Remarks on the Ineffective State of the Practice of Physic in Great Britain with Proposals for its Future Regulation and Improvement*. London: R. Bickerstaffe; 1806.

8. Loudon I. *Medical Care and the General Practitioner 1750–1850*. Oxford: Clarendon Press; 1986.

9. Parkinson J. *An Essay on the Shaking Palsy*. London: Sherwood, Neely, & Jones; 1817.

10. Abercrombie J. *Pathological and Practical Researches of Diseases of the Brain and the Spinal Cord*. Edinburgh: Waugh and Innes; 1828.

11. Metcalfe NH. The influence of the military on civilian uncertainty about modern anaesthesia between its origins in 1846 and the end of the Crimean War in 1856. *Anaesthesia* 2005;60(6):594–601.

12. Mackenzie J. *The study of the Pulse. Arterial, venous and Hepatic and of Movements of the Heart*. Edinburgh: Young J. Pentland; 1902.

13. Couch J. *A History of the Fishes of the British Islands*. Volume IV. London: Groombridge and Sons; 1865.

1 WILLIAM ROSE (1640–1711)

Phoebe Anderson

William Rose was born in 1640 in Mickleton, Gloucestershire, to Thomas Rose and Francesse Fisher. He was the eldest of nine children. Rose's brothers were amongst the first colonists of Jamaica, who patented land in order to establish plantations under the family name. The Rose plantations established in the 1670s would persist throughout the following century. Rose himself was noted to have invested in the Royal Africa Company, which is known to have been involved in slavery. He was a wealthy man who was thought to have acted as the family banker. In his brother's will it is noted that Burrows became in possession of £1500 on his behalf; this was an enormous sum of money with a relative value today of close to £3 million. Rose moved to London from his birth town in London and subsequently married in 1666. Following the death of his first wife, Elizabeth Denton, he married his second wife, Elizabeth Cross. Between the two marriages he fathered 10 children, though two of the children died before the age of 5 years old.

Despite acting in some respects as a family banker, Rose was in fact an apothecary. He first practised in an apothecary on St. Nicholas Lane, London. He was registered with the London Society of Apothecaries in 1680 and remained on their register until 1705. Rose was no ordinary apothecary for he was a member of a wealthy and influential group within the guild, the Liverymen, all of whom were Freemen of the City of London. In order to be accepted amongst the Liverymen, an apothecary was required to have money and powerful connections. Towards the end of his career Rose was ranked amongst the heads of this group, meaning he held a position at the forefront of a large and wealthy guild, alongside some of the most influential men in London.

In the late seventeenth century, when Rose was practising, it was common for the apothecary to provide medical services to the local population, as a consultation with a physician was far too costly for the poor. By providing medicines without a prescription, apothecaries were thought by some to undermine the authority of the physicians. The RCP, who were concerned for both their reputation and their income, would try to curtail the apothecaries through strict regulation of medication and frequent inspection of their premises. For many years, tensions between the two professions ran high and eventually culminated in a landmark case, in which Rose was prosecuted. The Rose case was heard in the House of Lords in 1704 and is considered by many to have established the legal foundation for general practice in England.

Rose was working as an apothecary in London when he was prosecuted by the RCP for practising physic illegally. He had visited John Seale, an impoverished butcher, in his home and prescribed and dispensed medicines for the treatment of a venereal disease. Subsequently, Rose delivered a very large bill to the patient. The butcher's condition did not improve, it only deteriorated. Seale was so irate, more likely about the large bill than his worsening condition, that he denounced Rose to the RCP. The RCP already had reason to pursue Rose as he had been distributing a handbill advertising his own special remedy under the name of 'Rose's Balsamick Elixir'. He had marketed his remedy as the 'most noble medicine that art can produce', much to the dismay of the physicians who did not approve of such advertising. Given the growing tension between the Society and the RCP, the RCP took this opportunity to prosecute Rose before the King's Bench. Initially, the RCP's argument was accepted and Rose was fined for misbehaviour. Despite the law supporting the argument against Rose, the judge and jury found an ambiguous verdict. It was found that Rose had only accepted payment for the mixing of drugs and not for providing advice, a writ of error was granted and the case was eventually reheard in the House of Lords.

Rose was represented throughout the proceedings by the Society of Apothecaries, who portrayed the physicians as monopolists and the apothecaries as essential providers of medical services who were practising where the physicians would not, amongst the poor. The House of Lords found in favour of Rose and the Society of Apothecaries, confirming their status as members of the medical profession who were able to prescribe. The case had legitimised a practice that had already become custom. The general consensus amongst historians is that this case established the legal foundation for the evolution of apothecaries into general practitioners. Following the judgment, there would continue to be substantial reform and regulation of the profession, with a great focus given to education and training towards the end of the eighteenth century. However, it was not until the mid-nineteenth century that the term 'general practitioner' would be widely used. It is thought that Rose, through no intention of his own, had played an instrumental role in the establishment of general practice in England.

Following the trial, Rose was left in an uncomfortable position. The RCP continued to denounce his work as ignorant and illegal and the Society of Apothecaries publicly distanced itself from his practice. He died several years later in 1711, aged 71 years old, and was buried in St. Dionis Backchurch in London, in the north aisle behind the altar. He died intestate but an inventory request submitted by his wife showed that he was barely solvent at the time of his death, suggesting that despite the importance of his trial, he had fallen from grace and no longer held a position amongst the powerful and wealthy men of the city of London.

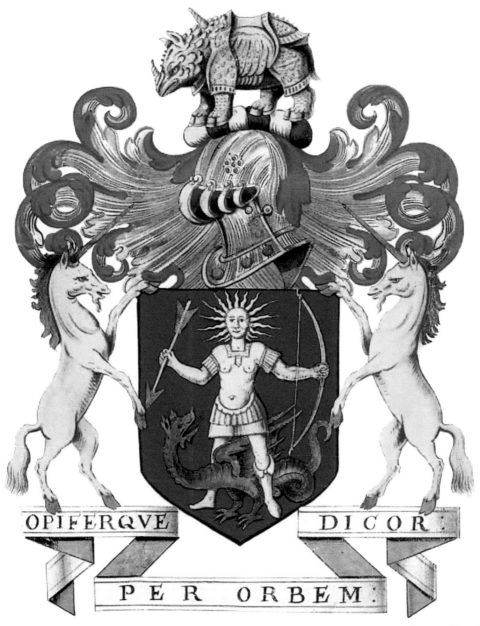

OPIFERQVE DICOR:

PER ORBEM:

The coat of arms of the Worshipful Society of Apothecaries of London. (Courtesy of the Worshipful Society of Apothecaries of London.)

Rose's impact on the establishment of general practice is still recognised today. The RCGP has commemorated him with a prize in his name, the Rose Prize. The prize also commemorates his namesake, Fraser Rose (1897–1972), who was instrumental in the foundation of the RCGP. The prize is an annual award for original work in the history of general practice in the British Isles.

Further Reading

Cook JH. The Rose case reconsidered: Physicians, apothecaries and the Law in Augustan England. *Journal of History of Medicine and Allied Science* 1990;45(4):527–55.

Elmer P, Grell OP (eds.). *Health, Disease and Society in Europe 1500–1800. A Source Book*. Manchester: Manchester University Press; 2004.

Hunt J. Echoing down the years: The tercentenary of the Rose case. *The Pharmaceutical Journal* 2001;266(7134):191–95.

2 GEORGE MAN BURROWS (1771–1846)

Krishma Kataria, Emma L. Vinton, Nathan Samuel and Neil Metcalfe

George Man Burrows was born in Chalk, Kent, in May 1771. The son of a medical practitioner who died when Burrows was still a child, he was raised by his young, widowed mother. Burrows attended Kings School, Canterbury, and when he was 16 years old he became an apprentice to Mr Richard Thompson, a respected surgeon in Rochester. In 1793, he moved to London to attend Guy's and St Thomas' Hospital Medical School and on completion of his medical degree he was admitted into the distinguished Corporation of Surgeons and The Society of Apothecaries, and he began practising as a general practitioner in Bloomsbury Square and Gower Street, London.

In July 1794, Burrows married his first wife, Mary Dale. Mary died the following year, when their daughter, Mary, was born. In March 1797, Burrows married Sophia, daughter of Thomas Druce, Law Stationer of Chancery Lane, London. They had five sons and four daughters but not all survived. Their eldest son was Sir George Burrows, First Baronet (1801–1887) who had a very eminent career, including becoming president of the BMA (1862–1863), a representative of the RCP to the GMC between 1860 and 1869 and, in 1870, he was appointed physician extraordinary to the Queen.

Some of Burrows' most celebrated work relates to his membership of the Society of Apothecaries, founded by Royal Charter in December 1617. The Society has a long, vibrant history: as early as 1704, apothecaries were permitted to become legal members of the medical profession, after the legal case of William Rose (1640–1711) was fought in the House of Lords. This case underpinned the legal foundations of English general practice and by the early nineteenth century apothecaries were becoming known as General Practitioners of Medicine or GPs. Dissatisfied with the lack of formal regulation for doctors a rise in tax on glass that had hard hit, Burrows formed at a meeting in the Crown and Anchor on the Strand on 3 July 1812 the Association of Surgeon-Apothecaries of England and Wales. His primary aim was to improve medical education and increase the respectability of the profession.

Under Burrows' diligent leadership, the association grew rapidly. Afterwards, he recollected that during this period (1812–1815), he personally responded to 1500 letters and attended 130 committee meetings. The association campaigned for an act to set up a regulatory body for general practice that was distinct from the Royal Colleges of Physicians, Surgeons and the Society of Apothecaries. Their persistence led to the passing of the Apothecaries Act on 1 August 1815. This Act was the first to introduce postgraduate medical qualifications and six-months' hospital experience for all general practitioners. Despite this, for numerous years the training remained piecemeal and many general practitioners were unsatisfied with the Bill, including Burrows himself, who was unhappy with the way the Society of Apothecaries enforced the Act. The Act was not well received by the RCP or the RCS nor the chemists and druggists to whom it applied. They conceded only when a clause was added, preserving their rights. Today, however, the Act is seen as instrumental in the advancement of postgraduate medical education. Without it, postgraduate medical education may not have become so well regulated.

The Worshipful Society of Apothecaries celebrated its 400th anniversary in 2017. It continues to offer specialist training and examination across its two distinct academic faculties. Remains the advancement of medical knowledge and they have recently introduced the 'International Advanced Assessment' course. Burrows was a member of the very first Court of Examiners at the Society; however, due to the misconduct of a court assistant he gave up this role, releasing a formal statement saying he was 'now content with the advancement of medical education and knowledge of general practitioners'.

Before giving up his Society role, Burrows co-founded *The London Medical Repository*, a collection of monthly medical science periodicals in January 1814, with colleagues David Uwins (1780–1837) and Anthony Todd Thomson (1778–1849). As co-editor, Burrows successfully negotiated the demands of work with frequent medical writing and publication. This enabled him to gain a strong reputation and influence in medical circles. However, soon after, his health started to deteriorate. He developed respiratory problems and gout, which ultimately contributed to him leaving general practice in 1816.

Burrows later turned his attentions to psychiatry. He visited asylums, observed how they were run and planned essential improvements. In 1817, he wrote *Cursory Remarks on a Bill for Regulating Madhouses*, and, in 1820, *An Enquiry into Certain Errors Relative to Insanity and Their Consequences, Physical, Moral and Civil*. They were novel in that they challenged common misconceptions about the mentally ill. Burrows was highly dedicated to improving outcomes for vulnerable patients and, in 1823, he opened a small private psychiatric establishment in Clapham called The Retreat, a licensed house in which he claimed 85 per cent of his patients were victims of an hereditary taint; mental illnesses were passed to them from their parents.

In 1824, Burrows became a full licentiate of the RCP (LRCP) and was awarded a Doctor of Medicine (MD) from St Andrews University. Four years later, he wrote *Commentaries on the Causes, Forms, Symptoms, and Treatment,*

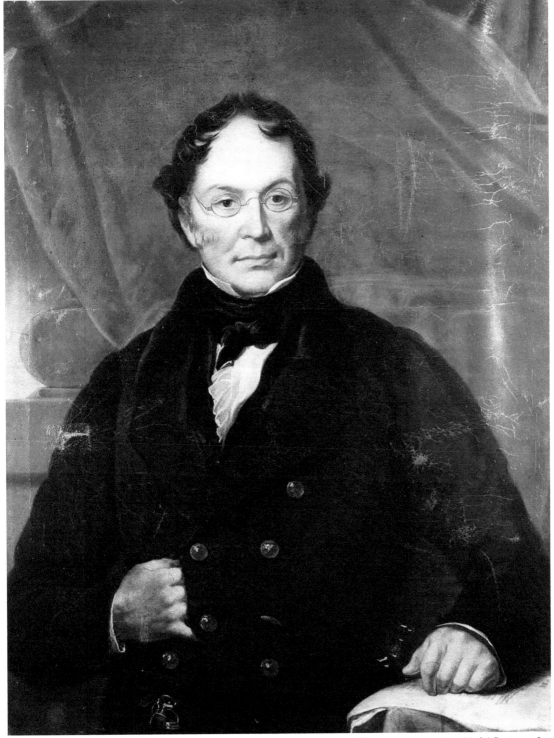

Portrait of George Burrows by J.G. Middleton, or after his portrait (with differences) in the Worshipful Society of Apothecaries of London. (Courtesy of Wellcome Library, London.)

Moral and Medical of Insanity (1828). This book was incredibly well received by professionals and the general public and it found acclaim across Europe and America. The *Edinburgh Medical and Surgical Journal* commended it as 'a treatise of high order; in fact, the most elaborate and complete general treatise on insanity that has yet appeared in the English language'. Every copy was sold and some German translations were distributed. The overwhelming success of his commentaries saw his reputation soar. He became popular with physicians from Europe and America who met him when the working party was appointed 'to inspect his hospitals for the "insane"'. Burrows received many diplomas and research funding proposals from all over Europe. As a result, his credibility grew exponentially. Naturally, this led to a rise in the number of patients at his Retreat.

In 1830, at the height of his career, Burrows' professionalism came under attack during two successive cases of wrongful confinement. The latter of these involved Lord Henry Brougham (1778–1868), Lord Chancellor to Earl Gray. Brougham supported the sanity of a gentleman under enquiry. Burrows opposed him but acted professionally and Brougham later apologised. However, he asserted that he had been given 'no choice, according to his instructions'. This left Burrows doubting his own credibility so he published a formal response with supporting evidence. This was successful and *The Times* later published the statement: 'Dr Burrows had been unfairly treated, and has succeeded in removing the most material of the imputations cast on his character in this affair'. Nevertheless, Burrows' reputation was badly tarnished following these incidents; the *Quarterly Review* coined the phrase '*burrowsed*' meaning wrongfully confined. Burrows' practice suffered and he gradually withdrew from psychiatric work.

In 1839, Burrows was elected onto the committee of the RCP by the Fellows. This confirmed to him that he had made significant contributions to medicine throughout his life. Satisfied with his success, in 1843, he started a private general practice, allowing others to manage the Clapham Retreat. Burrows spent much of his spare time supporting medical practitioners and their dependents through financial hardship in his role as vice-president of the Society of the Relief of the Widows and Orphans of Medical Men. His generosity was greatly received and after a long and vibrant career, Burrows died from bronchitis on 29 October 1846, at the age of 76 years old. He was buried in Highgate Cemetery, London.

He had a leading role in the movement that led to the passing of the Apothecaries' Act and in the reforms that led to the Medical Act in 1850. His legacy could permit him to be viewed as one of the most influential general practitioners ever with the previous description of him as 'the father of General Practice' to no longer be strangely neglected.

Further Reading

Anon. Attacks on Dr. Burrows. *London Medical Gazette* 1830;6:84–88.

Anon. Anderdon v. Burrows. *London Medical Gazette* 1830;6:183–87.

Anon. *Memoir of George Mann Burrows*, M.D., F.L.S. London: Wilson & Ogilvy; 1846.

Anon. The London Medical Directory. *The Lancet* 1845;46(1151):322.

Bettany GT. Burrows, George Man (1771–1846). In: Stephen L, Lee S (eds.). *The Dictionary of National Biography*. Volume 3. London: Oxford University Press; 1885.

Bettany GT. Burrows, George Man. In: Stephen L (ed.). *Dictionary of National Biography*. Volume 7. London: Smith, Elder & Co; 1886.

Burrows GM. *Cursory Remarks on a Bill for Regulating Madhouses*. London: Kings College; 1817.

Burrows GM. *Commentaries on the Causes, Forms, Symptoms, and Treatment, Moral and Medical of Insanity*. London: D.N. Shury; 1828.

Burrows GM. Letter to Sir Henry Halford. *London Medical Gazette* 1830;6:28–30.

Burrows GS. George Man Burrows and the anguished birth of General Practice. *British Medical Journal* 2017;359:454–55.

Porter R. *The Greatest Benefit to Mankind: A Medical History of Humanity from Antiquity to the Present*. New York: W. W. Norton; 1998.

Royal College of Physicians London. *A Letter to Sir Francis Milman, Bart. M.D., President of the Royal College of Physicians of London, on the Subject of the Proposed Reform in the Condition of the Apothecary and Surgeon-Apothecary*. London: D.N. Shury; 1813.

The National Archive. Will of Doctor George Mann Burrows, Physician, Doctor of Medicine of No. 46 Upper Gower. PROB 11/2044/192.

3 ROBERT MASTERS KERRISON (1776–1847)

Emma-Jane Jones

Robert Masters Kerrison was born in 1776 in London and began his working life as an apothecary. He commenced his training in 1790, attending anatomical lectures and demonstrations as part of his practical apprenticeship at the Hunterian School, Soho. Kerrison qualified as an apothecary at the beginning of the nineteenth century after being awarded MRCS. At that time, many apothecaries held the MRCS qualification; hence they were often referred to as surgeon-apothecaries.

The turn of the nineteenth century brought unease amongst apothecaries regarding high taxation on glass, described at the time as comparable to a second income tax. A group of apothecaries in London met to discuss this. However, concerns over an increasing number of 'quacks' within the profession took precedence. Kerrison described the quacks as tarnishing the reputation of apothecaries and that many were losing up to £200 a year as a consequence. During the late eighteenth and early nineteenth centuries, apothecaries were prescribers for those who were unable to afford physicians. Their knowledge was obtained from drug preparation and administration, although there was a lack of regulation regarding licensing and education. As a result of the concerns of apothecaries, an Association of Apothecaries and Surgeon Apothecaries was formed in 1812, motivated to improve regulation within the profession.

Kerrison joined the Association of Apothecaries and Surgeon Apothecaries in late 1812 after writing to them expressing his views of discontent at the treatment and disregard shown towards Apothecaries. This included those with appropriate education, and providing ideas of how to resolve the situation. The committee, chaired by George Man Burrows (1771–1846), were highly motivated for reform and consisted of 24 London members and seven from regions across England. Previous attempts to reform education and legislation for apothecaries had been met with resistance from the RCP and RCS. This was because apothecaries were not viewed as highly within society as physicians or surgeons. Ultimately, this committee became an influential group which authored and published a number of pamphlets to raise public awareness of the threats to the profession.

One of the most popular of these was Kerrison's *An Inquiry into the Present State of the Medical Profession*. This was a self-funded publication that he sent to every member of the Houses of Parliament to prove the necessity of legislative changes. The pamphlet was published in 1814 following the ever-growing frustration amongst the committee regarding treatment they had perceived from the RCP and the RCS after initial proceedings to pass the Bill had already been rejected, resulting in withdrawal. He wrote 'When the duly educated Surgeon-Apothecary shall be recognised in his proper character and protected by the operation of just and equal law [to the physicians] these abuses will cease to exist'. Kerrison reflected some years later in the *London Medical Gazette* about his concerns regarding the then heads of the RCP and RCS, stating that the Bill was in the best interests of the public by ensuring every apothecary was suitably trained.

Throughout the inquiry, Kerrison used the term 'general practitioner' to refer to the apothecaries. The use of the term was driven by apothecaries throughout London during the early 1800s; however, this was again met with resistance from the RCP and the RCS. The term had no legislative meaning until the 1820s but became popular through its use in pamphlets and Kerrison is one of those credited for this. He believed 'General Practitioner' was born more appropriate in describing the contemporaneous role of an apothecary as it encompassed medicine, surgery, midwifery and prescribing; up to 19 out of 20 patients were treated by general practitioners around 1814. His pamphlets were informative and provided detailed accounts of the events surrounding the Bill proposed for Parliament.

Kerrison also placed emphasis on the contemporaneous high ranking of physicians within the society. He illustrated how the rising prosperity of Great Britain from the early seventeenth century enabled physicians to continue charging high fees. This left the poorer classes unable to afford medical care, with desperation often leading them to more likely seek the help of unqualified pretenders, especially in areas outside of London. He used the example in Edinburgh, where the term apothecary was unknown, but surgeons practised dually as general practitioners. They were easily accessible and had more realistic expectations of payment, which removed the need for lower-class patients to seek help from those insufficiently qualified.

In 1815, Kerrison's second influential paper was published. It was titled *Observations and Reflections on the Bill now in Progress through the House of Commons, for Better Regulating the Medical Profession as far as Regards Apothecaries*. He documented the timeline of events leading up to the Bill being presented and the concern that the RCP may still oppose the Bill; however, it was finally passed into law in 1815 as the Apothecaries Act. The Act reflected the changing roles of apothecaries to general practitioners and brought in regulation for their training and education. A court of examiners was delegated and it was decided that an apprenticeship must be held before a licence to practise medicine may be granted, known as the LSA.

During his time as a practising apothecary, Kerrison also held the position as an editor for the *Surgeon-Apothecary's Journal and Review*. He also addressed the ongoing issue of water sanitation in London where improvements were

AN
INQUIRY

INTO THE PRESENT STATE OF

THE

MEDICAL PROFESSION IN ENGLAND,

CONTAINING

AN ABSTRACT OF ALL THE ACTS AND CHARTERS

GRANTED TO

PHYSICIANS, SURGEONS, AND APOTHECARIES,

AND

A Comparative View of the Profession

IN

SCOTLAND, IRELAND, AND ON THE CONTINENT

OF

EUROPE.

ALSO,

A COMPENDIOUS ACCOUNT OF ITS STATE AMONGST THE

𝕬𝖓𝖈𝖎𝖊𝖓𝖙 𝕲𝖗𝖊𝖊𝖐𝖘 𝖆𝖓𝖉 𝕽𝖔𝖒𝖆𝖓𝖘 :

TENDING TO ILLUSTRATE

The urgent Necessity of Legislative Interference,

AND THE

MERITS OF THE BILL

ABOUT TO BE PRESENTED TO PARLIAMENT

BY THE

APOTHECARIES AND SURGEON-APOTHECARIES

OF

ENGLAND AND WALES.

———◆———

TROS TYRIUSQUE MIHI NULLO DISCRIMINE AGETUR.—VIRG.

———◆———

BY ROBERT MASTERS KERRISON,

Member of the Royal College of Surgeons ; of the Society of Apothecaries ; Translator of Richerand's Physiology ; and one of the Editors of the Surgeon-Apothecary's Journal and Review.

═══════════

London :

Printed by J. Barfield, 91, Wardour-Street;

FOR LONGMAN, HURST, REES, ORME, AND BROWN, PATERNOSTER-ROW ; LUNN, SOHO-SQUARE ; LAING, EDINBURGH ; AND ARCHER, DUBLIN.

———◆———

1814.

Title page of Kerrison's 1814 publication *An Inquiry into the Present State of the Medical Profession.* (Courtesy of Wellcome Library, London.)

needed. Kerrison retired as an apothecary to train to be a physician in Edinburgh where he graduated MD on 1 August 1820 (D.M.I. de Neuralgia Faciei Spasmodica) and was awarded LRCP on 22 December 1820.

In 1841, Kerisson was elected Fellow of the Royal Society (FRS), perhaps somewhat of a surprise to him, as he wrote in the *London Medical Gazette* that those previously practising as surgeon-apothecaries did not gain such recognition. In the same piece, he acknowledged the improvements the Apothecaries Act of 1815 had established for general practitioners, although reform would extend deeper than education alone as he called for more equitable health care principles, through both physician payments and competition.

Kerrison died at his home on Upper-Brook Street on 27 April 1847, aged 71.

Further Reading

Association of Apothecaries and Surgeon Apothecaries. *A Letter to Sir Francis Milman, Bart. M.D., President of the Royal College of Physicians of London, on the Subject of the Proposed Reform in the Condition of the Apothecary and Surgeon-Apothecary: With an Appendix, Containing the Correspondence between the General Committee and the Three Corporate Medical Bodies*. London: D.N. Shury; 1813.

Kerrison RM. *An Inquiry into the Present State of the Medical Profession*. London: J. Barfield, Wardour-Street; 1814.

Kerrison RM. Observations and reflections on the Bill now in progress through the House of Commons, for better regulating the medical profession as far as regards apothecaries. *Pam* 1815;6:311–32.

Kerrison RM. State of the medical profession. *The London Medical Gazette* 1841;29(1):122–23.

Loudon I. *Medical Care and the General Practitioner 1750–1850*. Oxford: Clarendon Press; 1986.

RCP. *Lives of the Fellows: The Roll of the Royal College of Physicians of London*. Volume 3, 2nd edn. London: Harrison & Sons; 1878.

4 ANTHONY TODD THOMSON (1778–1849)

Atia Khan and Neil Metcalfe

Anthony Todd Thomson was born in Edinburgh on 7 January 1778. He was the youngest of four to Alexander Thomson, who was a British official in the Government of Georgia, Savannah, who retired to Edinburgh. Thomson attended the University of Edinburgh in 1795 but never took the degree of MD from there. In 1798, he became a member of the Speculative Society, forming strong, lifelong friendships with Lord Brougham and Lord Henry Cockburn. He also became a member of the Royal Medical Society in 1799. Soon after his father's death, Thomson moved to London setting up a large practice in Sloane Street, which quickly became exceptionally successful, earning him an estimated £3000 a year. He became noted for the kindness and care with which he treated all of his patients, gaining a medal from the Humane Society after resuscitating someone who had drowned. During his 20 years in London, Thomson gained a considerable reputation for skin expertise, his passion for medical botany and materia medica led to him lecturing extensively in this branch of medical science studying medicinal drugs and substances.

Thomson was awarded MRCS in 1800 and became instrumental in founding the Chelsea, Brompton and Belgrave Dispensaries. These institutions gained a good reputation for dermatology and are still active today. This is also when his first interest in skin diseases arose. At the time, he was also accredited for the establishment of an infant school in the parish of St Luke's, Chelsea and during this period he married Christina Maxwell, with whom he had one son and two daughters. He introduced dermatology as a special interest for general physicians and worked as a key physician in the first skin hospital in Great Britain called The London and Westminster Infirmary for the Treatment of Diseases of the Skin, which was founded in 1819. He worked in the hospital with Thomas Bateman (1778–1821) being his consultant, and found this significantly influenced his own clinical practice as he learnt the most contemporary methods of investigation, diagnosis and treatment. He also introduced dermatology to the dispensary and hospital which became the University College Hospital, and established the first notable teaching hospital school of dermatologists.

After the death of his first wife in 1820, Thomson remarried in the same year to Katharine Byerley. Together they had three sons and five daughters. Byerley, along with their two sons, often collaborated with Thomson by working as illustrators to his literary works.

Thomson was heavily involved in medical literature. He was a joint editor of the *London Medical Repository* alongside George Man Burrows (1771–1846) and William Royston (1761–1816). Thomson worked tirelessly for the publication house to become the voice of the Association of Apothecaries and the Surgeon-Apothecaries, personally contributing many articles on apothecary, medicine and therapeutics. His interest in botany was sparked after he attended a series of short courses in 1810 in London. The experiences of working for the *London Medical Repository* and the short courses led him to write his most notable work, *A Conspectus of the Pharmacopoeias* (1810). This gained worldwide recognition, running into 14 editions and being translated into several foreign languages. It was deemed to be the most important work on pharmacy and materia medica internationally and was also incorporated in the *British Pharmacopoeia* in 1887.

Thomson believed general practitioners had the unique opportunity of understanding patients holistically, which was one of the main reasons that he often spent hours in clinic consulting a wide spectrum of patients. This prompted him to document his findings within a section of Bateman's *Practical Synopsis of Cutaneous Diseases* (1829), which included an atlas and comprehensive illustrations by his son and wife. He also wrote *Elements of Materia Medica and Therapeutics* (1832), and further contributions to dermatology are found in his *Practical Treatise on Diseases affecting the Skin* (1850), which was completed after his death by his son-in-law Dr Parkes.

Thomson was a keen academic and believed general practitioners should take an active role in different medical societies in order to improve collaborative work and understanding of rarer diseases. He himself was very active in various medical societies such as the Ethnological Society, the Harveian Medical Society, the Linnean Society, the Medico-Chirurgical Society and the Westminster Medical Society. He played a major role in these professional societies and shared positive relations with other academics and Fellows, whilst his liberal cast of mind enabled him to take an active part in helping the creation of the Apothecaries Act of 1815. He had an interest in promoting the adoption of an improved system of education amongst apothecaries, and thus, lobbied for compulsory apprenticeships and formal qualifications for all medical practitioners. The Act required experience in anatomy, botany, chemistry, materia medica and 'physic', in addition to six months of practical hospital experience and thus was the beginning of regulation of the medical profession in the United Kingdom.

Thomson became a sought after lecturer, especially regarding botanical and medical matters, including at the Pharmaceutical Society where he was famously known as the Professor of Botany. Thomson's engaging lectures on botany at the Pharmaceutical Society and in the gardens of the Royal Botanical Society were popular amongst

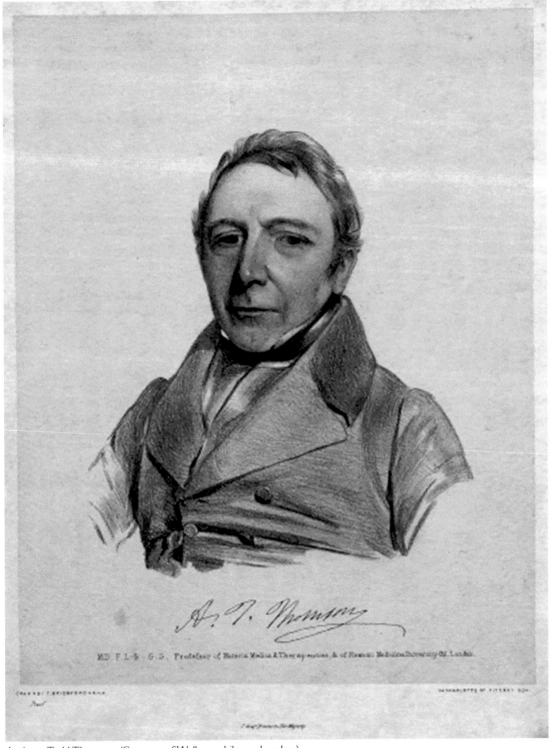

Anthony Todd Thomson. (Courtesy of Wellcome Library, London.)

medical students due to his pleasant nature as well as arranging for students to use the Royal Botanical Gardens in Regent's Park. He was a firm believer in the efficacy of drugs in the treatment of disease, and believed it was the role of the doctor to be able to convince patients to comply with their medication. To help with this, he is often credited with having helped design an ingenious device in the form of a spoon, which allowed the amount of fluid being administered to the patient to be controlled by partially occluding the lumen at the end of it. By controlling the quantity of medicine being administered, patient compliance with a treatment plan was thought to increase. The spoon became known as the 'Gibson spoon' due to the silversmith Charles Gibson who adapted Thomson's suggestion of a lumen and whose name was engraved on them.

In 1826, Thomson was awarded MRCP and retired from general practice. He focused thereafter on clinical teaching, dermatology and materia medica. He took an active part in promoting the London University (now University College London) and, in 1828, was elected as its first professor of materia medica and therapeutics. In 1832, he also became professor of medical jurisprudence alongside Andrew Amos; however, when Amos was appointed as a member of the governor-general's council in India in 1837, Thomson became sole professor.

Thomson's health deteriorated in 1835. Up to this point he had been notorious for his sheer workload: he used to rise at 5am every morning and start to write for three hours followed by making house calls for patients and lecturing students, returning home only to eat dinner and then continuing to work until the early hours of the morning. However, after his health declined he reduced his labours considerably. He continued to write, lecture and practise, focusing much of his attention to the diagnosis and treatment of skin diseases. He published two works of general interest: a translation of Eusèbe Baconnière de Salverte's *The Philosophy of Magic, Prodigies and Apparent Miracles* (1846) and an edition of James Thomson's *The Seasons* (1847). Thomson died at Ealing on 3 July 1849 at the age of 71 from pneumonia and pleurisy leaving behind his wife and 11 children, and is buried in Perivale churchyard, Middlesex. His fine collection of specimens of materia medica, with many illustrations, was purchased by the government after his death for the use of Queen's College, Cork.

Further Reading

Bartrip PWJ. Anthony Todd Thomson (1778–1849). In: Matthew HCG, Harrison B (eds.). *Oxford Dictionary of National Biography*. Volume 54. Oxford: Oxford University Press; 2004.

Johnston W. A Memoir of Anthony Todd Thomson. *The Lancet* 1849;2(54):46–47.

Williams DI. Anthony Todd Thomson and the rise of the General Practitioner. *Journal of Medical Biography* 2002;10(4):206–14.

5 THOMAS WAKLEY (1795–1862)

Neena Suchdev

Thomas Wakley was born on 11 July 1795 at Land Farm in Devon, the youngest son of 11 children to Henry and Mary Wakley. As a boy he took to farm life with enthusiasm and never forgot his humble beginnings long into his medical career. He gained a solid education at Chard in Somersetshire, and Honiton in Devonshire, which were some of the best grammar schools in the area.

At 15 years old Wakley became apprentice to an apothecary, Mr Incledon in Taunton. Prior to the Apothecaries Act, medical training was unstructured at best. In fact, no official training was required to practise; those that showed some promise and wished to qualify were sent to larger institutions to get a diploma. Wakley went on to gain two further apprenticeships: one with Mr Phelps who was his brother-in-law, the other with Mr Luke Coulson who belonged to a well-known medical family at Henley-on-Thames. Following these he later attended the United Hospitals of Guy's and St Thomas' in 1815.

Nineteenth-century medical education was plagued by nepotism. The leaders of the profession depended little on merit or outstanding ability to climb up the career ladder. Budding surgeons would undergo expensive apprenticeships or even have their fees waived if the teaching surgeon was a family friend. Such positions were desired for being highly lucrative. Preference was given to those who could afford it, and so true intelligence was rarely singled out. From the outset, Wakley's future lay in the 'rank and file' of the profession, a pathway that was almost predestined for those without money or position. He was, however, a keen anatomist, and developed sound dissection skills at the Webb-Street School in Southwark.

Wakley, who had spent his youth surrounded by people of integrity, felt the injustice and unfairness of such an education keenly. It would follow him throughout university as he watched those who progressed through purchase rather than merit to the more lucrative posts. Though the system angered him, his sympathy was directed at his peers; the community values inherent in general practice suited his character from the start. In 1817, he was awarded MRCS before embarking on a career in general practice.

Wakley was 24 years old when he married Elizabeth Goodchild, daughter to a governor of St Thomas' Hospital. Given Wakley's disdain of nepotism, it is interesting to note that it was with the help of his father-in-law that he secured a West End practice on Argyll Street. Here Wakley and his wife might have gone on to live a very comfortable life in a fashionable part of London, were it not for a brutal attempt on his life in 1820. In that year there was much in the way of political unrest, when a plot was made by Arthur Thistlewood and his gang to assassinate members of the Cabinet. The culprits were found, and sentenced to execution by being hung, drawn and quartered. The act of beheading was given to a masked man, who decapitated the deceased before raising the head to the crowd. The crowd did not take to him kindly as they abhorred the maiming of the dead, and it was several members of the crowd who made the assumption that he must have been part of the medical profession due to the skill with which he decapitated the assassins. It was stated in a newspaper article that the deed had been carried out by a 'young surgeon of Argyll Street'. This made Wakley the prime suspect to have been the executioner. Around three months later, a group of men came to his door in the middle of the night under the pretence of needing help and attacked him with a knife before setting fire to his house and practice. It is rumoured that the attempted murder was orchestrated by Thistlewood's gang; however, other theories suggest that he was targeted by jealous acquaintances who had sent him threatening letters in the past. Though his house and belongings were insured, the insurance company at first refused to pay him under the assumption that he was responsible for the fire. The matter was eventually brought before the King's Bench. When he was finally paid the full claim amount, however, there was nothing left of his practice to return to. He could see no option other than to start anew.

In the period that followed, Wakley met propagandist William Cobbett. Cobbett was the parliamentary candidate for Coventry, as well as being editor for the *Weekly Political Register* and *Cobbett's Evening Post*. He quickly became a source of inspiration for Wakley as someone who shared his tenacious sense of justice and morality. The dramatic events of Argyll Street were difficult to forget, and Wakley became consumed with a desire to get involved in something bigger. His friendship with Cobbett became a stimulus. Wakley knew the corruption that surrounded the medical profession and its teachings were very visible, and there needed to be a way of bringing it under public scrutiny. The idea of a weekly newspaper began to take shape, one that would be devoted to the interests of the medical profession.

The first edition of *The Lancet* was issued on Sunday 5 October 1823, costing sixpence. Wakley, the founding editor, had two objectives with his new paper: firstly the spread of knowledge and medical information amongst the medical profession; secondly how to combat the nepotism affecting hospital post appointments. For the next 10 years his paper became a campaign against the opponents of progress, making *The Lancet* one of a kind. Unlike the contemporary

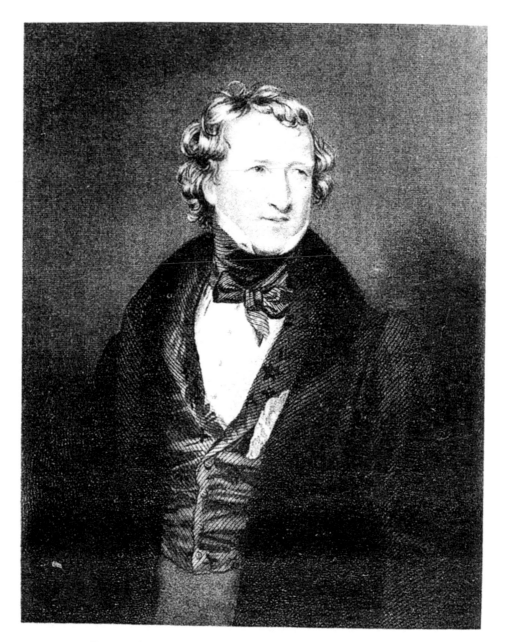

Engraved by W. H. Egleton, from a painting by K. Meadows, Esq.

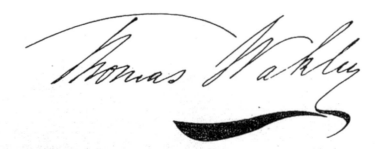

Portrait of Thomas Wakley. (Courtesy of Wellcome Library, London.)

medical press written to gratify the elite few, here was a journal that threatened to unveil the corruption of the whole institution. He referred to this in the preface to the first volume of *The Lancet*:

> Ceremonies and signs have now lost their charms, hieroglyphics and gilded serpents their power to deceive. But for these it would be impossible to imagine how it happened that medical and dietetical knowledge, of all other the most calculated to benefit Man, should have been by him the most neglected.

The first edition reported three medical cases. These were 'A Case of Anasarca', 'A Case of Hydrocephalus' and 'A Case of Hydatids of the Liver'. Also included was a lecture given by Sir Astley Cooper (1768–1841), Sergeant Surgeon to the King. A particular point of interest is the inclusion of letters between Cooper and Henry Earle (1789–1838), another surgeon of influence who responded to an accusation from Cooper. This set the precedent that levels of hierarchy had little place in *The Lancet*, and that incorrect or outdated information would be challenged regardless of who delivered it.

For the years that followed, *The Lancet* was met with both controversy and admiration. Wakley made it his duty to publish medical lectures from the great surgeons and physicians of the time, without their permission. Indeed, in 1824, John Abernethy (1764–1831), a surgeon of St Bartholomew's Hospital, tried to take legal measures to prevent *The Lancet* from publishing his lectures, a motion which was refused on the grounds that 'official lectures in a public place for the public good had no copyright vested in them'. Now any medical professional could read the lectures only delivered previously to those who could afford it.

Wakley was animated in his scathing reports of the nepotism rife in teaching hospitals, and, in 1828, he published the details of an operation with severe complications performed by Bransby Blake Cooper (1792–1853). In the report he made it clear that the only reason Cooper was a surgeon was because he was nephew to the aforementioned Sir Astley Cooper. Wakley was sued, but the damages were minor and easily paid off. By this point the journal had achieved a circulation of around 8000, which was twice the readership of that in 1825. The popularity of *The Lancet* continued to grow and achieved the largest circulation of any medical journal in United Kingdom of Great Britain and Ireland until it was overtaken by the *British Medical Journal* (*BMJ*) in the 1870s.

In the first 10 years of the journal's publication, Wakley's critics and defenders of the status quo fought bitterly against reform with lawsuits and slander. Some have criticised Wakley's writing style as being a little rough around the edges and far too blunt at times. Others argue that this is why *The Lancet* was able to thrive amongst such controversy and that a headstrong figure such as Wakley was needed to plant the seeds of medical reform.

Though he continued to edit *The Lancet* until his death, Wakley attempted another method of political change by becoming one of the two Members of Parliament (MPs) for Finsbury in 1835 as a radical. This was in the same year that saw Tory Prime Minister Robert Peel replaced by Lord Melbourne, a Whig. Wakley, caring for neither, was not attached to any political party. In addition, in 1839, he became Coroner for West Middlesex, a position previously held by lawyers rather than medical men. This appointment drove him to expose cases of suspicious deaths and industrial accidents, publishing them in *The Lancet* and campaigning for greater transparency.

Wakley died on 16 May 1862 of a pulmonary haemorrhage. He was buried next to his wife and daughter at Kensal Green cemetery. The editing of the journal was passed on to his son, James Wakley. Since Wakley's death *The Lancet* has continued to evolve into one of the most respected medical journals of the twenty-first century, but its founder's primary intention should be remembered as the spark that ignited a triumph of medical reform.

Further Reading

Bynum WF. Wakley, Thomas (1795–1862). In: Matthew HCG, Harrison B (eds.). *Oxford Dictionary of National Biography*. Volume 56. Oxford: Oxford University Press; 2004.

Gardiner W. *Facts Relative to the Late Fire and Attempt to Murder Mr Wakley in Argyll Street*. London: T. Gardiner and Son; 1820.

Sharp D. Thomas Wakley (1795–1862): A biographical sketch. *The Lancet* 2012;379:1914–21.

Sprigge SS. *The Life and Times of Thomas Wakley (facsimile of 1899 edition)*. New York: Robert E Krieger; 1974.

Wakley T. Preface. *The Lancet* 1823;1(1):1–2.

6 ROBERT RAINEY PENNINGTON (1766–1849)

Rashi Yadav

Robert Rainey Pennington was born in 1766 in England. Not much is known of his early years or personal life outside of his contributions to the medical profession. He worked as an apprentice at St Bartholomew's Hospital in London, under the supervision of Percivall Pott (1714–1788) who discovered that cancer could be caused by environmental factors. Whilst there, he and another student, John Abernathy (1764–1831), most well known for inventing the Abernathy biscuit to aid digestion, developed a rivalry. In the later years, he shared an anecdote in which during their time as students, each claimed precedence. During ward rounds one day, Pennington was closely following Pott who was giving a running commentary of a case Pennington found very interesting. Abernathy elbowed Pennington out of the way, which led to Pennington calling him out: 'The place of combat was in the corner of the ground which is near to the anatomical theatre, and thither we repaired, followed by our anxious and admiring confrères. I took off my coat and prepared for action. Jack did not follow suit, and began, like Bob Acres, to show unmistakable symptoms of not coming to the scratch. In fact, he declined the ordeal of battle, and I was for the future first'. Abernathy later claimed that 'the truth of the case was this – the moment I saw you uncover your biceps, I was certain I should be thrashed, and so, my boy, I surrendered at discretion'. He was awarded MRCS on 5 April 1787 with Pott one of the examiners.

Pennington practised in Lamb's Conduit Street, Bloomsbury, London for most of his life. Behind his house in Montagu Place he had a dispensary in Keppel Street where many of his medicines were concocted. Pennington was reported to have been a fantastic general practitioner and highly respected; his practice was arduous and grand. Not only did he have his patients in town, he also made frequent visits to the countryside where he would often stay the night and make his way back to London first thing in the morning in time to see his home patients. Whilst most contemporary doctors were earning £2000–3000 per annum, it was rumored that Pennington was making up to £10,000 per annum. He also claimed to have tended to every member of the cabinet and every judge on the bench. In addition to this, before Great Ormond Street ever existed, the London Foundling Hospital, established in 1739, took into its care abandoned children in the days before contraception and abortion relieved the desperation of forsaken, sick, or destitute mothers. Pennington was the visiting doctor who was described as having a 'kindly face' by the staff at the time and dutifully tended to his patients with the extensive supply of medicine for which he was well known.

The origin of the role of a general practitioner directly leads back to 1704, when the Worshipful Society of Apothecaries of London won a legal suit known as the Rose case named after William Rose (1640–1711), which allowed apothecaries to prescribe and supply medicine. Over a century later, the Apothecaries Act of 1815 was passed establishing the need for formal qualifications and practical experience for apothecaries or general practitioners. This was the start of the medical profession being regulated. The teaching, however, still remained disparate with it ranging from studying at Oxbridge to an apprenticeship at an apothecary's shop. This lack of consistency led to many general practitioners feeling underappreciated and demoralised. On 11 December 1843, Pennington was awarded FRCS. A year later, in 1844, a Bill was drawn up for the 'better regulation of medical practice throughout the United Kingdom' emphasising the need for a 'body' with the power to elect a representative council for general practitioners. At this time, Pennington stated 'that manifestly nothing would effectually secure the public interests, as the establishment of a College of General Practitioners in Medicine, Surgery and Midwifery'.

Later that same year Pennington founded the National Association of General Practitioners and was elected President with the eventual aim of inaugurating the College of General Practitioners, Surgery and Midwifery. Within a few months thousands of general practitioners had registered. The initial plan was to set up an exam to anyone wanting a career in the medical field, which would be overseen by surgeons and physicians, followed by a period of study and a second exam for the specific college, which would lead to their final registration; this would allow general practitioners to be taught and examined by their own peers. However, the RCS vehemently opposed this. In 1848, after lengthy discussions, a compromise was reached with the order of exams for general practitioners reversed. Rather than the preliminary exam being administered by physicians and surgeons, it would be taken as a final exam. However, at the last minute, negotiations broke down and the RCS refused the agreement.

The formation of a college for general practitioners remained in limbo after this. Despite being president, Pennington, who was in his eighties at this stage, no longer had the same conviction and stamina that he had in his youth. He would later sell his practice to a Mr Hillier, who was unable to keep it going. In the last couple of years of his life Pennington practised in Portman's Square where he died on 8 March 1849. During his lifetime, the face of medicine changed with the progressive separation of general practitioners from surgeons and physicians; these doctors were working without a governing body and without much support. Although the College of General Practitioners wasn't founded until over a hundred years after his death, in 1952, the campaigning Pennington did initiated the need to bring about an academic body that would oversee and support this group of doctors. Described as very sociable and hospitable and often referred to as the originator of 'homeopathy', he was highly venerable and recognised for being a good diagnostician and prescriber.

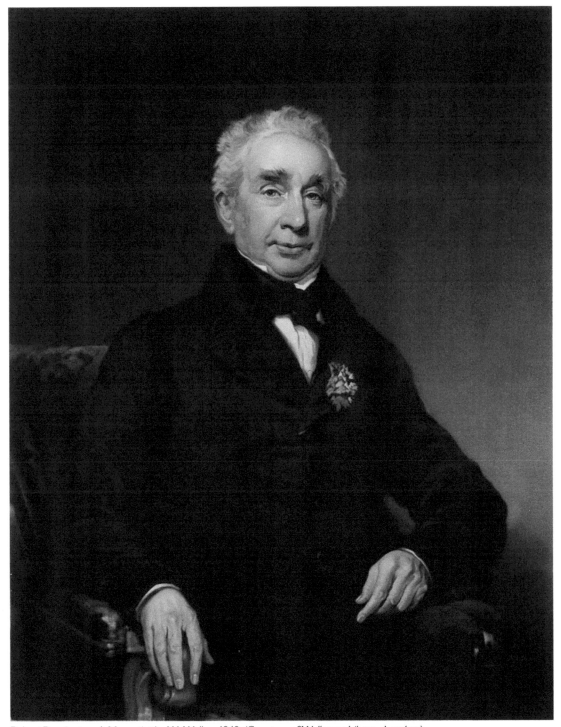

Robert Pennington. A Mezzotint by W. Walker, 1849. (Courtesy of Wellcome Library, London.)

Further Reading

Clarke JF. *Autobiographical Recollections of the Medical Profession*. London: J. & A. Churchill Publishing; 1874.

Holloway SWF. The Apothecaries' Act, 1815: A reinterpretation. *Medical History* 1966;10(2):107–29.

Hunt JH. The foundation of a College. The conception, birth, and early days of the College of General Practitioners. *The Journal of the Royal College of General Practitioners* 1973;23(126):5–20.

Loudon IS. James Mackenzie Lecture: The origin of the general practitioner. *The Journal of the Royal College of General Practitioners* 1983;33(246):13–23.

McConaghey RM. Proposals to found a Royal College of General Practitioners in the nineteenth century. *The Journal of the Royal College of General Practitioners* 1972;22(124):775–88.

Richardson R. Friends of the foundlings. *The Lancet* 2012;380(9850):1299.

7 JOHN HUXHAM (1692–1768)

Martha Kate Nicholson

John Huxham was born in the village of Harberton, Devon, in 1692. The eldest son of a butcher, he inherited his father's property in the nearby parish of Staverton after being orphaned early in life. Following his father's death, he was entrusted to the care of Thomas Edgley, a local minister who shared his father's nonconformist religious views. He received a classical education from the grammar school of Isaac Gilling, one of his guardian's fellow dissenting Presbyterian ministers, in the town of Newton Abbot. Despite a lack of application to his studies, it was evident that Huxham had a prodigious memory, and proved to be a very able student.

Following further schooling at the dissenting academy at Exeter, at 17 years old Huxham embarked on a medical education. Due to limitations on the rights of religious dissenters put into place after the restoration of the English monarchy, the universities of Oxford and Cambridge were closed to Huxham. This led him to begin his studies in the Netherlands at Leiden, under the instruction of Herman Boerhaave (1668–1738). Despite selling his father's house, Huxham only completed around a year and a half of the medical course at Leiden before exhausting his inheritance. Undaunted, he was able to finish his degree at Rheims in France where fees were considerably less, and was awarded MD in 1717.

Upon his return to England, Huxham first began to practise close to his birthplace, in the town of Totnes, Devon. It became evident, however, that greater opportunities awaited him in Centres in Plymouth, where he moved soon afterwards. Thanks to Edgley's recommendation, Huxham soon found friends amongst the dissenters of Plymouth. Although their patronage allowed him to develop a modest practice, Huxham was dissatisfied, and wished to see his practice grow much quicker.

Also, in 1717, Huxham married Ellen Corham, the daughter of a wealthy family. It was noted by his contemporaries that he began to affect an air of gravity and importance following his marriage, dressing in a ruffled scarlet coat, carrying a gold-headed cane and employing a footman to carry his gloves when visiting patients. This appearance was allegedly accompanied by various ploys aimed at convincing potential patients of his popularity, such as riding out of town and arranging to be called out of church to see fictional patients.

In his spare time, Huxham would fill his hours with study of the medical classics, and was notably a great admirer of Hippocrates. After the most prominent physician in Plymouth, Dr Seymour, was taken ill with what was described as a 'madness' contemporaneously, Huxham was already very well read. Due to his knowledge, he was well positioned to take over Seymour's case load and increase the size of his own practice. Around this time, Huxham also defected from the nonconformist church, accepting the Church of England.

In 1723, the Royal Society appealed for records of weather observations. In response, Huxham began to keep meteorological records. He measured wind speed and direction, barometric pressure, temperature and volume of rainfall. He published these records along with the monthly prevalence of epidemic diseases in Plymouth as two volumes, in 1739 and 1752, under the name *Observationes de aere et morbis epidemicis*. From then on Huxham continued to publish regularly, including his most famous work, *An Essay on Fevers and their Various Kinds* (*An Essay on Fevers*) in 1750. This latter work brought together Huxham's observations of various fevers which were prevalent at the time, including the conditions under which they appeared, their natural courses and characteristics and his own proposed treatments. Included in this work were accurate, early descriptions of typhoid, typhus, bronchitis and smallpox, amongst others. In the prevention of smallpox, Huxham was an early advocate for inoculation, considering the disease in its natural form to be far more dangerous.

In his clinical practice, Huxham was influenced heavily by the works of Thomas Sydenham (1624–1689), using mostly his own observations of patients to inform his treatment. Although regarded as a moderate and careful prescriber, Huxham was known to attempt 'heroic measures' in the treatment of some of his patients, including his own wife in July 1742, who subsequently died from what was described as a 'dropsy', despite his intervention using emetics, cathartics and diuretics, amongst other drugs available at the time. A tincture of quinine, consisting of cinchona bark, bitter orange peel, serpentary root, saffron and cochineal was formulated by Huxham as a treatment for specific fevers, and was listed in the *British Pharmacopoeia* as *Huxham's tincture*, and later tinc. chiconae B.P.

Thanks in part to Huxham's work, Mariana Victoria of Spain was cured of a life-threatening fever, and in gratitude her husband, King Joseph I of Portugal, arranged for *An Essay on Fevers* to be translated into Portuguese, with an intricately-bound copy gifted to Huxham. In addition to this, *An Essay on Fevers* was translated into Latin, French and Italian, and during his lifetime Huxham's writings were published throughout Europe in Amsterdam, Bremen, Lisbon, Munich, Naples and Paris, as well as in his native Kingdom of Great Britain. In addition to his work on fevers, Huxham was known for recommending the provision of fruit and vegetables to sailors to prevent scurvy, albeit in the form of

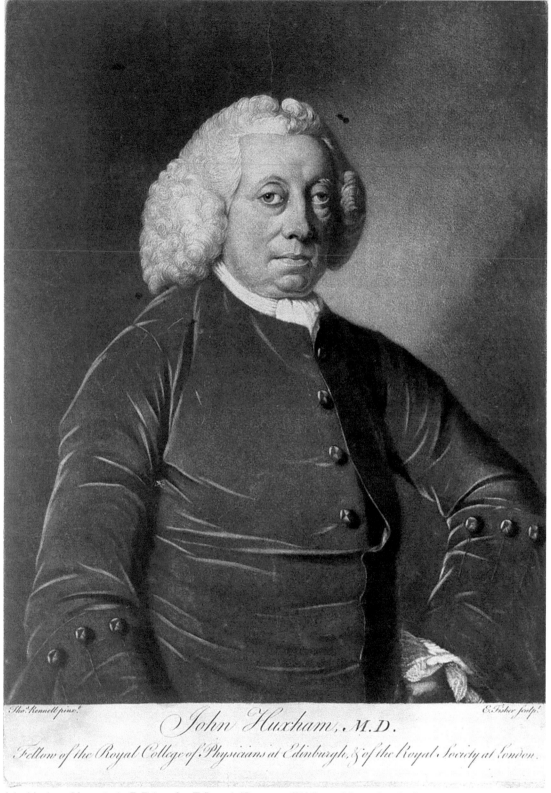

John Huxham. Mezzotint by E. Fisher after T. Rennel. (Courtesy of Wellcome Library, London.)

cider as well as apples, oranges and lemons. These recommendations, as well as Huxham's account of scurvy seen in Plymouth sailors, were published in 1766 in his book, *De scurbuto*.

Huxham was elected to the Royal Society as a fellow in 1739. He was later awarded the same Society's most prestigious award, the Copley Medal, for his observations on antimony in 1755, and the same year was also awarded FRCP of Edinburgh. Over the years, he submitted many communications to the Royal Society, on topics as diverse as anatomy, astrology and natural history, demonstrating the breadth of his reading and expertise.

Visiting patients in a sedan chair, Huxham continued to practise medicine in Plymouth until his death on 11 August 1768. He was predeceased by his second wife, Elizabeth Harris, and left two daughters and a son. His eldest child, John Corham Huxham, followed in his father's footsteps and also became an FRS, later going on to edit new editions of his father's publications.

Further Reading

Blewitt O. *The Panorama of Torquay: A Descriptive and Historical Sketch of the District Comprised Between the Dart and Teign*. London: Simpkin and Marshall; 1832.

Curtis C. John Huxham (1692–1768) Devonshire Physician. *Journal of the American Medical Association* 1965;192(1):56.

Huxham J. *An Essay on Fevers: To Which Is Now Added, a Dissertation on the Malignant, Ulcerous Sore-Throat (Classic Reprint)*. London: Forgotten Books; 2016.

McConaghey RMS. John Huxham. *Medical History* 1969;13(3):280–87.

8 EDWARD JENNER (1749–1823)

Olivia Sjökvist

On 17 May 1749, Edward Jenner was born in the town of Berkley, Gloucestershire. His natural abilities as a keen observer and his inquisitive predisposition allowed him to become a great scholar and general practitioner. His meticulous methodology led to numerous scientific breakthroughs, the most significant being that of the relationship between cowpox and smallpox. His work led to the discovery and implementation of a vaccine against smallpox, one of the leading causes of death and disfigurement during his time, laying the foundation for the total eradication of the disease in 1980. Jenner's legacy is as a patriarch to modern immunisation.

Reverend Steven Jenner, vicar in Berkley and rector of Rockhampton, was Jenner's father. His mother, Sarah Jenner, died in childbirth when Jenner was five years old. Two months later his father also died, leaving him in the care of his eldest brother Stephen, who succeeded his father as rector of Rockhampton, along with his three sisters.

Jenner's family wanted him to pursue a career in medicine. When he was 14 years old, Jenner started an apprenticeship with surgeon-apothecary Mr Daniel Ludlow (b.1720) of Chipping Sodbury in Gloucestershire where he remained for seven years until he moved to St George's Hospital in London to further his medical training under John Hunter (1728–1793). Hunter, at the time, was thought to be the leading teacher of surgery as well as an avid biologist, creating a teaching museum of more than 14,000 animal and human specimens. In contrast to other leading surgeons of his time, Hunter strongly believed in the intimate relationship between anatomy and physiological function, which he aimed to ingrain into the minds of his students.

When he was 23 years old, Jenner re-established himself in Berkley and pursued his interest in the natural world, keeping meticulous notes of his observations and frequently corresponded with Hunter about his various hypotheses. Hunter encouraged Jenner's passions and famously once wrote 'Why think? Why not try the experiment?' Hunter gave him a thermometer, a rare instrument at the time, allowing Jenner to study the hibernation of hedgehogs by measuring their body temperatures during different seasons. Other subjects that caught Jenner's interest included the lifecycle of the eel and the migration of birds. In 1778, Jenner's letter to Hunter was published in the *Philosophical Transactions of the Royal Society of London* entitled 'Observations on the natural history of the cuckoo'. This describing the nesting habits of the cuckoo, for which he was elected an FRS in 1788.

Jenner's inquisitive nature extended to medicine. He helped establish the Fleece Medical Society in Rodborough, Gloucestershire, where a group of doctors would meet on a monthly basis to discuss recent medical advancements and freely hypothesise on their own observations in the field. Jenner contributed to the meetings with his own papers on angina pectoris and its relation to coronary heart disease, ophthalmia and valvular disease of the heart, in particular mitral stenosis. The link between cowpox and smallpox was often discussed during these meetings and may have served as a springboard for Jenner's experiments.

In Jenner's local community, it had long been believed that milkmaids who contracted cowpox from cows were not affected by the smallpox virus. The common 'treatment' for smallpox during this time was a process called *variolation* by which young children were infected with the virus by inhaling dried smallpox scabs. This method carried a one to two per cent mortality rate compared to the 30 per cent mortality rate in individuals contracting the virus by natural means. Jenner, however, thought to act on his hypothesis that individuals who had been infected with the cowpox virus would be immune to the smallpox virus.

In 1796, Jenner tested his theory. He infected a small eight-year-old boy named James Phipps with pus taken from the cowpox blister from a local milkmaid called Sarah Nelmes. Jenner then took pus from the blister produced by smallpox and inoculated Phipps, who did not produce any post-exposure symptoms of smallpox. Jenner continued his experiments on other individuals and, in 1798, he published his findings in a book entitled *An Inquiry into the Causes and Effects of the Variolae Vaccinae; a Disease Discovered in some of the Western Counties of England, Particularly Gloucestershire, and Known by the Name of The Cow Pox*. He further published two books detailing his continued observations from his trials, confirming his theory that cowpox inoculation protected against smallpox, entitled *Further Observations on the Variolæ Vaccinæ, or Cow-Pox* (1799) and *A Continuation of Facts and Observations Relative to the Variolæ Vaccinæ, or Cow-Pox* (1800).

Jenner's theories on vaccination were met with scepticism from many. It must be remembered, however, that vaccination was introduced into a society where little was known about the spread and cause of disease. Some parents objected as vaccination involved scoring the flesh of their children's skin; some religious officials believed the vaccine to be 'unchristian' as it was derived from an animal. Other medical professionals were also doubtful as to the efficacy of the vaccination as vaccinated individuals would still become infected with smallpox, mainly due to cross-contamination between cowpox and smallpox or poor vaccination technique.

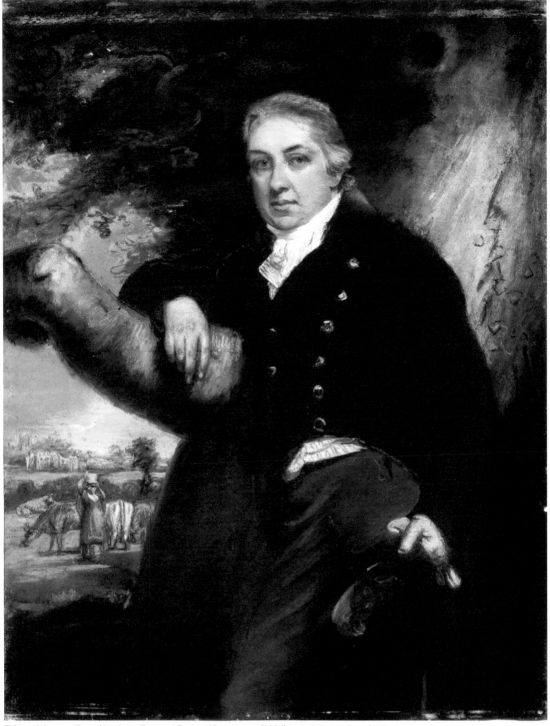

Edward Jenner. Pastel by John Raphael Smith. (Courtesy of Wellcome Library, London.)

In a column of the *Lancaster Gazette* in February 1821, Jenner outlined his ultimate aim with vaccination: 'let the country be ever so extensive, ever so populous, where vaccination has been solely and universally propagated, smallpox has been wholly got rid of, and never brought back again…' Eventually, Jenner's wishes were made true and on 8 May 1980 the World Health Organization (WHO) announced it 'declares solemnly that the world and its peoples have won freedom from smallpox' after a successful worldwide vaccination programme.

With regards to his family life, Jenner married Catherine Kingscote in 1788 and had three children. Jenner enjoyed the reputation of a respectable country general practitioner seeing patients in both his home, the Chantry and riding great distances to see patients in their own homes.

On 26 January 1823, at 73 years old, Jenner passed away in the Chantry having suffered a stroke and was buried at Berkley Church. He is celebrated as the father of vaccination and immunology and is thought to have saved more lives than any other human being ever.

Further Reading

Fisher R. *Edward Jenner, 1749–1823*. London: André Deutsch; 1991.

Glynn I, Glynn J. *The Life and Death of Smallpox*. New York: Cambridge University Press; 2004.

Jenner E. Observation on the natural history of the cuckoo. *Philosophical Transactions of the Royal Society of London* 1788; 78:219–37.

Jenner E. *An Enquiry into the Causes and Effects of the Variole Vaccinae, a Disease Discovered in Some of the Western Counties of England, Particularly Gloucestershire and Known by the Name of the Cow Pox*. London: Sampson Low; 1798.

Smith J. *The Speckled Monster*. Chelmsford: Essex Record Office; 1987.

Williams G. *Angel of Death*. Basingstoke: Palgrave Macmillan; 2011.

9 JAMES PARKINSON (1755–1824)
Aidan Lee

James Parkinson was born on 11 April 1755 at No. 1 Hoxton Square, Shoreditch, Middlesex. He was raised in Hoxton with his parents, John and Mary Parkinson, and two siblings, William and Mary Parkinson. His father, John Parkinson (1725–1784), was an accomplished general practitioner who received the Grand Diploma of the Corporation of Surgeons of London in 1765. From 1775 to 1776, John Parkinson was the anatomical warden (lecturer in anatomy) to the Company of Surgeons, which, when it received its Royal Charter in 1800, became the RCS.

Little is known of Parkinson's early education but based on his own writings he was well versed in Greek and Latin and also studied mathematics, the natural sciences and some French. His understanding of Greek and Latin was critically important in his understanding of the ancient medical authorities. He was also an expert in shorthand, allowing him to write at great speed. More is known of Parkinson's medical education. He began his medical education as an apprentice surgeon to his father. Parkinson became one of the earliest medical students at the London Hospital Medical College when he studied there for six months in 1776.

During his apprenticeship in 1781, Parkinson married Mary Dale with whom he had six children between 1783 and 1794. Following the death of his father, Parkinson was examined and received the diploma of the Company of Surgeon's on 1 April 1784 and continued the family practice.

Parkinson cared for the people of Hoxton as a general practitioner until his death in 1824. Parkinson's third child, John Key Williams Parkinson (1785–1838) qualified and joined his father's practice in 1806. It can be assumed that the 'Parkinson and Son' practice was large in the early nineteenth century. It is estimated that the population of Shoreditch increased quickly from 30,000 in 1801 to 50,000 in 1811. This population was cared for by half a dozen qualified practices.

'Parkinson and Son' was appointed 'Surgeon, Apothocary, and Man-midwife' to the poor of St. Leonard Shoreditch Workhouse Infirmary in 1813. It was their duty to care for the workhouse paupers that their places of works as well as their homes and to care for their children. For over 25 years, Parkinson was also a medical attendant at Holly House, one of the three madhouses in Hoxton. Holly House was a private institution which accepted both paying and pauper patients.

Parkinson was a member of many medical societies, including the Medical Society of London, Medico-Chirurgical Society of London, Hunterian Society, Society for the Relief of Widows and Orphans of Medical Men and Association of Apothecaries and Surgeon-Apothecaries of England and Wales of which he was the chairman from 1817 to 1820, immediately after the resignation of George Man Burrows (1817–1820). His time at the association included him helping prepare the Apothecaries Act of 1815, which led to the requirement of examinations for the diploma of LSA and enabled prosecution in cases of malpractice. Away from medicine, he was a member of the radical London Corresponding Society and, in 1794, was examined under oath before the Privy council in connection with the 'popgun' plot to assassinate King George III.

Parkinson's most famous piece of writing was published in 1817, *An Essay on the Shaking Palsy*. The essay was published on an octavo volume containing 66 pages over five chapters. In this work, he was the first to describe and discuss the disease *paralysis agitans* (shaking palsy). The essay defined and illustrated six cases of paralysis agitans. He described the pathognomonic symptom as an involuntary tremor of the limbs, and a 'propensity to bend the trunk forwards, and to pass from a walking to a running pace'. He attempted to distinguish the disease from other diseases that involved tremors. Parkinson hypothesized that the pathology arose from the medulla. Considering the limited contemporaneous understanding of neurology and the fact that none of his patients underwent an autopsy, it is impressive that Parkinson was able to come so close to today's understanding of the disease. The essay was well received at the time and demonstrated Parkinson's excellent clinical acumen and descriptive skills. The disease was renamed posthumously in the 1860s by Jean-Martin Charcot (1825–1893), calling it Parkinson's disease.

Parkinson, possibly influenced by the French revolution, was a pacifist and a political reformer. Under the pseudonym 'Old Hubert', he advocated the reformation of representation in the House of Commons, the implementation of annual parliaments and the establishment of universal suffrage. He published numerous pamphlets as Old Hubert expressing his desire for change by peaceful means. Parkinson was a member of the London Corresponding Society and the Society for Constitutional Information.

After his aforementioned political endeavours, in 1794, his interests shifted to less controversial topics, which included chemistry, geology and palaeontology. Parkinson was an avid writer and in addition to his numerous journal articles and political pamphlets, he published many books in various fields. These works included *Medical Admonitions for Families* (1799), *Chemical Pocket Book* (1799), *Hospital Pupil* (1800), *Villagers Friend and Physician* (1800), *Dangerous Sports* (1800), *The Ways to Health* (1802), *Hints for the Improvement of Trusses* (1802), *Organic Remains of a Former World* (1804) and *Observations on the Nature and Cure of Gout* (1805).

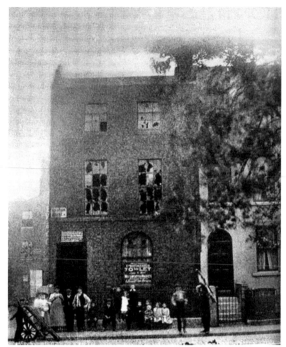

A picture of No. 1 Hoxton Square. (From Rowntree LG. James Parkinson. *Bulletin John Hopkins Hospital* 1912;23:33–34. Courtesy of Wellcome Images, London.)

AN

ESSAY

ON THE

SHAKING PALSY.

BY

JAMES PARKINSON,
MEMBER OF THE ROYAL COLLEGE OF SURGEONS.

LONDON:
PRINTED BY WHITTINGHAM AND ROWLAND,
Goswell Street,

FOR SHERWOOD, NEELY, AND JONES,
PATERNOSTER ROW.

1817.

Title page of Parkinson J. *An Essay on the Shaking Palsy*. London: Sherwood, Neely, and Jones; 1817. (Courtesy of Wellcome Images, London.)

Parkinson died on 21 December 1824 in Hoxton aged 69 years old. He was buried where he was baptised and married, at St. Leonard's Church, although no tombstone is present. Whilst there is no known portrait of Parkinson, a description from his friend Gideon Mantell (1790–1852) exists: 'Mr Parkinson was rather below middle stature, with an energetic, intelligent, and pleasing expression of countenance, and of mild and courteous manners; readily imparting information either on his favourite science or on professional subjects'.

Parkinson was a general practitioner who spent his career establishing new views on both the social and scientific aspects of life. His work on this palsy was unprecedented and ultimately led to others acknowledging his work by naming this condition eponymously after him. He developed a strong foundation for the modern understanding of Parkinson's disease, and in doing so contributed invaluably to the medical field.

Further Reading

Jefferson M. James Parkinson 1755–1824. *British Medical Journal* 1973;2(5866):601–3.

Morris AD. James Parkinson, born April 11, 1755. *The Lancet* 1955;265(6867):761–63.

Morris AD. *James Parkinson: His Life and Times.* Boston: Birkhäuser; 1989.

Parkinson J. *An Essay on the Shaking Palsy.* London: Sherwood, Neely, and Jones; 1817.

10 JOHN ABERCROMBIE (1780–1844)
Saadiyah Khan

John Abercrombie was born in Eastchurch, Aberdeen on 12 October 1780. He was the only child of the Reverend George Abercrombie of East church. His education began at Aberdeen Grammar School and then continued at Marischal College, Aberdeen where at 15 years old, graduated Master of Arts (MA). In 1800, he began studying medicine at the University of Edinburgh with his contemporaries including philosopher and poet Thomas Brown (1778–1820). Both Abercrombie and Brown were awarded MD in 1803. After one year of postgraduate study at St George's Hospital, London, he returned to Edinburgh and began work as a general practitioner. He worked at 8 Nicolson Street next to Edinburgh Riding School. Later, in 1832, this building became the Playfair Building, which currently belongs to the RCS of Edinburgh.

Abercrombie was awarded MRCS of Edinburgh and, in 1805, was appointed surgeon to the Royal Public Dispensary in Richmond Street. The dispensary provided free medical care to the sick and poor and provided opportunities for work for many new apprentices in general practice. In 1815, Abercrombie attained the role of senior surgeon at the New Town Dispensary in Thistle Street. However, his extraordinary care, sociability and time spent with patients led to increasing recognition and following the death of physician James Gregory (1753–1821) Abercrombie was considered Edinburgh's leading general practitioner. He was awarded FRCP in 1824.

Following several of his papers being published in the *Edinburgh Medical and Surgical Journal*, Abercrombie moved on to more comprehensive writing. Two books were published in 1828 and received wide commendation. They were translated into French and German, and went through a number of editions. *Pathological and Practical Researches on Diseases of the Brain and Spinal Cord* (1828) was considered the first textbook in neuropathology, a subject first defined by Abercrombie as a separate entity. His second book, *Researches on the Diseases of the Intestinal Canal, Liver and Other Viscera of the Abdomen* (1828), incorporated the first clinical descriptions of duodenal and perforated duodenal ulcers confirmed by post-mortem. There was limited resource during this period for associating clinical features with pathology. This was particularly a time before the emergence of radiological interventions and abdominal surgery. The first specimen of a perforated duodenal ulcer is on display at present in Surgeons' Hall Museum, Edinburgh.

As Abercrombie's abilities as a doctor became well known he began treating patients from across the British Isles and various countries. He became medical adviser to, and developed a good friendship with, novelist and historian Sir Walter Scott (1771–1832). As his reputation increased further, he was then appointed by King George IV as physician to the King in Scotland. He increasingly published works on philosophical ideas as opposed to medicine. In 1830, he published his *Inquiries concerning the Intellectual Powers of Man and the Investigation of Truth* (1830). By 1833, a sequel was published, *The Philosophy of the Moral Feelings* (1833). Both writings were appreciated widely at the time of their publication but were fast to be replaced by more original works. In 1834, The University of Oxford presented to him an honorary degree of MD. Within the previous 50 years there had been just one other honorary doctorate of Medicine, that being Edward Jenner (1749–1823).

Abercrombie wrote a number of essays on topics of everyday use which when accumulated were referred to as *Elements of Sacred Truth for the Young* (1844). He became dedicated to the study of religion and as an elder of the Church of Scotland published *The Man of Faith: Or the Harmony of Christian Faith and Christian Character* (1835). In 1835, his *alma mater* awarded him Rectorship of Marischal College, Aberdeen. In this year Abercrombie was designated vice-president of The Royal Society of Edinburgh and a member of The Royal Academy of Medicine of France.

Charitable by nature, Abercrombie supported the Edinburgh Association, which provided medical services in many countries. The association expanded to become the Edinburgh Medical Missionary Society. In 1841, Abercrombie was partially paralysed, yet continued his role as a general practitioner. During the Disruption of 1843, he joined the evangelical party, which secured a majority in the General Assembly and formed the Free Church of Scotland.

Abercrombie died at his home, 19 York Place, Edinburgh, on 14 November 1844. The cause of death was confirmed on autopsy as rupture of a coronary artery with haemopericardium. He is buried alongside the east wall of St. Cuthbert's Churchyard beside the entry to Princes Street Gardens. He had a collection of over 900 books, which after his death his family handed to the RCS of Edinburgh. Large volumes of papers were contributed to the library of the RCP of Edinburgh. A year after his death in 1845, his book on religious ethics simply called *Essays* was published.

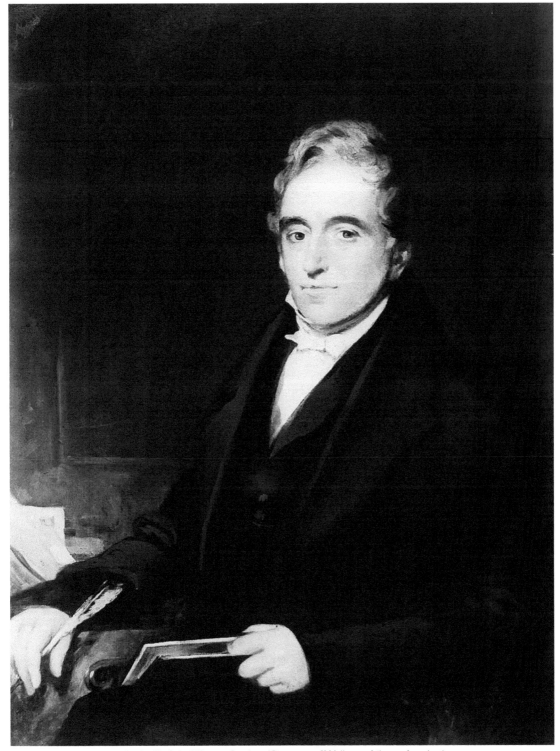

Portrait of John Abercrombie by Sir John Watson Gorden. (Courtesy of Wellcome Library, London.)

Further Reading

Abercrombie J. *Pathological and Practical Researches of Diseases of the Brain and the Spinal Cord.* Edinburgh: Waugh and Innes; 1828.

Drake D, Yandell, LP. *The Western Journal of Medicine and Surgery,* Volume 3. Louisville, Kentucky: Prentice & Weissinger; 1845.

Maclagan D. *Sketch of the Life and Character of Dr. Abercrombie.* Edinburgh: Neill; 1854.

11 JACOB AUGUSTUS LOCKHART CLARKE (1817–1880)

Neil Metcalfe

Jacob Augustus Lockhart Clarke was born in 1817. Due to his father dying early, Clarke was brought up by his mother in France until he was 13 years old. He gave no early indications of a successful career when young and it was commented that he was regarded by his family as lazy. On returning to England he chose the medical profession, to which his elder brother and grandfather belonged, and studied at Guy's and St Thomas' Hospitals. Clarke was known as a retiring, quiet and modest man who was of 'noble independence, honest and just and intellectually keen'. He did not initially graduate from the University of London but was awarded LSA in 1842.

On obtaining the diploma of the Apothecaries' Society, Clarke straight away moved into general practice starting at Pimlico, London, living with his mother. However, at the same time as working as a general practitioner, he became devoted to microscopical research on the brain and nervous system. He was a pioneer of a histological technique in studying the nervous system, using diluted spirits of wine for 24 hours and then in pure spirit of wine, changing the spirit every five to six days for a period of about 14 days. Transparency was induced by placing the sections in a 1:3 or 1:5 mixture of strong acetic acid and spirit for 2–10 minutes, according to their thickness. The sections were then floated in turpentine to clear them and mounted in Canada balsam under a thin glass slide. This method was later described in *The Lancet* as having 'revolutionised histological research'.

Clarke undertook much research. This was done with extreme care and thoroughness and he went on to establish many new facts of structure that had important bearings on the physiology and pathology of the nervous system. Clarke was the first to establish the location of the dorsal nucleus of the spinal cord and describe the posterior vesicular columns. Today, the dorsal nucleus is eponymously known as Clarke's nucleus and the posterior vesicular column as the column of Clarke. He also described the nucleus intermediolateralis and differentiated the medial cuneate nucleus from the lateral cuneate nucleus.

Similarly, Clarke became widely published. This included in French and in German. His first paper, 'Researches into the Structure of the Spinal Cord', was received by the Royal Society on 15 October 1850 and published in their *Transactions* for 1851. This paper was illustrated, like many of his subsequent papers, by particularly accurate and appreciated drawings which he drew, and these have been subsequently reproduced in numerous works. Some of his titles included 'The Development of Striped Muscle in Man, Mammalia, and Birds', 'The Intimate Structure of the Brain Human and Comparative on the Structure of the Medulla Oblongata' and 'On the Structure of the Optic Lobes of the Cuttle-Fish'. Together with the neurologist Hughlings Jackson (1835–1911) he wrote 'On a Case of Muscular Atrophy with Disease of the Spinal Cord and Medulla Oblongata'. He also wrote an early account of account of syringomyelia shortly after the work of Charles-Prosper Ollivier d'Angers (1796–1845). Further work on diabetes paraplegia, epilepsy, hysterical paroxysms and the treatment of neuralgia by iodine were carried out. However, one of his major achievements, though not particularly well noted contemporaneously or in the annals of history, is his detailed clinico-pathological description of a case of amyotrophic lateral sclerosis (ALS). His written account, published with Charles Bland Radcliffe (1822–1889) in the *British and Foreign Medico-Chirurgical Review*, in 1862, was three years ahead of Jean-Martin Charcot's (1825–1893) description of this disease and 12 years before Charcot's first use of the term ALS. Other journals he wrote for included the *Medico-Chirurgical Transactions*, *Transactions of The Microscopical Society & Journal* and the *Archives of Medicine*. He later contributed to *System of Surgery* (1870), edited by Timothy Holmes (1825–1907), when writing of the separate sections of the muscular system, diseases and injuries of nerves and on locomotor ataxy. Throughout he was as successful in general practice as the 'distractions necessitated by the scientific work allowed'.

Recognition of his achievements eventually followed. He was elected an FRS in 1854 and, in 1864, received the Queen's Medal of the Royal Society, also known as the Royal Medal and the society's highest honour. This was for 'his researches on the intimate structure of the spinal cord and brain, and on the development of the spinal cord, published in five memoirs in the *Philosophical Transactions* and in other writings'. In 1867, he was elected an Honorary Fellow of the King and Queen's College of Physicians in Ireland in recognition of his scientific work. He was awarded MD from the University of St Andrews in 1869. For this examination he was allowed a 'dispensing clause', seemingly excused from the section 'on Medical Anatomy and on the Principles of Medicine'.

Clarke left general practice in 1871. In the same year he was awarded MRCP under the 'Dispensing Clause'. He became physician to the Hospital for Epilepsy and Paralysis in Regent's Park but it was felt that he did not have a lot of success in this appointment, probably due to a combination of retired habits, and his having published no book by which the public could judge his work. His obituary in the *BMJ* mentioned that his professional success there 'was in no way commensurate to his deserts'.

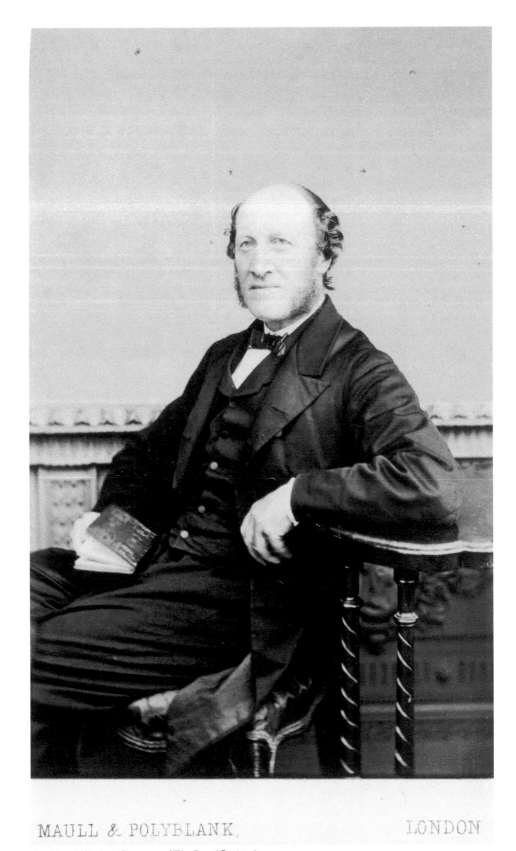

MAULL & POLYBLANK,   LONDON

Photograph of Jacob Clarke. (Courtesy of The Royal Society.)

Having had a severe attack of pleurisy in 1870, Clarke's health later deteriorated significantly in 1879. He was attended in his last illness by the aforementioned Jackson and Stephen Mackenzie (1844–1909). *The Medical Times and Gazette* recorded on 31 January 1880 that 'many friends would have been glad of the privilege of serving him, but he was, though kind-hearted and generous, very reserved, and few knew of his illness'. He died on 25 January 1880 of phthisis at his sister's house at 3 Endlesham Villas in Balham. *The Lancet* described him as 'a man single of purpose, of noble independence and honesty, wholly free from ambition, and wanting in that knowledge of the world necessary for making way in it'.

Further Reading

Anon. J. Lockhart Clarke, M.D., F.R.S. *The Lancet* 1880;115(2944):189.

Anon. Obituary. J. Lockhart Clarke, M.D., F.R.S. *British Medical Journal* 1880;1:188.

Bettany GT. Clarke, Jacob Augustus Lockhart (1817–1880). In: Stephen L, Lee S (eds.). *The Dictionary of National Biography*. Volume IV. London: Oxford University Press; 1887.

Lockhart Clarke J. Researches into the structure of the spinal chord. *Philosophical Transactions of the Royal Society of London* 1851;141:607–21.

Lockhart Clarke J. Further researches on the grey substance of the spinal cord. *Philosophical Transactions of the Royal Society of London* 1859;149:437–67.

Lockhart Clarke J, Hughlings Jackson J. On a case of muscular atrophy with disease of the spinal cord and medulla oblongata. *Medico-Chirurgical Transactions* 1867;50:489–98.

Radcliffe CB, Lockhart Clarke J. An important case of paralysis and muscular atrophy with disease of the nervous centres. *The British and Foreign Medico-Chirurgical Review* 1862;30:215–25.

Turner MR, Swash M, Ebers GC. Lockhart Clarke's contribution to the description of amyotrophic lateral sclerosis. *Brain* 2010;133(11):3470–79.

12 THOMAS HUNT (1798–1879)

Jean-Claude Massey

Thomas Hunt was born on 18 February 1798 in Watford, Hertfordshire. He was the eldest son of a non-conformist Baptist minister Reverend Thomas Hunt (1763–1844) and his wife Maria Edwards (1763–1848). Little is known regarding Hunt's childhood but it is assumed that he followed his father from one parish to the next; these include Ridgemount, Dunstable and Tring.

As a non-conformist Baptist at this time, a place at the medical schools of Oxford and Cambridge it was difficult for Hunt to obtain. However, undeterred from entering the medical profession, he started an apprenticeship as a surgeon because such a position at the time did not require a university education. He began his training around 1812 whereby he received a grant from the John Bankes Trust. John Bankes was one of Hunt's ancestors whom was a Master of the Haberdashers' Company and a Freeman of the City of London and claims to the Trust were permitted to descendants of Bankes on the occasion of marriage, apprenticeship or setting up a business. During his training as an apprentice surgeon he took courses in anatomy and surgery at Guy's and St Thomas' Hospital in London.

Hunt was awarded MRCS in August 1820. The work he did was as a contemporaneous general practitioner, performing simple operations and treating certain conditions in the community that did not require hospitalisation.

In 1826, Hunt was practising in Upper Clapton. He later moved in 1829 to Herne Bay in Kent with his new wife Martha Mary Colam (1808–1861) whom he married on 8 August 1827. This marriage produced a total of 13 children (of which at least eight survived him). Amongst his children were Arthur Ackland Hunt (1841–1914) who later became a celebrated artist, and Thomas Hunt Jr. (baptised 1837–died circa 1875) who was awarded MRCS in 1859.

Hunt's greatest contribution to medicine perhaps came in 1846 whereby he pioneered a new plan for the advancement of medical sciences submitted to the South Eastern Branch of the Provincial Medical and Surgical Association (which later became the BMA) at its annual meeting. For this plan he had collected and collated observations in a new method that would bring about a more standardised approach in how to undertake research. In Hunt's report 'Memoir on the medicinal action of arsenic' (1849) a questionnaire had been sent out to association members and also non-members. What was original about this was that Hunt made the observers aware of the fact that they were taking part in the investigation. All previous attempts to gather information from other professionals at this time had been done without warning by asking for their observations. How Hunt's method differed is that he asked the participants to note the use of arsenic over the time period and respond back with the results in the form of a questionnaire. Previously, the observations given were described in a *BMJ* supplement 'The B.M.A. and collective investigation' as being 'very incomplete and not capable of rigid analysis'. By taking the initiative, Hunt had pioneered the start of a new method for collectively investigating throughout the medical profession. This method of collective investigating is the basis of a lot of modern day medical research, and this form of communication between medical colleagues on how to best produce a collective investigation has led to the betterment of medical treatment around the world.

During his time in Herne Bay, Hunt's interest in dermatology developed, and his first book, *Practical Observations on the Pathology and Treatment of Certain Diseases of the Skin Generally Pronounced Intractable*, was published in 1847. Hunt practised at Herne Bay for approximately 20 years before taking residence in London at 26 Bedford Square before 1850. Several years after moving to London Hunt was awarded FRCS in 1852 where he lectured on skin conditions at the Hunterian School of Medicine. He later published different editions of his book including *A Guide to the Treatment of Diseases of the Skin: with Suggestions for their Prevention. For the Use of the Student and General Practitioner* in 1861 and showing the intended audience very much included general practitioners. His commitment to dermatological studies, publishing articles and books led to positive reviews of his book on diseases of the skin being commented on in *The Lancet* as 'Mr Hunt has transferred these diseases from incurable class to the curable'.

Hunt was also a keen member and doctor of the Western Dispensary for Diseases of the Skin (founded in 1851) from at least August 1852. The dispensary originally occupied 21A Charlotte Street in Fitzroy Square before later moving to 179 Great Portland Street in London in 1879. There, Hunt was listed as one of the consultant surgeons of the dispensary. The dispensary's aim was to provide affordable medical care for those who would be unlikely to afford treatment otherwise. However, it is unclear whether this service received any charitable contributions, as it still cost the patients a shilling a week, meaning the average member of society would have been unlikely to afford these services at this time. The services provided included the treatment of scorbutic and other eruptions, ringworm, scald head and baldness. The dispensary was known to have a good record with patients with advertisements stating that 'not one patient in a thousand had been discharged incurable'. In addition to this, the dispensary boasted that in 1857, they dealt with 9317 cases, an incredible feat seeing as the dispensary only opened for five and a half hours each week.

A

GUIDE TO THE TREATMENT

OF

DISEASES OF THE SKIN:

WITH

SUGGESTIONS FOR THEIR PREVENTION.

FOR

THE USE OF THE STUDENT AND GENERAL PRACTITIONER.

Illustrated by Cases.

BY

THOMAS HUNT, F.R.C.S.,

Surgeon to the Western Dispensary for Diseases of
the Skin.

"In chronic diseases, the entire system has been altered ; and to effect a
cure, the entire man must be remodelled."—SYDENHAM.

NINTH EDITION.

LONDON :

T. RICHARDS, 37, GREAT QUEEN STREET.

M.DCCC.LXXI.

Image of the title page of one of Thomas Hunt's books. (Courtesy of Wellcome Library, London.)

Hunt was one of the more vocal supporters for the use of arsenic in medical practice in the nineteenth century. He argued that discreet use of the substance could have a place in the treatment of skin diseases, neuralgia, syphilis and cancer to name a few. During his life he published several papers in journals enthusiastically endorsing the use of arsenic; however, little follow-up came of his work and the use of arsenic diminished. Despite this, it can still be found to be used in specific cases such as all-trans retinoic acid resistant acute promyelocytic leukaemia, showing that Hunt's thoughts on the use of arsenic as a treatment for cancer were not unfounded.

For a time Hunt served as vice-president of the Medical Society of London. In addition to this, Hunt was an active member of the Epidemiological Society and stood in a position of high standing by acting as the Medical Officer of Health (MOH) in the district of St. Giles, in which he resided.

Hunt died at the age of 81 on 26 November 1879. He dedicated his entire working life to medicine, dying shortly after being made a consultant surgeon at the dispensary in 1879. His reputation in the medical field led to Hunt obtaining many highly regarded positions in medical societies and in the public eye. Hunt's pioneering record collecting has resonated through to the modern day in which Hunt's ideas can be seen to have heavily impacted on the use of collective investigation.

Further Reading

Hunt T. *Practical Observations on the Pathology and Treatment of Certain Diseases of the Skin Generally Pronounced Intractable*. London: J. Churchill; 1847.

Hunt T. *Medicinal Action of Arsenic; Collected from the Reported Experience of the Members of the Provincial Medical and Surgical Association, and Other Sources*. Worcester: Deighton & Co; 1849;XVI(Part II):402–4.

Hunt T. *A Guide to the Treatment of Diseases of the Skin: with Suggestions for their Prevention. For the Use of the Student and General Practitioner*. London: T. Richards; 1861.

McConaghey R. The B.M.A. and collective investigation. *British Medical Journal* 1956;1(4964):59–61.

13 WILLIAM BUDD (1811–1880)
Zoe Shipley

William Budd was born on 14 September 1811 in the small town of North Tawton in Devon. He was born into a large family of 10 children of which William was the sixth child to parents Samuel Budd and Catherine Wreford. Six of their children went on to graduate from university in medicine. His father, Samuel Budd (1775–1841), previously worked as a naval surgeon during the war against France (1792–1802) in 1794 and was also a local doctor in the town. Five of Budd's brothers and himself followed their father into medicine with three studying at the University of Edinburgh, including Budd, and three studying at the University of Cambridge.

Budd first began his medical career as an apprentice at his father's country practice in North Tawton. He then worked alongside some influential figures over the next four years studying medicine in Paris. He observed the work of Pierre Louis (1787–1872), who was an anatomical pathologist and clinical investigator, and the work of French doctor Pierre Bretonneau (1778–1862) who was known for successfully performing the first tracheostomy in 1825 as well as for his work on scarlet fever, diphtheria and observations on infectious outbreaks in 1826 in Tours, France. Louis had a particular interest in putrid fever, also known as Typhus, and he discovered that the body's natural defence mechanisms of the small intestine called Peyer's patches were inflamed and ulcerated in patients with putrid fever. Bretonneau also reported an outbreak of a similar communicable disease in a military school with the same Peyer's patches findings in those who had died from it. This medical exposure in Paris together with having himself contracted typhoid fever that year sparked his interest in how these communicable diseases were being spread.

After Paris Budd went to the University of Edinburgh to finish his medical studies where he qualified in 1838 and obtained his MD. He was awarded a gold medal from the University of Edinburgh for his work on acute rheumatism, which he produced whilst studying there.

After graduating Budd went to work as a general practitioner in North Tawton. Shortly after this there was an outbreak of typhoid fever (1839) in a nearby village where most of the patients that he cared for lived. With his recent experience of typhoid fever and the new local outbreak, he was intrigued even further to research his interest of typhoid fever and communicable diseases. He observed each of the first few cases and followed their interaction with family and visitors. This led him to note that people coming into contact with infected patients were also becoming part of the typhoid fever epidemic. He wrote his findings on how people in the village became infected with typhoid fever through close contact with infected family and friends in an essay in 1839 entitled 'The investigation of the sources of the common continued fevers of Great Britain and Ireland, and the ascertaining of the circumstances which may have a tendency to render them communicable from one person to another'. This essay was unsuccessfully submitted by Budd to a medical competition and therefore was not recognised as one of his great pieces of work.

Budd's next medical role was on the naval hospital ship *HMS Dreadnought* at Greenwich in 1840, where he served a very short time treating ex-members of the merchant navy. However, he was forced to resign only weeks into working there due to contracting typhoid fever himself once again.

It was not until Budd had settled in Bristol after moving there in 1842 that he would find the answer to his typhoid fever work. He became a physician to both St. Peter's Hospital and the Bristol Royal Infirmary in his early years in Bristol. He then worked as a general practitioner in Clifton, a suburb of Bristol. In 1847, he diagnosed another small epidemic of typhoid fever present in a terrace of houses called Richmond Terrace which contained 34 households. Thirteen of these households had at least one case of typhoid fever and Budd realised that the only link between these houses was the use of the same well, whilst the other houses without typhoid fever had a separate water supply. This link sparked his hypothesis that transmission was spread through water. Budd realised that contaminated water supplies were the breeding ground for many communicable diseases and that the infected patients had a certain intestinal discharge in their faecal matter that was then being ingested by others. He believed that this was also the source of cholera transmission and noted this down whilst preparing his own work. However, John Snow (1813–1858), beat him to publication of this theory with his book *On the Mode of Communication of Cholera* (1855). This was one month before Budd's paper on 'Mode of propagation of cholera' was published in 1856 in *The Lancet*.

Budd's typhoid fever hypothesis, described in his 'On intestinal fever' paper published in *The Lancet* 1859, was initially disputed by many contemporaries due to his contagion hypothesis. It split fellow country doctors into two groups: one who believed typhoid fever was a disease spread directly between humans and the other who believed that the disease was transmitted through bad drainage systems just like in Richmond Terrace. After also researching the typhoid fever outbreak at the Convent of Good Shepherd near Bristol in 1863, Budd confirmed in his later work of 'Typhoid fever: It's nature, mode of spreading and prevention', published in 1873, that this fever was propagated through a certain organism being discharged from the intestine of infected people.

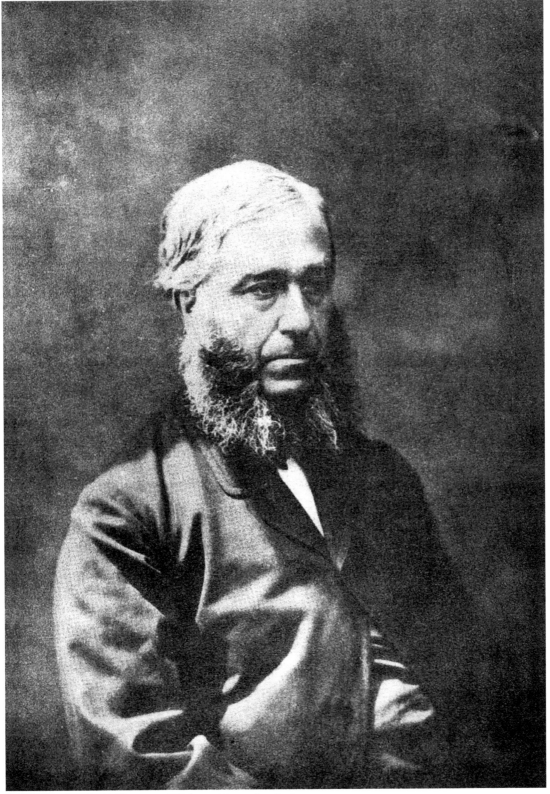

Portrait of William Budd. (Courtesy of Wellcome Library, London.)

Throughout his time in Bristol Budd worked in ensuring that the waterworks became cleaner. He was also committed to preventing epidemic disease within Bristol, especially as they had the third highest mortality rate in England. By 1849, he prompted changes in the new Bristol Water Company and influenced new public health measures to help keep water supplies to houses clean and not contaminated by sewage works even before he had full support that this was the main source of typhoid fever transmission. The improvements in sewage works proved to be successful as it was thought to have limited the number of deaths during three cholera epidemics spanning from 1849, when there were 1979 deaths, compared to 29 deaths in 1866. He devised the use of disinfectants consisting of chloride of lime and perchloride of iron to be used in the drains and privies of areas with an epidemic. Budd's findings changed Bristol's quality of water for good; his ground-breaking work was a cornerstone to modern society.

Budd carried on his post as a physician at Bristol's hospitals and went on to lecture at Bristol Medical School. He also continued his research on infectious diseases in humans such as scarlet fever and in animals such as smallpox. His interest in the study of animal epidemics made him differ from many of his contemporaries but it was key for his hypotheses testing, the ideas from which he then transferred to epidemics in humans. For his work on epidemics and infectious diseases, he was awarded FRS in 1871.

In 1873, Budd's health deteriorated after what he believed was another round of typhoid fever and he had to retire from his work later that year after becoming hemiplegic following a stroke. He died in Walton-in-Gordano, Somerset, in 1880. He became acknowledged as one of the pioneers of modern epidemiology and his great influence on Great Britain and Ireland's view on clean water supplies and sewage drainage fulfilled his deep interest in the prevention of disease. He truly prevented many more epidemics of communicable diseases, which were common in that era. Whilst working as a general practitioner, he was well respected by the community in which he worked and furthermore, he was able to witness first-hand the conditions his patients lived in. This knowledge, combined with his medical research, gave him the platform to create and become a leading advocate for preventative strategies in the community, demonstrating the importance of clean water supplies for people's health.

Further Reading

Bettany GT. Budd, William (1811–1880). In: Stephen L, Lee S (eds.). *The Dictionary of National Biography*. Volume III. London: Oxford University Press; 1885.

Budd W. Mode of propagation of cholera. *The Lancet* 1856;1:379.

Budd W. On intestinal fever. *The Lancet* 1859;ii: 4–5, 28–30, 55–6, 80–2.

Budd W. *Typhoid Fever: It's Nature, Mode of Spreading and Prevention*. London: Longmans, Green and Co; 1873.

Dunnill MS. Commentary: William Budd on cholera. *International Journal of Epidemiology* 2013;42:1576–77.

Moorhead R. William Budd and typhoid fever. *Journal of the Royal Society of Medicine* 2002;95:561–64.

Pelling M. Budd, William (1811–1880). In: Matthew HCG, Harrison B (eds.). *Oxford Dictionary of National Biography*. Volume 8. Oxford: Oxford University Press; 2004.

Reeves C. Budd, William. In: Bynum WF, Bynum H (eds.). *Dictionary of Medical Biography*. London: Greenwood Press; 2007.

Snow J. *On the Mode of Communication of Cholera*. London: Churchill; 1855.

14 JOHN SNOW (1813–1858)
Samuel Wood

Born on 15 March 1813 in North Street, York, then one of the poorest parts of the city, John Snow was the son of William, a coal yard labourer. Despite his humble beginnings, he was schooled at St. Peters in York and showed an aptitude for mathematics and the natural sciences. When he was 14 years old Snow made his first steps towards a medical career through an apprenticeship to Mr William Hardcastle (1794–1860), an apothecary-surgeon in Newcastle upon Tyne. During this apprenticeship Snow was fortunate to be in the inaugural class of the Newcastle Medical School of 1832 and attended a number of lectures at the fledgling institute.

It was during his time in Newcastle that Snow first came in contact with the disease that stands at the forefront of his legacy. The cholera epidemic of 1831 started in Sunderland and spread throughout the Northeast of England. Hardcastle, as a prominent doctor in the area, was key in the medical treatment of the people in his and neighbouring parishes and at his side was Snow. Upon finishing his apprenticeship in 1833, Snow had two further assistantships in general practice, first in Burnopfield, County Durham, with Mr John Watson (1790–1847), and then with Mr Joseph Warburton (1786–1846) in Pateley Bridge in Nidderdale, Yorkshire.

To make the next step in his career, Snow moved to London in 1836, but due to his meagre means he walked the 200 mile journey from York to enrol in formal medical education at the Hunterian Medical School, Soho. At this time Snow lodged with Mr Joshua Parsons (1814–1892), a fellow student, with whom he developed a strong friendship. They regularly debated Snow's belief in vegetarianism, leading to contests of physical strength and vigour. In one such contest they raced to St. Albans and back on foot, Snow ultimately admitting defeat and catching a horse-drawn bus home from Edgware Road.

He was awarded MRCS in 1837 and LSA in 1838 and enrolled at the Westminster Hospital. Following this, he found quarters at 54 Frith St., Soho and started his general practice. Snow worked tirelessly to develop his reputation, visiting the outpatients of Charing Cross Hospital and caring for four sick clubs, eventually amassing a busy patient load. Alongside these efforts in general practice, he continued to further his medical education and standing amongst local doctors. This he achieved through research into respiratory and circulatory physiology, producing numerous papers and subsequently being awarded Bachelor of Medicine (MB) in 1843 and MD with Honours in 1844 from the University of London.

Snow's first published report was on 'Asphyxia and on the resuscitation of newborn children' in 1841, but his works spanned a range of subjects from capillary circulation to scarlet fever. Anaesthesia became a major interest of his and his work in the field was stimulated by the discovery of the modern anaesthetic agents, ether and chloroform, in 1846 and 1847, respectively. This interest led him to design a new inhaler for the administration of anaesthesia, which was adopted into common use in infirmaries throughout Great Britain and Ireland. Snow's noted work in the field led to his invitation to administer chloroform to Queen Victoria during the birth of Prince Leopold in 1853 and of Princess Beatrice in 1857, for which he was highly commended.

Alongside this, Snow continued his general practice in Soho and through his work he again encountered the devastating effects of cholera during the epidemic of 1848. Snow's scientific curiosity led him to doubt the prevailing opinions on the transmission of cholera; he questioned why a disease supposedly spread by foul air would cause only gastrointestinal symptoms, deducing that it must instead be spread by contaminated water. In 1849, Snow outlined his ideas in a pamphlet, *On the Communication of Cholera*, in which he explained his theory of the faecal-oral mode of transmission.

Frustratingly for Snow, there was little acceptance of his theory until the epidemic of 1854. At this time, Snow made an astute observation regarding the local water supply: between the outbreak in 1848 and the present epidemic, the Lambeth Water Company had moved its supply upstream of where sewers emptied into the River Thames. Noting this change, Snow found that the death rates from cholera in the areas supplied by the company had dropped dramatically compared to those of other companies whose supply had not moved. Further to this, the final proof of his theory came from his own local area. In August 1854, an outbreak of cholera occurred in Soho which resulted in over 500 fatal cases in just 10 days. Snow mapped the cases and found that the highest incidences were in close proximity to the Broad Street pump. Having presented this information to the parochial council the handle of the pump was removed and the epidemic waned within days. Snow published an expanded second edition of *On the Communication of Cholera* in 1855, and in that same year was elected as the president of the Medical Society of London.

Throughout his adult life, Snow struggled with tuberculosis and renal problems. As years passed his health continued to decline until, at 45 years of age, he died from a stroke on 16 June 1858. Whilst a man of a shy and retiring nature, Snow made a great impression on many who received his care. He was never known to discriminate and he treated everyone from paupers to royalty with the same respect, professionalism and tireless enthusiasm. This sentiment is perhaps best recorded in a quote from a letter by Hooper Attree (1817–1875) published in

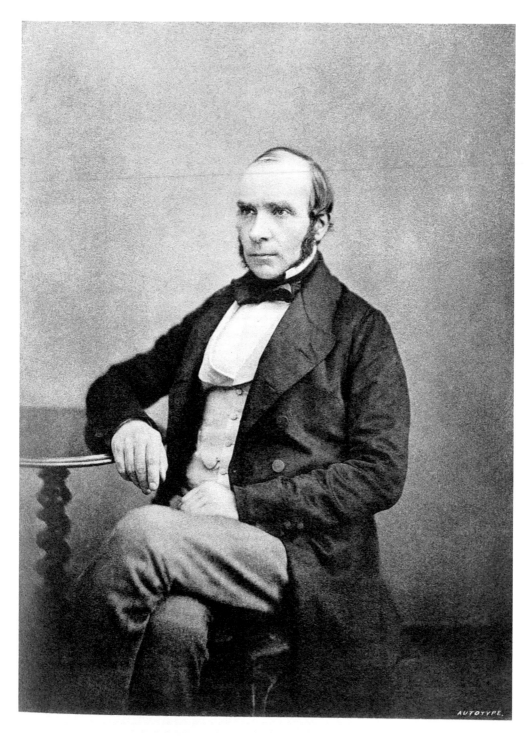

John Snow

(Autotype from a Presentation Portrait, 1856, and Autograph facsimile.—B. W. R.)

John Snow in 1856. (Courtesy of Wellcome Library, London.)

The Lancet following Snow's obituary: 'Who does not remember his frankness, his cordiality, his honesty, the absence of all disguise or affectation under an apparent off-hand manner? Her Majesty the Queen has been deprived of the future valuable services of a trustworthy, well-deserving, much-esteemed subject, by his sudden death. The poor have lost in him a real friend in the hour of need'. In 2003, a poll of British doctors ranked Snow as the greatest doctor of all time.

Further Reading

Ashcroft A. John Snow – Victorian physician. In: Hargreaves A, Lazenby E, Gardner-Medwin D (eds.). *Medicine in Northumbria. Essays on the History of Medicine in the North East of England*. Newcastle-upon-Tyne: Pybus Society for the History and Bibliography of Medicine; 1993.

Leaman A. John Snow MD – His early days. *Anaesthesia* 1984;39(8):803–805.

Richardson B W. The life of John Snow, MD: Appended as an introduction to: Snow J. *On Chloroform and other Anaesthetics*. London: John Churchill; 1858.

Snow J. *On the Mode of Communication of Cholera*. 2nd ed. London: John Churchill; 1855.

Snow SJ. John Snow MD (1813–1858). Part II: Becoming a doctor – His medical training and early years of practice. *Journal of Medical Biography* 2000;8(2):71–77.

15 CHARLES HARRISON BLACKLEY (1820–1900)

Emma L. Vinton, Neil Metcalfe and Eleanor Morris

Charles Blackley was born in Bolton, Lancashire, on 5 April 1820. His father died when he was three years old and his mother relocated to Manchester to raise and educate him. He had a simple education in Bolton and on leaving school he worked as an apprentice printer and engraver at Bradshaw and Blacklock's of Brown St. Manchester, where George Bradshaw's celebrated railway guides originated. He long had a passion for homeopathy and after leaving school he devoted much of his time to evening classes in botany, chemistry and greek. In his early twenties, Blackley travelled to Manchester, Jamaica, and married his wife Mary Mills there in 1844. They had three children together, John Galley in 1846, Charles in 1849 and Bertha Mary in 1856, several years after their return to Hulme, Lancashire.

Blackley had left the printing business in 1855 and enrolled at Pine Street Medical School, Manchester. He was awarded MRCS in 1858 and practised as a general practitioner in Hulme whilst supporting his growing family. Blackley suffered with asthma and hay fever for many years and regularly noticed his own symptoms amongst his patients. He used several homeopathic remedies in the absence of mainstream treatments but this was often scorned by colleagues, who discredited his approaches. He remained undeterred and he dedicated many hours researching the true nature and mechanisms of hay fever, commencing his experiments on hay fever in 1859. Like his peers Morrill Wyman (1812–1903) and George Beard (1839–1883), he was keen to limit symptoms and find a cure. Hay fever had been isolated as a condition in 1819 by John Bostock (1773–1846). Existing theories at the time identified dust, ozone, benzoic acid, light and heat as possible causes of hay fever. Blackley performed experiments on himself with various substances, and even performed controls for each experiment. For example, he applied benzoic acid to one nostril and a solution containing only diluted alcohol to the other.

Using a microscope, Blackley discovered that the samples of dust which brought on hay fever attacks contained pollen. Blackley investigated pollens from over 80 different types of plant and discovered that grasses caused the greatest reaction. He experimented with fresh and dry extracts of pollen, administered to the nose, mouth, eyes and lacerated skin. By exposing himself and his patients to each agent systematically he discovered which would give the strongest reaction. By inoculating the upper and lower limbs with the fresh moistened pollen, Blackley gave a classic description of a positive skin test: 'In a few minutes after the pollen had been applied the abraded spot began to itch intensely; the parts immediately around the abrasion began to swell... the swelling seemed to be due to effusion into the subcutaneous cellular tissue'. With higher doses he found that even more severe symptoms began to occur, including a rapid heartbeat, fever and sweating for up to 48 hours. Blackley also took air samples at different altitudes by flying kites adorned with glycerine sticky slides and later added a clockwork mechanism so slides could be exposed for a set time. The number of pollen grains collected could be counted under the microscope and Blackley correlated these results with the severity of his own symptoms. He further added a carbolic acid infused glycerin sampling solution to deter insects and concluded that at times of the year associated with elevated pollen much higher levels existed at 1000–2000 feet than at ground level. This explained why people in cities far away from pollen sources still experienced hay fever symptoms. Drug treatments did not prove effective and Blackley concluded that sufferers should spend summers in suitable low-pollen areas.

Charles Darwin was fascinated by Blackley's experiments on whether pollen could be carried large distances in the upper regions of the atmosphere. He wondered if pollen would lose its potency if boiled and dried, but Blackley confirmed that it did not. Darwin asked Blackley why he had not considered the distinction between plants fertilised using wind as a vector (entomophilous) and those that used insects as a vector (anemophilous). Darwin wrote in a letter to Blackley dated 5 July 1873: 'Perhaps where grass is cut and dried; some pollen of the entomophilous division may be blown about; but naturally hardly any would thus be blown. Whereas the pollen of anemophilous plants cannot fail to be largely blown in every direction'. Blackley replied on 7 July 1873. He mentioned that his high-altitude experiments had been inspired by Darwin's discussion of collecting atmospheric dust at Porto Praya in his *Journal of Researches*. Darwin asserted that coniferous pollen could be carried several hundred miles and be deposited on ships, explaining why some sailors experience hay fever whilst at sea. Blackley's response, dated 11 July 1873, wrote that it had 'a very important bearing upon the subject, and I very much regret that it should have escaped my attention'. He added that 'investigations have had to be made with the hourly recurring demands of a moderately large practice pressing upon [him]'. Despite increasing general practice demands, Blackley was eventually successful in being the first known person to identify pollen as the true cause of allergic rhinitis (hay fever), and published his findings in his book *Experimental Researches on the Causes and Nature of Catarrhus aestivus* (1873).

Blackley knew that asthma could be precipitated by the inhalation of pollen and had invoked an attack of asthma during a number of his experiments. He differentiated between different types of asthma which had or had not been induced by pollen, but also believed that there was a progression in the disease state from hay fever to asthma. He thought that both conditions were due to mucosal changes brought about by pollen, which caused dilation and,

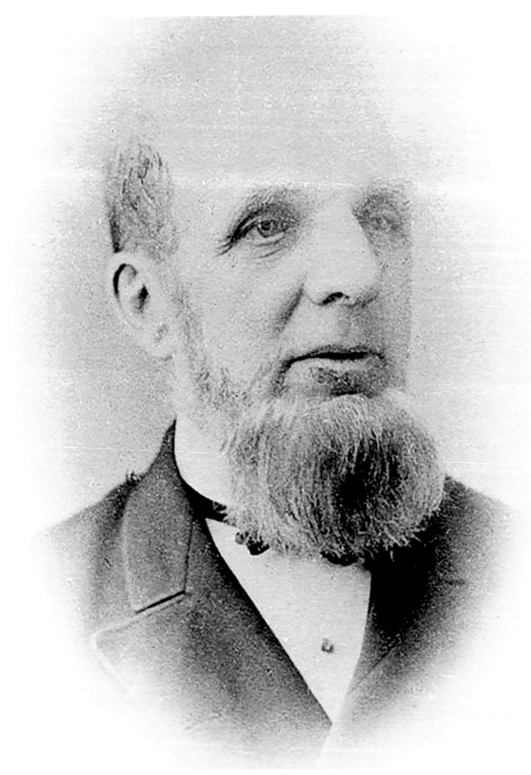

Charles Harrison Blackley. (Courtesy of Wikimedia Commons.)

therefore, exudation from the capillary vessels of the connective tissue. This theory resulted from an experiment he carried out in which he breathed by mouth through rubber tubes of differing diameters. He could not produce in himself any asthmatic sensation unless the tubes were very narrow, so concluded that the major bronchi or trachea would have to reduce their diameter excessively in order to produce symptoms.

In 1873, Blackley was affiliated to the British Homeopathic Society and became an Honorary Member of the Manchester and Salford Homeopathic Dispensary. For a time, he acted as president of the British Homeopathic Society. He also edited the *Manchester Homeopathic Observer* and published articles across a range of medical and scientific journals. He completed his MD at the University of Brussels in 1874 and his later work isolated the smallest possible pollen sample needed to induce and maintain hay fever symptoms. This required him to weigh pollen grains using a dilution method. Darwin was very impressed with Blackley's work and in his letter dated 9 March 1877 he wrote: 'Your calculation of the weight of pollen grains is wonderful'. Blackley had commented in an earlier letter that: 'the problem of cure has still to be solved and really resolves itself principally into a question of prophylaxis. I fear it will prove to be the most formidable and difficult part of the task I originally set myself'.

Blackley was praised for his rigorous and methodical approach to collecting, measuring and recording his findings. Some of his peers, including the aforementioned Beard and William Young (1843–1900), did not accept his explanation of hay fever, instead linking germ theory or the role of nasal secretions or lifestyle factors as potential sources. Blackley's focus on pollen was later supported by William T Dunbar (1863–1922), an American doctor and Director of the State Hygiene Institute in Hamburg, Germany.

In January 1900, Blackley suffered a hemiparesis. He subsequently died from a short terminal illness on 4 September 1900 aged 80 years old and was buried in Ormskirk, Lancashire.

John Galley Blackley (1846–1919), son of Charles Harrison Blackley, also qualified as a doctor, being awarded MB and MRCS. Inspired by his father's work, John became a physician for diseases of the skin and the senior physician at the London Homeopathic Hospital. He was also president, treasurer and Honorary Secretary of the British Homeopathic Society.

Further Reading

Blackley CH. *Experimental Researches on the Causes and Nature of Cattarrhus Aestivus (Hay-fever or hay-asthma)*. London: Baillière, Tindall and Cox; 1873.

Blackley CH. *Instruments and Text for Measuring Effect of Breath on Pollen*. London: Baillière, Tindall and Cox; 1873.

Blackley CH. *Hay Fever: Its Causes, Treatment, and Effective Prevention: Experimental Researches*. London: Baillière, Tindall and Cox; 1880.

Crameri R (ed.). *Allergy and Asthma in Modern Society: A Scientific Approach*. London: Karger; 2006.

Davidson J. *A Century of Homeopaths: Their Influence on Medicine and Health*. London: Springer; 2014.

Taylor G, Walker J. Charles Harrison Blackley, 1820–1900. *Clinical Allergy* 1973;3(2):103–8.

Waite KJ. Blackley and the development of hay fever as a disease of civilization in the nineteenth century. *Medical History* 1995;39(2):186–96.

6 HUGH OWEN THOMAS (1834–1891)

Kayleigh Jones

Hugh Owen Thomas was born in 1834 in Anglesey. When Thomas was 19 years old, his family relocated to Liverpool where Evan Thomas (1804–1884), descendant of a long line of bonesetters whose skills were passed down between generations. The family were widely known as the 'meddygon esgyrin' (bone doctors). When 19, the Thomas family relocated to Liverpool when Evan Thomas set up a practice that treated injuries sustained by the sailors at the docks. At the time of Thomas birth, his father's bone setting skills were under much scrutiny, as he was an unqualified practitioner, so Evan Thomas decided that when the time came that his sons went to medical school rather than follow his path in order to avoid the disadvantages that he had perceived to have suffered from having not followed that medical path. In 1854, when 21 years old, Thomas attended Edinburgh Medical School where he witnessed the surgeons performing numerous amputations. During his three years there, he was greatly influenced by his professor of medicine, John Hughes Bennett (1812–1875), who had theories behind the beneficial use of fresh air to treat individuals, a practice that Thomas would later adopt in his own patient management.

Thomas missed his final exams, as his father was ill. This meant that he had to take a conjoint diploma, and was awarded LRCP MRCS instead of a Bachelor of Medicine, Bachelor of Surgery (MBBS). Thomas spent some time in Paris but he returned in 1858 to join his father at his practice in Liverpool. Thomas was always supportive of his father's bone setting skills even when he faced prosecution for malpractice but his father's reluctance to introduce new medical practices into his work frustrated Thomas. This led him to leave and set up on his own at 24 Hardy Street in Garston, Liverpool. His medical knowledge combined with the traditional skills of bone setting, meant he was sought by shipwrights and deck hands that had fractures and dislocations and that he became legendary; surgeons from America would visit to learn his techniques.

By 1866, Thomas had moved his practice to 11 Nelson Street, an area that was quickly becoming known as Chinatown. As a result of having never applied for a surgical fellowship, he was not subject to the rules and regulations of an institution. This allowed him to develop his own methods and innovations.

Whilst his expertise in setting bones and treating trauma became renowned amongst the dockers, Nelson Street was located in a part of Liverpool where disease, particularly tuberculosis, was rife, leaving numerous children crippled. At the time there were great advancements in the use of anaesthesia but Thomas was appalled by the attitude of surgeons to the amputation of limbs. Having studied the work of Thomas Sydenham (1624–1689), who believed in the importance of working with nature, Thomas used the skills he had acquired as a bonesetter to develop contraptions and splints to immobilise joints and limbs to assist with reducing inflammation and promote healing.

Thomas was a busy general practitioner at Nelson Street and he was dedicated to his patients. In 1873, Thomas nephew, Robert Jones (1857–1933), also a doctor, wrote an account of Thomas typical day. He stated that it would begin at 6am and continue until midnight. Thomas would do his rounds in the morning, visit patients at home to adjust any of their splints or treatments, see patients in his consulting rooms and perform surgery during the afternoon; he would see urgent cases in the early evening before spending hours in his workshop developing new ideas and methods. Thomas could see up to 160 patients a day. During this time he developed the Thomas splint and Thomas test, his most significant contributions to orthopaedics. The Thomas splint consisted of two rigid rods attached to a ring that fitted around the thigh, used to immobilise the thigh to treat fractures of the femur. The Thomas test determined whether there was flexion contracture of the hip.

During the 1870s, a hospital was built in the Welsh town of Rhyl. The hospital had balconies for the patients and it used fresh air as an integral part of treatment. This hospital provided Thomas with the opportunity to try out ideas he had learned from Bennett, about the importance of fresh air for patients. Back in Liverpool, he had already started treating children on improvised beds outside their homes. His work was recognised officially by the hospital's committee: 'The committee would also express their best thanks to Dr Thomas of Liverpool in the way.... he frequently visited the hospital in order to illustrate the working of surgical appliances invented by himself which have proved the greatest benefit to the patients'. This was one of the only times that Thomas work was commended during his lifetime. He very rarely attended any meetings which he was invited to and his background in bone setting was considered to be eccentric and lacking in any qualification by the orthopaedic surgeons of the time. He did, however, have a loyal supporter in Rushton Parker (1847–1932), a young surgeon who had witnessed a young boy walking on crutches despite having his hip immobilised by a Thomas splint.

As he aged Thomas began to realise that, as many of the medical professions' views towards his work were less than supportive, it was quite possible that all his innovations and methods would die with him. Urged by Parker he began to write books about his practices. In 1878, Thomas published his first book, *Diseases of the Hip,*

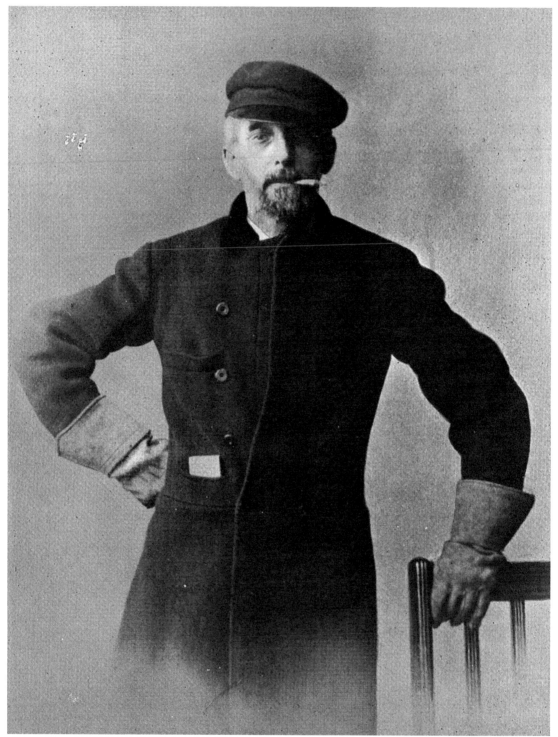

Hugh Owen Thomas. (Courtesy of Wellcome Library, London.)

Knee and Ankle but it did not gain much support due to the tone he used. He condemned developments in surgery and the surgeons who readily turned to amputation to treat the poor. His second book, *Past and Present Treatment of Intestinal Obstructions* (1879), a subject completely unrelated to his work in orthopaedics, recommended that in cases of obstruction of the bowel, the bowel should be rested prior to any unavoidable surgery. However, *Intestinal Obstruction* (1884) by Frederick Traves (1853–1923), recommended various other types of treatment for obstruction failed to mention Thomas or any of his methods. Traves stated that this was due to the fact that he believed that Thomas methods were already a recognised treatment. This led to a dispute between them as Thomas was infuriated that his methods and ideas would never be attributed to him. By then the majority of the medical world and even his supporters had turned against him.

Thomas died of pneumonia at 57 years of age. Although he had faced much opposition during his lifetime, his work as a general practitioner had made him a hero amongst the common people. Thousands lined the streets of Liverpool at his funeral, with his obituary in *The Lancet* remarking: 'The toilers at our docks and warehouses are not sensitive beings… to see thousands of these stirred to their depths… in passionate sobs and tears… gaze into an open grave, proves that its silent occupant had won his way to their hearts'. Following his death, his nephew continued running the Nelson Street surgery and became responsible for bringing the world's attention to his uncle's innovations. It was his quiet, diplomatic method rather than Thomas outspoken nature that ensured Thomas developments did not die with him. Later, when Jones was director of military orthopaedics during the First World War (1914–1918), he introduced the Thomas splint to the battlefield, a move that saved countless men from death due to femoral fractures. Furthermore, he oversaw the opening of various open-air hospitals across the country that used Thomas splints to immobilise and rest the patient. Jones saved Thomas work and this helped establish Thomas to become known as 'the father of British orthopaedics'.

Further Reading

Carter AJ. Hugh Owen Thomas: The cripple's champion *The British Medical Journal* 1991;303:1578–81.

Cope Z. Some famous general practitioners and other medical historical essays. *The Journal of the College of General Practitioners* 1962;5(1):148–49.

Hagy M. 'Keeping up with the Joneses' – The story of Sir Robert Jones and Sir Reginald Watson-Jones. *Iowa Orthopaedic Journal* 2004;24:133–37.

Jones AR. The influence of Hugh Owen Thomas on the evolution of the treatment of skeletal tuberculosis. *The Journal of Bone and Joint Surgery* 1948;30-B:547–50.

MacNab DS. Hugh Owen Thomas 1834–1891 (the founder of orthopaedic surgery). *The Canadian Medical Association Journal* 1941;45:448–52.

Wren S, Ashwood N. The life and times of Hugh Owen Thomas. *Trauma* 2010;12:197.

17 CHARLES MACMUNN (1852–1911)

John Anthony Doherty and Neil Metcalfe

Charles Alexander MacMunn was born at Seafield House, Easkey, county Sligo in Ireland. He was born on 11 April 1852 as the son of James MacMunn, a medical practitioner. MacMunn was educated at Dromore School where he subsequently enrolled at Trinity College, Dublin, in 1867 to study medicine. He obtained BA (with Honours) in 1871, MB the following year and proceeded to MD in 1875 and MA in 1884.

Soon after graduating in medicine, MacMunn decided to move to Wolverhampton, England. There he joined his cousin James MacMunn (1822–1873) at his practice at 14 Waterloo Road. However, the following year his cousin passed away leaving MacMunn to take over the practice. The following year, in 1874, he married Laetitia MacMunn, an artist, who was his cousin James' daughter and they had three children together. One of their children, Lionel Alexander, later went on to follow his father's footsteps and also decided to study medicine. MacMunn later remarried (1908) to Beatrice Webb, the sister of Captain Matthew Webb who was the first man to ever swim the English Channel.

MacMunn was very keen on research and to help fulfil his passion he built a laboratory in the loft over his stables. He found that his day-to-day medical work limited his time available to do research but his wife Beatrice later recalled that when he was out and about on his rounds he would scrawl ideas onto the cuffs of his shirts. Other accounts have also said that he had a pipe built into his home laboratory and an eyepiece drilled through the wall of his study so that he could scrutinise the patients who were coming and whether they were worth interrupting his research for. MacMunn's loft-laboratory was equipped with a wide range of instruments, which he was able to purchase as a result of funding from various societies, including the Birmingham Philosophical Society and The Royal Society. His new equipment allowed him to perform the research he wanted and after a few years he published a seminal paper called 'Studies in medical spectroscopy' which was published in the *Dublin Journal of Medicine* (1877). He then recorded his key findings in a book which he wrote called *The Spectroscope in Medicine* (1880). In 1889, MacMunn was made the first ever honorary pathologist to the Wolverhampton Royal Hospital.

When MacMunn was a student in Ireland he was encouraged by William Stokes (1804–1878) at Meath Hospital, Dublin, to study Spectroscopy, something that has already mentioned became a large part of his research and publications. The spectroscope is an optical device used for observing spectrums of light from a particular source and in MacMunn's case, tissue samples. He replaced the eyepiece of a microscope with a spectroscope and using this device he was able to analyse the spectra of absorption bands emitted from living tissues. One of the key findings from his work revolutionised medicine and our understanding of the human body. His work on molecules, which he called histohaematins, that are found in tissues, and myohaematin, found in muscles, gave a better understanding of the molecular mechanism of respiration in human cells. His accounts of these molecules were published in the *Philosophical Transactions of the Royal Society* (1886) and the *Journal of Physiology* (1887). Prior to his discovery it was believed that the process of respiration was carried out in the blood but MacMunn's work changed this thinking and he was able to show that this process actually took place intracellularly in the histohaematins and myohaematins of tissue and muscle.

However, MacMunn's published work was denounced by German scientist Felix Hoppe-Seyler (1825–1895). Hoppe-Seyler then claimed that he was not able to replicate MacMunn's work and suggested that the molecules. Hoppe-Seyler tried to demonstrate that the molecules that MacMunn found were simply breakdown products of haemoglobin, a product found in blood. This attack on his work left MacMunn greatly deflated and demoralised. Consequently he decided to take a step back from research and to concentrate more on his medical practice and later decided to work for the armed forces in the Boer War (1899–1902). He volunteered for service with the South Staffordshire regiment and performed medical work for the 3rd (Wolverhampton) volunteer battalion between 1899 and 1902. For his contribution to the forces he received the Queen's South Africa Medal with three clasps. He also received a medal for his long service and the King Edward VII Coronation Medal. He contracted malaria during his time in South Africa with the forces. His health deteriorated slowly from this point and he decided to retire in 1909. MacMunn passed away on 18 February 1911 in Wolverhampton.

Posthumously, MacMunn's work was vindicated. Work by the Polish scientist David Keilin (1887–1963), in 1925, showed that the molecules myohaematin and histohaematin, which MacMunn had discovered, were in fact what are now know as cytochromes. Cytochromes are important intracellular structures which form part of the energy-producing mitochondria and play a key role in cellular respiration. This meant that the research that MacMunn had performed and that had been dismissed by Hoppe-Seyler had in fact been correct and his work is consistently referred to in the key events leading to the discovery of mitochondria. In 2014, a new €17 million science building was opened in honour of MacMunn in Sligo, highlighting the importance of his work and his contribution to medicine. The 80-station

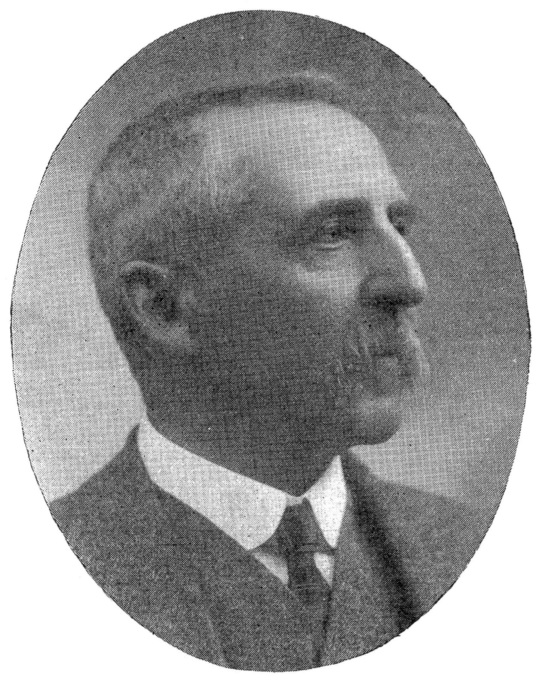

DR. C. A. MacMunn.

Photograph by]   *[Bennett Clark, Wolver hampton.*

Portrait of Charles MacMunn in *BMJ* on 4 March 1911. (Courtesy of Wellcome Library, London.)

foundation laboratory, seven teaching laboratories and four research laboratories are no doubt more conducive for research than MacMunn's hayloft and, at the time of its opening, were described by the head of science as likely to have met with MacMunn's approval. MacMunn was not able to see the importance of his discoveries but his work has proved to be beneficial in the understanding of the human body.

Further Reading

Keilin D, Keilin J. *The History of Cell Respiration and Cytochrome*. Cambridge: Cambridge University Press; 1966.

MacMunn C. Studies in medical spectroscopy. *Dublin Journal of Medical Science* 1877;63(6):515–28.

MacMunn C. *The Spectroscope in Medicine*. London: Churchill; 1880.

18 SIR PATRICK MANSON (1844–1922)

Alexandra Macnamara

Patrick Manson was born on 3 October 1844 in Oldmeldrum, 18 miles north of Aberdeen. He was the second eldest of nine children, with four brothers and four sisters. His father, John Manson, was a yeoman farmer as well as a manager of a local Linen Bank. His mother, Elizabeth Livingstone, was a distant relative of the great explorer and Christian missionary of Africa, Mr David Livingstone. Sir Patrick, who used to mock himself as a 'Scandinavian pirate' owing to his Norwegian descent, was described as a dull but curious child. Amongst his Presbyterian family, he was noted to have a good memory of church sermons when five years old. He enjoyed the countryside, carpentry, mechanics, cricket and was known to be good at shooting. Once, after shooting a fierce cat, he pulled a long tapeworm from the cat's remains, which he found particularly interesting. This was perhaps Sir Patrick's first attempt at parasitology.

Sir Patrick's parents moved to Aberdeen where he attended grammar school and proved to be very good with carpentry and metal work. Two years later he became an apprentice at Blaikie Bros, ironmasters of Aberdeen. However, Sir Patrick was unable to continue his work due to a spinal condition, which required him to lie on his back for six months. During this time, he developed an interest in natural history and after discovering that these studies would count towards a medical curriculum, he decided to become a doctor.

Sir Patrick was admitted to the University of Aberdeen in 1860 to study medicine, and also supplemented his studies at the University of Edinburgh. In October 1864, when he was 20 years old, he passed his final exams but was too young to practise medicine. He graduated from the University of Aberdeen with MB in October 1865.

Sir Patrick's first job was in Durham, working as an assistant medical officer at a 'lunatic asylum'. As well as his work with patients, he also worked performing dissections, and noticed some changes in the internal carotid artery in certain patients. These observations led to him producing a paper, which was accepted as a thesis for his MD from the University of Aberdeen, which he was awarded in July 1866.

Inspired by his older brother who had travelled to Shanghai, Sir Patrick decided to travel. He obtained the post of a medical officer for Formosa, where he worked for five years in the customs service. During this time he was able to document his observations on local diseases, including leprosy and elephantiasis. In 1871, he was appointed medical officer to the Imperial Maritime Customs in Amoy and found his work was in great demand. Here he had his own general practice through which he made many positive changes. He was one of the first to introduce vaccination, which was of great importance due to the high prevalence of smallpox. Although his general practice meant he experienced and excelled in many areas of medicine, including obstetrics, it could be argued that he made a greater impact with his surgical skills. He created several new operations, for example draining liver abscesses and removing elephantoid tumours.

In order to answer many of the questions that he had contemplated whilst working abroad, Sir Patrick decided to return to the Great Britain and Ireland to undertake further study. In 1875, he returned to Scotland, but finding little information of help to him, he travelled to London and studied Ophthalmology at the City of London Hospital. In March 1875, in the British Museum in Bloomsbury, he discovered the writings of Timothy Lewis (1841–1886). Lewis described a minute nematode worm found in human blood, which he named *Filaria sanguinis hominis*. This inspired Sir Patrick to find a suitable microscope and conduct his own research. Later that year, on 21 December 1875, Sir Patrick married Henrietta Isabella Thurburn, with whom he would go on to have three sons and a daughter. Shortly after his wedding, in February 1876, he returned to Amoy.

From further observation of the *Filaria* parasitic worm, and studying the blood of his patients that had been affected by the parasite, Sir Patrick discovered several characteristics of the worm which led him to believe it was transmitted by an insect, most likely the brown mosquito. Firstly, he noticed that it would escape from its covering in cooler temperatures, suggesting that it had been associated with a cold-blooded creature. Secondly, it was only seen in the blood of his patients during the night. Finally, he noticed individual cases could be seen developing at some distances from each other.

Sir Patrick's further experiments revealed the role of the female mosquito in 'nursing' the parasite and he had his work read out on 7 March 1878 at the Linnean Society of London before being published in the journal of the same society a year later. Although the fellows of the society were reported not to have been impressed, he was not perturbed and went on to repeat his experiments. He went on to publish a book in 1883, which was then combined with further information to be published as *The Metamorphosis of Filaria sanguinis hominis in the Mosquito*.

Despite his many successes, Sir Patrick acknowledged the difficulties of maintaining his general practice whilst trying to continue his research. In a letter to Spencer Cobbold (1828–1886) in 1879, he wrote, 'Men like myself in general practice are but poor and very slow investigators, crippled as we are with the necessity of making our daily bread'.

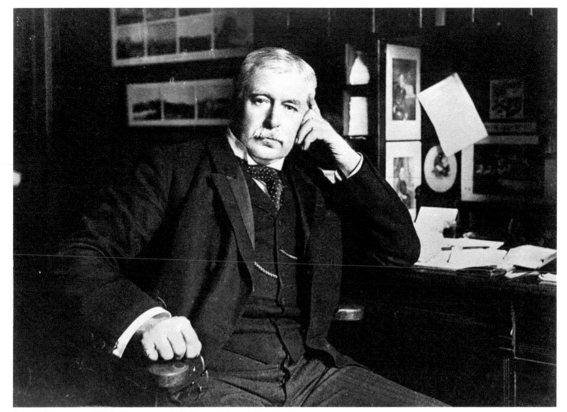

Patrick Manson in 1904. (Courtesy of Wellcome Library, London.)

In 1883, Sir Patrick travelled to Hong Kong with his family and set up a private practice. He formed the Hong Kong Medical Society and helped build the Hong Kong College of Medicine, where he became the first Dean of the college. Sir Patrick received some recognition for his work in 1886 in the form of an honorary Doctor of Laws (LLD) degree from the University of Aberdeen, Sir Patrick later returned to London in 1890 for financial reasons and started a consulting practice near Harley Street.

After his first year in London, Sir Patrick was awarded MRCP and a year later became physician to the Seaman's Hospital Society in Greenwich. It was here in 1893 that he had the chance to study the malaria parasite. He felt that there were similarities between the malaria parasite and the *Filaria* he had studied in Amoy and subsequently produced his mosquito–malaria hypothesis and published this in the *BMJ* in December 1894. This hypothesis greatly influenced the research of Ronald Ross (1857–1932), who would go on to 'solve' the problem of the life cycle of the malaria parasite.

By 1900, Sir Patrick's ideas had been widely accepted and on 14 June 1900 he was elected an FRS in recognition of his research. He went on to be knighted in 1903 and, in 1904, he was awarded an honorary degree of Doctor of Science (DSc) by the University of Oxford.

As well as his better-known work, Sir Patrick also researched and contributed to medical knowledge of many other tropical diseases such as schistosomiasis, leprosy, beriberi, African sleeping sickness and yellow fever. He summarised all this research in his book *Manson's Manual of Tropical Diseases* (1898).

Whilst in London, Sir Patrick began teaching on the subject of tropical medicine and gave several lectures. However, he felt that this teaching would not be adequate and campaigned for a separate School of Tropical Medicine to be created. After many letters and meetings, the London School of Tropical Medicine was opened on 2 October 1899.

Away from medicine, it has been suggested that Sir Patrick contributed greatly to the future of China. In 1896, he helped James Cantlie (1851–1926) in saving Yat-Sen Sun (1866–1925) from kidnap and imprisonment by secret agents of the Ching Dynasty in London. It has been argued that had it not been for their effort, Sun might have been executed and China may not have been liberated from the feudal Ching Dynasty in 1911.

Sir Patrick retired to Ireland in 1914 where he enjoyed spending his time fishing. However, he still continued to see patients and contribute to the School of Tropical Medicine. In February 1921, he received an honorary degree of LLD by the University of Cambridge. Sir Patrick died on 9 April 1922, aged 78 years old, after suffering from several heart attacks.

With Sir Patrick's lifetime of contributions to tropical medicine, he is now often referred to as the 'father of tropical medicine'. His contributions to medical science have helped shape the modern teaching and understanding of tropical medicine and his work will have both directly or indirectly helped or will help vast numbers of patients in the past, present and future.

Further Reading

Cope Z. *Some Famous General Practitioners: And Other Medical Historical Essays*. London: Pitman Medical; 1961.

Kelvin KW, Kwok-Yung Y. In memory of Patrick Manson, founding father of tropical medicine and the discovery of vector-borne infections. *Emerging Microbes and Infection* 2012;1(10):e31.

Manson P. On the development of *Filaria sanguinis hominis*, and on the mosquito considered as a nurse (communicated by Dr. Cobbold, F.R.S., F.L.S.). *Journal of the Linnean Society of London* 1879;14:304–11.

Manson P. On the nature and significance of cresenteric and flagellated bodies in malarial blood. *British Medical Journal* 1894;2(1771):1306–8.

Manson-Bahr PH, Alcock A. *The Life and Work of Sir Patrick Manson*. London: Cassell; 1927.

Stephens JWW. Manson, Patrick (1844–1922). In: Matthew HCG, Harrison B (eds.). *Oxford Dictionary of National Biography*. Volume 36. Oxford: Oxford University Press; 2004.

Venita J. Sir Patrick Manson. *Archives of Pathology & Laboratory Medicine* 2000;124:1594–5.

19 SIR JAMES MACKENZIE (1853–1926)
James Clark

James Mackenzie was born on 12 April 1853 on Pictstonhill Farm in the small village of Scone in Scotland. This was near the ancient abbey where, from remotest antiquity, the Kings and Queens of Scotland were crowned. He grew up on a farm with his parents and six siblings. His education started locally at Perth Academy where he hardly excelled. He struggled to memorise some areas of the curriculum and found learning easier by association and reasoning. When 15 years old he requested to leave school and began an apprenticeship at a chemist in Perth, Scotland. During this time he developed a keen interest in literature and science and convinced himself that he had the intellect to go to university.

Sir James started studying medicine at Edinburgh University when he was 21 years old. He struggled with the scientific years but enjoyed the clinical parts of the course, at one point studying under Joseph Lister (1827–1912), the pioneer of antiseptic surgery. Having qualified, he started his medical career as a general practitioner in Burnley, Lancashire, where he would practise for over 25 years. Immediately, he realised that university had not prepared him for his new work. He felt that whilst clinical research focused on the end-stages of diseases, it was missing accurate descriptions of the early signs and symptoms of illness that might present to a general practitioner.

Having witnessed the death of pregnant patient due to heart failure, Sir James' inquisitive nature prompted him to begin studying the heart and its rhythms. He designed his own polygraph to record the heart's pulses. This consisted of hermetically sealed funnels connected by tubing to a tambour (rubber tubing) and lever that could be made to write on a revolving cylinder. One receiver recorded the radial pulse, one the jugular venous pulse and one the apex beat of the heart in the chest. He used the polygraph to record pulses and rhythms of many of his patients with different heart conditions and used the varnished traces to describe and explain different types of arrhythmias.

By 1902, Sir James' first book, *The Study of the Pulse*, which documented 28 years of his personal research in Burnley, had become one of the most important publications in cardiology. It also made him a leading world authority on the subject. His book *New Methods of Studying Affectations of the Heart* (1905) described and explained first-degree heart block for the first time, labelling it an arrhythmia due to a depression in the heart's conductivity. He discovered sinus arrhythmias and extra-systolic beats and was able to described their origins.

Importantly, Sir James' would follow up on his patients, in some cases for over six years, enabling him to comment on their prognosis. As a result he was the first to suggest that the contemporaneous management of months of bed rest for sinus arrhythmias was unnecessary and that these patients could carry on with their lives normally. He also studied hearts extensively at post-mortem. Observing the physical changes in cardiac tissue helped him to explain the causes of certain arrhythmias and heart conditions.

In a series of papers to the *BMJ*, Sir James also demonstrated the effects of digitalis on cardiac tissue in atrial fibrillation. He suggested that the heart was slowed due to the drug acting on the vagus nerve. This belief caused a disagreement with a former colleague Sir Thomas Lewis (1881–1945), then editor of *Heart*. Lewis, whose work on atrial fibrillation had been rejected by Mackenzie in the past, believed that digitalis acted directly on the atrioventricular bundle and so refused to publish Sir James' work. Sir James was furious, asking whether all research submitted to the *BMJ* would not be published simply because the editor temporarily disagreed with it. In Sir James' obituary, Lewis later wrote: 'He was an exceptionally vigorous and strong personality... but open never the less to conviction on all questions without reserve. He saw, as few or none of his day saw, where clinical knowledge ends and ignorance begins'.

Others had previously described atrial fibrillation but Sir James was the first to understand the condition pathologically using his polygraph. He noticed that a certain type of rhythm irregularity caused the atrial 'a' wave to disappear from his polygraph recording and any pre-systolic murmurs could not be heard. At first he thought the cause of these changes was a nodal rhythm where the heartbeat was initiated at the atrioventricular node due to atrial paralysis. However, after consulting with Arthur Cushny (1866–1926), who had replicated fibrillation on dogs in a laboratory, they found that it was a fibrillating atrium that caused the abnormal rhythm. These findings are documented in his 1908 textbook *Diseases of the Heart*.

In 1907, Sir James moved to London to further his research and defend it from opposition. As a general practitioner he was a firm believer that a diagnosis should be made by observing the patient as a whole and felt that a doctor that only studied one organ was at a disadvantage. This belief often did not sit well with his specialist colleagues who respected his ingenuity but doubted his intelligence. His work was often subjected to ridicule when discussed in physiological circles, and often his medical education and generalist background were called into question. Despite this, he co-founded with Lewis, in 1909, a cardiology journal called *Heart* and became a respected consultant and was awarded MRCP in 1915. In the same year he was knighted by King George V.

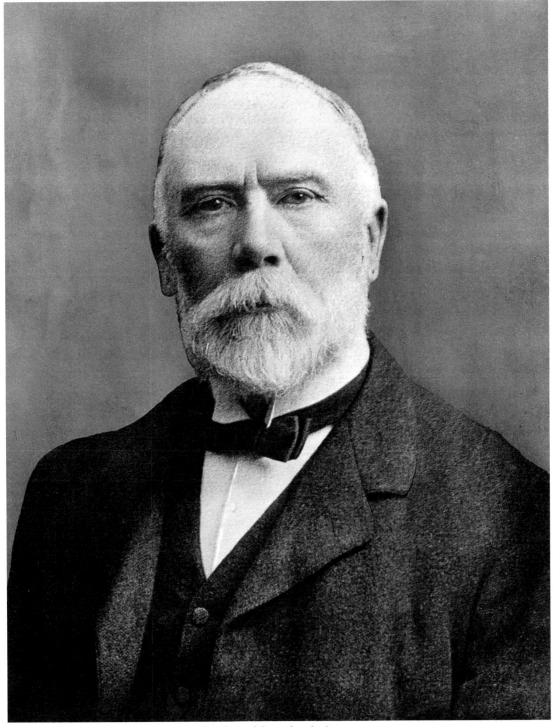

Portrait of Sir James Mackenzie. (Courtesy of Wellcome Library, London.)

When 65 years old, whilst suffering from angina, Sir James returned to Scotland to embark on a new venture. It was his dissatisfaction with his education in preparing him for general practice and his ideas about how clinical research should be carried out that prompted him to found the St Andrews Institute of Clinical Research. He wanted to change research from an individual-based activity to one that involved general practitioners collating information about disease and illness to improve diagnosis. The aims of the institute were to study the minor signs and symptoms of early disease that presented to general practitioners in an attempt to recognise illness earlier. The general practitioners would keep a record of every patient they saw and would document details of diet, employment, living conditions and smoking habits. This can be seen as one of the first attempts to study risk factors of disease. Local general practitioners would spend a significant amount of time at the institute studying and entering data on the patients they had seen recently.

The institute was not entirely successful. Over time its funding diminished and it did not produce enough new research. Eventually, in 1944, 19 years after its founder's death, it was closed. The institute did, however, pave the way for the future of general practitioner led clinical research; many of its ideals and methods were well before its time and are still used today. It also left behind a body of records that are still in use today.

On 26 January 1926, Sir James died from a heart attack. In accordance with his wishes, his heart was removed and sent to the Anatomy Department of the University of St Andrew, and the resulting pathological description was published in the *British Heart Journal*. The research that began in Burnley became vital for his career and is seen as revolutionary in the way it was conducted. He was prophetic in his views on medical teaching and the future of general practice. He is regarded as a founding father of cardiology as well as a pioneer of general practice based research.

Further Reading

Grant ID. The third James Mackenzie Lecture. Our heritage & our future. *Research Newsletter* 1957;4:7–23.

Lewis T. Sir James Mackenzie. *British Medical Journal* 1925;i:245.

Mackenzie J. *The Study of the Pulse. Arterial, Venous and Hepatic and of Movements of the Heart*. Edinburgh: Young J. Pentland; 1902.

Mackenzie J. *Diseases of the Heart*. London: Henry Frowde, Hodder & Stoughton; 1908.

Mackenzie J. *Symptoms and their Interpretation*. London: Shaw & Sons; 1909.

Mackenzie J. *Principles of Diagnosis and Treatment in Heart Affections*. London: Henry Frowde, Hodder & Stoughton; 1916.

Mackenzie J. *The Future of Medicine*. London: Henry Frowde, Hodder & Stoughton; 1919.

Mackenzie J. *Heart Disease and Pregnancy*. London: Henry Frowde, Hodder & Stoughton; 1921.

Mackenzie J. *Angina Pectoris*. London: Henry Frowde, Hodder & Stoughton; 1923.

McConaghey RMS. Sir James Mackenzie, M.D. 1853–1925. General practitioner. *The Journal of the Royal College of General Practitioners* 1974;24(144):497–98.

Moorhead R. Sir James Mackenzie (1853–1925): Views on general practice education and research. *Journal of the Royal Society of Medicine* 1999;92:38–43.

Osborne T. James Mackenzie, General Practitioner: A modest contribution to the archaeology of clinical reason. *Sociology of Health & Illness* 1993;15(4):525–46.

20 FRANCIS ADAMS (1796–1861)

Fiona Cowie

Francis Adams was born on 13 March 1796 in Auchinhove, Lumphanan, in Aberdeenshire. He was the son of James Adams, a farmer and labourer, and Elspet Black. Having been educated in his early years at his local parish school, he continued his studies at Aberdeen Grammar School. In 1809, he won a bursary to attend King's College in Aberdeen. It was here, from the age of 15 years old, that Adams began teaching himself Latin and Greek. He would spend 17 hours a day studying Virgil and Horace, who were classical Roman poets, as he felt his early education had not been completely sufficient.

In 1813, Adams graduated from King's College with an MA and then went on to study medicine at the University of Edinburgh. Once he had completed his degree in 1815, he moved to London to ultimately be awarded MRCS in December 1815. In 1819, when 23 years old, Adams returned to the North East of Scotland to Banchory, where he married Elspeth Shaw. They lived in the Old Manse house and had seven children.

Adams was the first resident doctor in Banchory, where he would go on to practise for 42 years and become a well-regarded doctor in the area. His most notable papers included the construction of the placenta, post-partum haemorrhage, foetal auscultation, malignant disease of the face and knee dislocations. Adams also wrote and translated several papers on club foot. He often visited the surgical wards in Aberdeen Royal Infirmary and was the first doctor to realise that dividing the Achilles tendon was a key error when trying to correct the deformity and also carried out research into the causes of club foot.

As well as being a prominent general practitioner, Adams was also a well-renowned classical scholar and was offered the position of chair in Greek at the University of Aberdeen. He declined the post and remained as Banchory's general practitioner. He was first introduced to the classics by George Kerr (1771–1826), a surgeon who was one of the founders of the Aberdeen Medico-Chirurgical Society. Adams bought Kerr's collection of Greek medical authors after the latter's death.

His passion for Greek literature led Adams to translate and write extensively on the subject. One of his earliest works was *Hermes Philologus* (1826) in which he wrote about the differences between Latin and Greek grammar. He translated the Byzantine Greek medical writings into English, including the *Nervous System of Galen* (1829). Between 1827 and 1829 he also translated the writings of Paul of Aegina, which was published by the Sydenham Society in three volumes as *The Seven Books of Paulus Aeginata* (1844–1847). The translations also included the commentaries of Adams on the on the writings, which encompass a comprehensive insight into the medical and surgical knowledge possessed by the Greeks, Romans and Arabians. Professor Charles Singer (1876–1960), a prominent doctor and medical history lecturer from London, was a great admirer of Adams' work. He called this translation 'the finest venture in pure historical medical research in the English language'. The Sydenham Society then asked Adams to translate the *Genuine Works of Hippocrates* (1849), which only took Adams four months to complete. This was described by Singer to be 'probably the most widely read of any work on medical history in the language'. In 1856, Adams' translation of the *Extant Works of Aretaeus, the Cappadocian* (1856) was published, which contained the Greek text along with the English translation. He also contributed to several other classical studies, which included the following: Dunbar and Barker's *Greek and Latin Lexicon* (1831), Lemprière's *Classical Dictionary* (1838) and Green-Hill's *Theophilus* (1842). In terms of poetry, he translated several poems from English into Latin and Greek including Charles Wolfe's poem on Sir John Moore and poems from Greek into English including *Hero and Leander* from the Greek of Musaeus (1820).

Adams received several honours. He was elected Presidential Chair of the Aberdeen Medico-Chirurgical Society, which he held from 1844 to 1845, highlighting how highly he was regarded as a doctor. This is further shown through him being awarded an honorary LLD from the University of Glasgow in 1846, and an MD honoris causa from the University of Aberdeen in 1856.

In 1845, Adams' wife died, meaning that he had his children to look after, as well as continuing his medical practice and his studies of the Classics. Being an avid scholar of Greek and Latin, Adams taught his children about the classical studies and also educated them about nature. His passion for nature and botany was passed on to his second son, Andrew Leith Adams (1827–1882). Together, they wrote a paper entitled 'On ornithology as a branch of liberal education' (1859) which was read in front of the British Association of Botany in Aberdeen. Andrew also studied to become a surgeon, first being awarded MB from the University of Aberdeen before later being awarded MRCS in 1848.

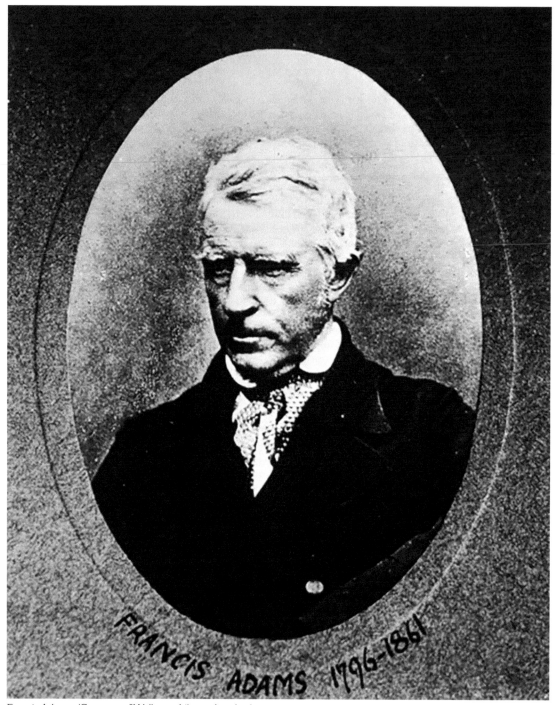

Francis Adams. (Courtesy of Wellcome Library, London.)

Adams was a dedicated and diligent general practitioner right up until his death. He contracted pneumonia after a long journey home after visiting a patient in winter and died on 26 February 1861 in Banchory 64 years of age. He was buried in Banchory churchyard. In 1996, a memorial was unveiled in Banchory to commemorate the 200th anniversary of his birth.

Throughout the majority of his life, Adams devoted over 10 hours of each day to translating every piece of Greek medical knowledge he could find into English. He was driven by the desire to enhance the education of medical students and doctors about the history of medicine. His translations were still being used by medical students in the 1970s. Without his dedication and passion for medicine and the classical studies, it is unlikely that the knowledge of ancient Greek medicine would be preserved in English today. Despite such energies, however, his real devotion was to general practice, as 'his first love and his last', wrote Singer, 'was his practice, his patients and the poor'.

Further Reading

Anon. Francis Adams (1796–1861). *Nature.* 1942;150(3801):286–87.

Craig J. Francis Adams 1796–1861: *The Lancet.* 1961;1(7174):441–42.

Dobbs M. Morcuende J, Gurnett C, Ponseti I. Treatment of idiopathic club foot: An historical review. *The Iowa Orthopaedic Journal* 2000;20:59–64.

Ford J. Medical Memorials, Francis Adams (1796–1861): Banchory, Aberdeen, UK. *Journal of Medical Biography* 2008;16(1):56.

Mackintosh J. *History of the Valley of the Dee, From the Earliest Times to the Present Day.* Aberdeen: Taylor and Henderson; 1895.

Payne JFP. Adams, Francis (1796–1861). In: Stephen L, Lee S (eds.). *The Dictionary of National Biography.* 4th ed. London: Oxford University Press; 1950.

Porteus H. A most learned country doctor. Francis Adams (1796–1861). *The Journal of the Royal College of Practitioners* 1969;17(82):277–81.

21 SIR ARTHUR CONAN DOYLE (1859–1930)

David M. Smith and Neil Metcalfe

Arthur Ignatius Conan Doyle was born on 22 May 1859 in Edinburgh, Scotland. He was the eldest of 10 children born to Charles and Mary Doyle. The 'Conan' in his name was one of his given names rather than part of his surname, and arose from his godfather and maternal uncle, Michael Conan. Despite coming from a family with no strong tendency towards medicine, Sir Arthur began studying towards the joint degree of MB, Master of Surgery at Edinburgh University in 1876.

In 1879, whilst a third year medical student, Sir Arthur was published in the *BMJ*. This publication took the form of a letter to the editor which detailed his self-experimentation with increasing doses of the drug gelsemium. These experiments only stopped due to the ingestion of such a high quantity of the drug to cause exceptional diarrhoea. The quality of the experimental observations were such to earn him publication.

Coming from a modest background and wishing to pay his own way as much as possible, Sir Arthur worked several medical jobs during his medical education. The most illustrious of these jobs was during 1880, when he spent seven months as a ship's surgeon aboard the arctic whaling vessel *SS Hope*. He would later recollect how he was very lucky that none of the crew had any serious complaints that the then third year medical student would have been responsible for attending to. His own account of his exploits on the *SS Hope* would some 132 years later be published in a book, *Dangerous Work: Diary of an Arctic Adventure* (2012). This would be regarded as one of Sir Arthur's earliest ventures onto the path that would lead him to be a world-renowned writer. His experiences in the arctic were liberating and in stark contrast to the regimented march through medical school. Sir Arthur commented in a letter to his mother 'I just feel as if I could go anywhere or do anything. I'm sure I could go anywhere and eat anything'.

Sir Arthur began writing whilst at medical school. Some examples can be found in the margins of his textbooks. One particular therapeutics book contains this mnemonic, regarding opium:

I'll tell you a most serious fact,
That opium dries a mucous tract,
And constipates and causes thirst.
And stimulates the heart at first,
And then allows its strength to fall,
Relaxing the capillary wall,
The cerebrum is first affected,
On tetanus you mustn't bet,
Secretions gone except the sweat.
Lungs & sexuals don't forget.

During his studies, Sir Arthur was put under the tutelage of Joseph Bell (1837–1911). Bell was a senior surgeon at Edinburgh Royal Infirmary and impressed Sir Arthur with his ability to both diagnose and to describe a patient's nationality, background and occupation, all without the patient opening their mouth, a trait he would bestow upon his famous detective some years later.

After medical school Sir Arthur spent some time working various jobs including another stint at sea as a surgeon and assistant to a medical school colleague George Budd (1855–1889), who had recently set up on his own. In the summer of 1882, when 23 years old, Sir Arthur started his own general practice in Southsea.

There is much negativity written of Sir Arthur's experiences at the practice. Many claim he was a poor general practitioner with few patients. Originally the practice only contained the medical contents of Sir Arthur's suitcase: a rigid, conical-shaped stethoscope; a few medical books; a brass name sign and some drugs he had purchased on tab from a local merchant. In the first six months patients were few and far between for Sir Arthur, with only one or two per week. However, eventually the patients came more frequently and the practice began earning money. After three years the practice was earning around £300 per month, a reasonable figure considering his parents had provided for a family of twelve on £280 a month.

November 1887 saw the publication of that year's *Beeton's Christmas Annual*. This issue of the magazine featured a story called *A Study in Scarlet*. This was the first publication to include Sir Arthur's character Sherlock Holmes and his friend and colleague Dr Watson. Holmes is a fictional private detective, known as a 'consulting detective' in the stories, and is known for a proficiency with observation, forensic science and logical reasoning that borders on the fantastic, which he employs when investigating cases for a wide variety of clients, including Scotland Yard. *A Study in Scarlet* was also the first time a magnifying glass is used as an investigative tool in crime fiction. Sir Arthur received £25 for the

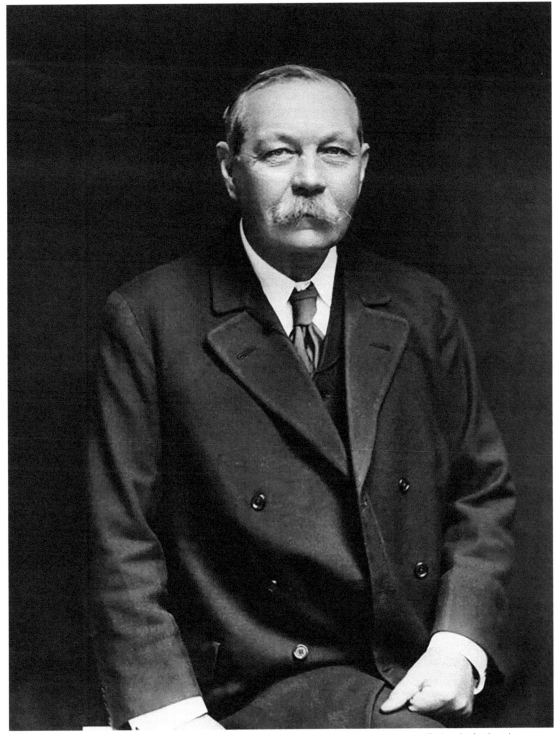

Sir Arthur Conan Doyle. (Courtesy of Lebrecht Music and Arts Photo Library. Credit: Mirrorpix/Lebrecht Authors.)

full rights to the novel and it was republished in July 1888 with illustrations by Sir Arthur's father. The novel took Sir Arthur three weeks to write whilst still practising as a general practitioner. There are 11 known original copies of this volume in the world which has not just made it a rare collectable but also is considered the most expensive magazine in the world, with a *Beeton's* 1887 selling for $156,000 at Sotheby's in 2007. In total Sir Arthur wrote four novels and 56 short stories. The final Sherlock Holmes story, *The Adventure of Shoscombe Old Place*, was published in *The Strand Magazine* in April 1927.

By 1891, Sir Arthur had dissolved his practice to retrain as an ophthalmologist in Vienna. He opened his offices in London and subsequently closed them within 12 months of his retraining, citing the fact that his earnings from writing and his lack of patients now made English literature a sounder career choice.

Sir Arthur's legacy is one of more than simply a great storyteller. In the Boer War (1899–1902) he championed the use of clean water in replenishing the troops: 'If bad water can cost us more than all the bullets of the enemy, then surely it is worth our while to make the drinking of unboiled water a military offence'. In 1907, he came across the curious tale of George Edalji (1876–1953), an Anglo-Indian solicitor convicted to seven years of hard labour for the maiming of several animals in 1903. A part of the case that interested Sir Arthur was with regards to the gentleman's eyesight. He wrote letters to both the *BMJ* and to *The Lancet* giving Edalji's eye measurements and asking for opinions on whether it was physically possible for the gentleman to have committed the crimes, without glasses, under the pitch black night sky. He also actively petitioned the pardoning of Edalji, in the daily newspapers, using his considerable sway as a prominent author of the time to rally public opinion. Edalji was eventually pardoned and the case was cited as being instrumental in the formation of the Court of Appeals in England and Wales.

Sir Arthur was a family man. He married his first wife Mary Louise Hawkins (1857–1906) in 1885 and they had two children together. She later died of tuberculosis. He then remarried in 1907 to Jean Elizabeth Leckie (1872–1940). He had been in love with Jean for some time prior to Mary's death although he never acted upon his feelings towards Jean whilst Mary was alive due to his loyalty to Mary. Jean bore three children for him.

In addition, Sir Arthur was a keen sportsman. While living in Southsea, he played football as a goalkeeper for Portsmouth Association Football Club, under the pseudonym A. C. Smith. He played in 10 first-class cricket matches for the Marylebone Cricket Club, with his one first-class wicket being that of his fellow general practitioner W. G. Grace (1848–1915). He was also a keen golfer, elected captain of the Crowborough Beacon Golf Club in Sussex.

There were a number of honours and awards for Sir Arthur. He was awarded the Queens South Africa Medal in 1901. In 1902, he was knighted as a Knight Bachelor but King Edward VII also raised Sir Arthur to the rank of Knight of the Most Venerable Order of the Hospital of St John Jerusalem. He also received the Order of the Medjidie, second class of the Ottoman Empire, in 1907.

Discussion could be made of Sir Arthur's ruminations on the psychic world, a topic he devoted much of his final years to. However, it seems apt to conclude with a mention of Sir Arthur's death due to a heart attack when at his house at Crowborough on the morning of 7 July 1930. Sir Arthur died surrounded by his family and sitting upright in his chair, gazing out towards the East Sussex scenery. His final words, directed at his second wife, summed up his feelings of adoration for this woman whilst giving her the strength to continue in his absence, and were delivered with the eloquence and grace the world had come to expect from him 'you are wonderful'.

Further Reading

Chong A. Dr Arthur Conan Doyle: The first portfolio GP? *British Journal of General Practice* 2013;63(616):597.

Cirillo VJ. Arthur Conan Doyle (1859–1930): Physician during the typhoid epidemic in the Anglo-Boer War (1899–1902). *Journal of Medical Biography* 2014;22(1):2–8.

Conan Doyle A. A study in scarlet. *Beeton's Christmas Annual* 1887;28:1–95.

22 JONATHAN COUCH (1789–1870)
Sophie Moriarty

Jonathan Couch was born on 15 March 1789 in the small Cornish village of Polperro. He was the only child of Richard and Philippa Couch. The family were residents of Polperro for many generations and Couch himself remained an active pillar of the community until his death in 1870. His father was a fish merchant, which initially sparked Couch's interest in ichthyology (the zoological study of fish), something for which he would later be renowned.

Following a modest education at local schools in Lanasalloes, Pelynt and later at Bodmin Grammar School, Couch apprenticed with two local medical men. He spent five years under Mr John Rice of East Looe and Mr Lawrence Liskeard, before leaving Polperro for London in 1808 to further his medical studies. He attended the United Medical Schools of Guy's and St Thomas' to take the diploma of surgeons where he was profoundly influenced by some of the contemporaneous high ranking physicians and surgeons. This paved the way for others from his village to pursue medical studies in London. In the times of religious, economic and scientific turbulence during the nineteenth century, he followed his own intellectual path and turned his back on a prosperous London career to return to Polperro. Loyal to his home but nonetheless incredibly forward thinking, he was not afraid of medical innovations, practising the then newly introduced and still contemporaneously controversial method of smallpox inoculation. He was a general practitioner and trusted village advisor of Polperro for 60 years and was proud to have known and served six generations of families throughout his career.

Medicine was not where Couch's interests ended. He is best known for his contributions to ichthyology. From a young age he made a habit of putting in writing all he found interesting. Polperro was a fishing village, and his constant contact with fishermen led him to focus his attention towards the study of fish. His meticulous observation and dissection skills, which he had developed during his surgical training, made him a great naturalist and he was one of the first to give an accurate description of amphioxus, also known as a lancelet. Couch trained and enlisted many of the local fishermen to aid him in his studies and was in regular correspondence with leading naturalists of the time including Thomas Bewick (1753–1828) and William Yarrel (1784–1856), whose works on British fish benefitted greatly from his significant contributions. Couch also produced many of his own ichthyological works and, in 1835, was awarded a prize for the best natural history of the pilchard. His most notable work was the four volume illustrated *History of the Fishes of the British Islands* (1862–1865). This work was as highly regarded for its artistry as much for its contribution to science. Each of the 256 illustrations were hand drawn and painted with watercolours by Couch himself, some of which are displayed in the Polperro Heritage Museum today. Considered an authority on ichthyology, he was consulted by the government regarding the habitats and behaviours of local fish and he has been described as a leading nineteenth century naturalist.

However, ichthyology was not the only subject to develop from Couch's work. He had a keen interest in many different subjects and was a member of numerous different societies. He produced works, both published and unpublished, on birds and natural history, folklore and local history and even a treatise on dreams. One of his unpublished works was the 12 volume *Journal of Natural History*. Remarkably, 10 of the 12 volumes were lost for over a century. In terms of articles on folklore and local history his main work in this area was *The History of Polperro* (1871), although it was not published until after his death of his son Thomas. He was also interested in Cornish geology, and did useful work in developing the difficult subject of Cornish fossil remains. From 1848 onwards, he was curator of the Royal Geological Society of Cornwall and contributed many papers and reports via its *Transactions*. He cared deeply about Polperro and those who called it home and had as much concern for the economics of the fisheries and the welfare of the fishermen as he did for his zoological pursuits. Couch contributed many short papers and articles to various important magazines and journals of the time, including *Annals of Natural History, Journal of the Royal Institution of Cornwall*, the *Reports of The Royal Cornwall Polytechnic Society* and *The Zoologist*. In total, he contributed 170 separate submissions, which are medical, biological and theological in nature.

Couch married three times. His first wife, Jane Prynn, died in childbirth in 1810 when Couch had just returned from his studies in London. His second wife was Jane Quiller, with whom he had six children. Following her death in 1870, Couch, then 70 years old, married Sarah Lander Roose, a 22-year-old local girl. Couch was succeeded by generations of intellectuals; three of his sons, Richard Quiller (1816–1863), Thomas Quiller (1826–1884) and John Quiller (b.1830), also became surgeons. Thomas Quiller, like his father, published works on local folklore and history, and Thomas' son was noted Cornish writer Sir Arthur Quiller-Couch (1863–1944), a novelist and literary critic whom influenced many writers. Couch's eldest son, Richard, was highly regarded in his own right for his work on improving the welfare of metal miners.

Couch, like his father before him, was a loyal Methodist. His religious views touched everything he pursued, as well as his writing and social conduct. His observations of nature were as loving and appreciative as they were analytical and objective. *The Dictionary of National Biography* described him as 'A local naturalist whose conscientious and loving observations of nature has made a lasting impression on science, he deserves to rank beside Gilbert White'.

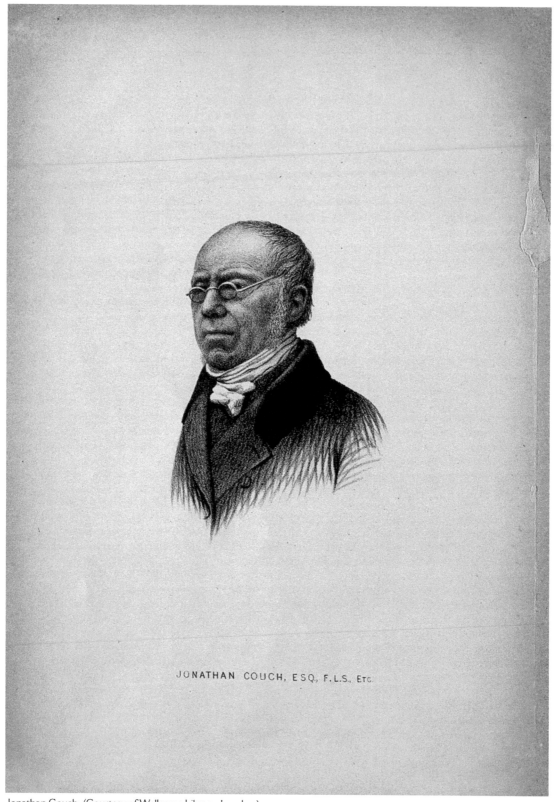

JONATHAN COUCH, ESQ, F.L.S, ETC.

Jonathan Couch. (Courtesy of Wellcome Library, London.)

Further Reading

Boase GC, Courtney WP. *Bibliotheca Cornubiensis*. London: Longmans, Green, Reader & Dyer; 1882.

Couch J. *A History of the Fishes of the British Islands. Volume IV.* London: Groombridge & Sons; 1865.

Couch J. *The History of Polperro.* Truro: W. Lake; 1871.

GTB. Couch, Richard Quiller (1816–1862). In: Stephen L, Lee S (eds.), *The Dictionary of National Biography.* Volume IV. London: Oxford University Press; 1950.

Johns JR. *Doctor by Nature. Jonathan Couch: Surgeon of Polperro.* Worcestershire: Polperro Heritage Press; 2010.

Wheeler A. Couch, Jonathan (1789–1870). In: Matthew HCG, Harrison B (eds.). *Oxford Dictionary of National Biography.* Volume 13. Oxford: Oxford University Press; 2004.

23 GIDEON ALGERNON MANTELL (1790–1852)

Rebecca Dunphy

Gideon Algernon Mantell was born on 3 February 1790 in Lewes as the third son of a shoemaker. He had an unconventional route through schooling, being taught to read, memorise and recite biblical passages at home before entering Dame's school at the age of 6 years old. He was not permitted to enter the usual public schools as his father, Thomas Mantell, was a Methodist and radical Whig. He then moved to a grammar school and latterly to Swindon where he was taught by his pastor uncle, developing his skills in public speaking, something which became very useful to him in his later life.

When aged 15 years old, Mantell entered an apprenticeship with James Moore. Moore was a local general practitioner and lover of natural history and botany who inspired Mantell to start his fossil collection. He then studied at St Bartholomew's and was awarded MRCS and LSA in 1811. He was unsuccessful in obtaining an assistantship in London, so he bought Moore's practice for £95 in 1818, alongside two large houses, using one for his practice and another for his fossil collection, already numbering several thousands of specimens.

Mantell became a well-respected figure in Lewes, being both a parish doctor and army surgeon at Ringmer Hospital. The latter role was despite voicing opposition to military floggings. He was dedicated to his patients, regularly conducting home visits to up to 40 patients per day and following up their progress. He was also skilled in obstetrics, delivering up to three babies on average per week, with a reportedly low mortality rate. He delivered 2410 women over a 15-year time span, with only two deaths: one from haemorrhagic complications, the other an undiagnosed maternal syncope. This is in comparison to contemporaneous maternal mortality rates of 1 in 10 births in London, 1 in 30 in Paris and 1 in 100 in Edinburgh. He also drew attention to the use of ergot in delayed labour.

In 1826, Mantell also intervened in the case of Hannah Russell who was accused of plotting and committing the murder of her husband, Benjamin Russell. Their 19-year-old lodger, Daniel Leney, who had been with Mr Russell when he collapsed and died whilst stealing corn, was also accused of murder. Arsenic poisoning was proposed to be the route of the husband's demise but Mantell stated this was unlikely, attributing it to angina pectoris instead. This was upheld by several experts including Professor William Brande (1788–1866), meaning Russell received a pardon from the King. This was too late to save Leney who had already been executed.

Mantell's interest in fossils was further cemented after a meeting in Hoxton Square in 1811 with James Parkinson (1755–1824) who as well as being a general practitioner with an interest in neurology was also a keen palaeontologist. The young Mantell was unable to afford the expensive books written by Parkinson but was nevertheless inspired, leading him to write his first book in 1812 entitled *A Systematical Arrangement of Secondary Fossils*.

In 1822, Mantell was involved in a famous discovery in the Tilgate Forrest, Sussex. His wife initially found several large fossil teeth before Mantell found several more nearby. Mantell realised the significance of the find, discussing it with the eminent palaeontologist Baron Georges Cuvier (1769–1832), who mistook the teeth as belonging to a rhino. Mantell, however, noted a resemblance between an iguana jaw bone skeleton in the Hunterian Museum and his discovery, naming the creature Iguanodon (iguana-tooth). This led to his being awarded FRS in 1825. His deductions about the origins of Iguanadon were further verified in 1877 when 23 further Iguanodon skeletons were discovered in a Belgian mine. Their presence in a mine proved his initial theory about the freshwater habitat of the Iguanadon. Iguanadon was not described as a dinosaur until 1844, when the term was coined by Richard Owen (1804–1892).

Mantell had an illustrious palaeontological career alongside his medical one. He published 67 books and described the dinosaur reptiles *Hylaeosaurus*, *Pelorosaurus*, and *Regnosaurus*, and Triassic reptile *Telerpeton elginense*. He was an avid fossil searcher who would conceal his finds from perceived rivals; he was known to return to private estates from where he had been previously ejected in pursuit of a find. His major works include *The Fossils of the South Downs: or, Illustrations of the Geology of Sussex* (1822) and *Medals of Creation* (1844). However, his dream of creating his own museum were shattered when the Sussex Scientific Institution failed to raise the necessary funds to allow the museum that had been founded in 1836 to continue. Consequently, 25-year-old specimen collection that was valued at £7000 ended up being sold to the Trustees of the British Museum for £4000. The British Museum holds between 20,000 and 30,000 of his exhibits.

In addition Mantell authored many medical papers. One included a very early description of greenstick fracture and another paper foretold the germ theory, later reviewed by *The Lancet*. He was a regular lecturer at the Clapham Athenaeum, a society for advancing both literary and scientific knowledge, and was also awarded LLD by Yale College in 1835.

In terms of family life, Mantell married Mary Ann Woodhouse in 1816. With Mary he had five children, though three died in infancy. His oldest son, Walter (1820–1895), became a surgeon and emigrated to New Zealand, later donating Mantell's personal papers to the Alexander Turnbull Library, New Zealand. He moved his family and medical practice several times in his later years, initially to Brighton in 1831 to 20 The Steyne. Later, due to declining

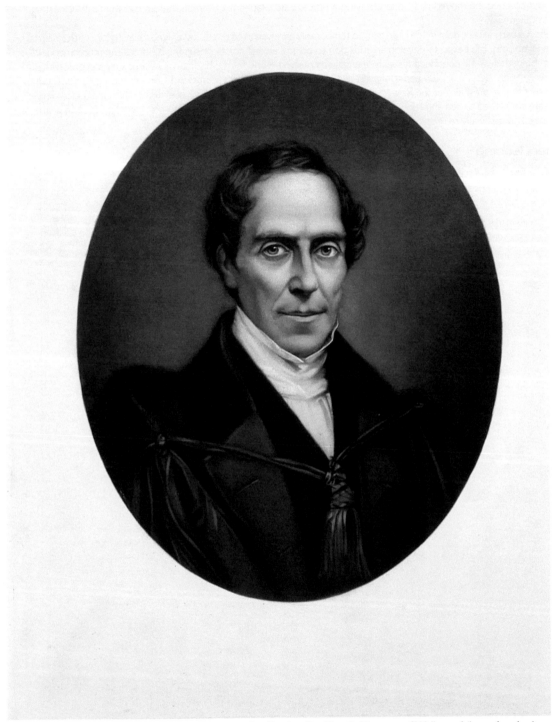

Mezzotint of Gideon Algernon Mantell by W.T. Davey after Sentier after Mayall. (Courtesy of Wellcome Library, London.)

health and practice, he moved to London, buying a practice at Clapham Common, before moving to 19 Chester Street in Belgravia.

A serious carriage accident in 1841 had caused temporarily paralysis in Mantell's lower limbs, leaving him with severe back and limb pain. He began to develop an addiction to opium, at one point consuming 32 times the recommended amount. Nonetheless, he continued his lecture engagements and work, feeling his financial status was too precarious for his resignation, despite a £100 pension given by Queen Victoria, on the recommendation of William Parsons, the third Earl of Rosse, president of the Royal Society. He delivered a lecture on 8 November 1852 whilst in an incredibly weak state but retired to bed and subsequently passed away two days later. His post-mortem gave his cause of death as 'opium taken medically to relieve pain but proving fatal from the weak state of the deceased'.

Further Reading

Dean DR. *Gideon Mantell and the Discovery of Dinosaurs.* Cambridge: Cambridge University Press; 1999.

Dell S. Gideon Algernon Mantell's unpublished journal, June–November 1852. *The Turnbull Library Record* 1983;16:77–94.

Mantell GA. *The Fossils of the South Downs: or, Illustrations of the Geology of Sussex.* London: L. Relfe; 1822.

Mantell GA. Remarks on partial fracture of the radius. *Boston Medical and Surgical Journal* 1841;25:217–18.

Mantell GA. *Thoughts on Animalcules: or, A Glimpse of the Invisible World Revealed by the Microscope.* London: Murray; 1846.

Swinton WE. Outside medicine: Gideon Algernon Mantell. *British Medical Journal* 1975;1(5956):505–7.

24 HENRY FAULDS (1843–1930)
Hiba Khan

Henry Faulds was born on 1 June 1843 in Beith, Ayrshire, into a family of modest means. His mother Anne Cameron was the wife of local grocer William Pollock Faulds, both of whom were of Scottish descent. His education began when he joined the local school Beith Academy but was forced to leave at 12 years of age to work as a clerk for his uncle Thomas Corbett, in Glasgow, in order to support his family. He subsequently found employment at a dress manufacturer where one of his tasks included classifying the huge variety of shawl patterns, which he later attributed to inspiring his fingerprint research. At 21 years old he enrolled at the Faculty of Arts at Glasgow University, where he read classics, logic and mathematics, before spending four years as a medical student at Anderson's College. He was awarded a licentiate of the Faculty of Physicians and Surgeons of Glasgow in 1871.

Religion was of great importance to Faulds. This led him to enlist as a foreign missionary through the Church of Scotland where he was posted to Darjeeling, India, to work at a hospital for the poor. He returned to Scotland in 1873 and married Isabella Wilson (1843/1844–1928), daughter of innkeeper Anthony Wilson. Later that year, Faulds received a letter of appointment from the United Presbyterian Church of Scotland to found a medical mission in Japan. Together with Isabella they sailed to Japan in December 1873 where they lived in a foreign concession at Tsukiji near Tokyo. Faulds worked in a prominent mission hospital, which was later bought by Ludolph Teusler and became St Luke's International Hospital. By 1876, he had established a medical school where he regularly lectured on surgery and physiology in Japanese and introduced the concept of aseptic technique to medical practice. He also founded the Rakuzenkai, which was Japan's first society for the blind, and he was assigned the position of honorary surgeon superintendent by the Japanese government.

During his time in Japan, Faulds became involved in archaeological excavations and was particularly interested in the fingerprint impressions that had remained on shards of ancient Japanese pottery. He began to study the fingerprints of his students and concluded that fingerprints had to be unique to each individual and could, therefore, be used for identification. In early 1880, he wrote to Charles Darwin about his theory, who forwarded the letter to his cousin Sir Francis Golton (1822–1911), who then forwarded it to the Anthropological Society of London. All avenues were unreceptive to his theory which led Faulds to publish a letter on 28 October of that year in *Nature* entitled 'On the Skin-Furrows of the Hand' where he described his studies on human and animal fingerprint, the racial differences and the practical application of his findings in criminology and forensics. In this paper, Faulds made two ground-breaking statements: firstly, 'When bloody finger-marks or impressions on clay, glass etc., exist, they may lead to the scientific identification of criminals'; secondly, 'A common slate or smooth board of any kind, or a sheet of tin, spread over very thinly and evenly with printer's ink, is all that is required [to take fingerprints]'.

There were two instances when Faulds used fingerprinting for identification, a technique known as dactylography, to assist in solving crime. The first was when his hospital in Tokyo was burgled and a close friend and colleague became a key suspect. Faulds compared his friend's fingerprints to those at the scene of the crime to vindicate him of the blame. The second involved tracing the fingerprints on a bottle of surgical alcohol to one of his employees who had been siphoning the hospital supply.

In 1855, Faulds repeatedly entreated Scotland Yard to set up a fingerprint bureau which he even offered to pay for himself. However, his pleas were recurrently denied and it was not until 1902 that a fingerprinting system was finally established for use by the police, with all credit being given to the aforementioned Galton and Police Commissioner Richard Henry (1850–1931), with no acknowledgement of Faulds' work.

During this time, Faulds' claim over fingerprints as a method of identification had come under much contention. Sir William Herschel, a British civil servant based in India, wrote to *Nature* shortly after Faulds' work was published, claiming that he had been using fingerprinting as a method of identification of criminals since 1860. This was followed by 17 years of correspondence between Faulds and Herschel with Faulds demanding proof in 1894 of Herschel's official use of fingerprints and resulted in Faulds publishing various books and pamphlets attempting to prove that he had been denied credit for his own theory. It has been suggested that there was a conspiracy between Galton and Herschel to discredit Faulds and take credit of the breakthrough for themselves.

After his final return to the United Kingdom of Great Britain and Ireland, Faulds first worked as a medical assistant in London and Staffordshire, then became a general practitioner and police surgeon in Stoke-on-Trent. He spent a substantial amount of time writing to and meeting with government officials in order to gain certified acknowledgement for his work. He also petitioned Winston Churchill, the then Home Secretary, to decorate him with a Knighthood. When these attempts were unsuccessful he issued questions for his local MP to raise in the House of Commons for an explanation into what he believed to be an injustice. There were reports from his close friend George Wilton that Faulds' actions were prompted by Galton's elevation to a Knighthood.

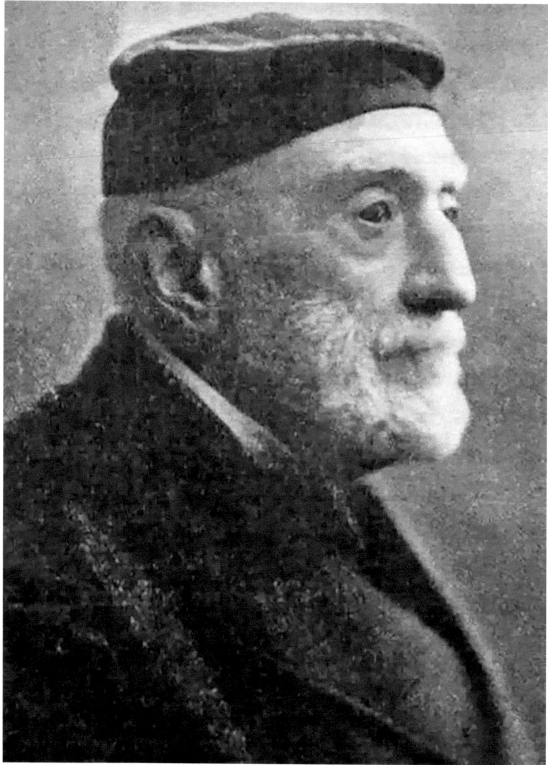

Henry Faulds. (Courtesy of Wikimedia Commons.)

Despite the fact that his earnings were meagre, Faulds continued to work for over 30 years until 1922, when 80 years old, he sold his practice and moved to James Street, Wolstanton. He died on 24 March 1930, at 86 years old, after suffering from years of increasing deafness and ill health, bitter at the lack of recognition he had received for his work. On 12 November 2004, a plaque was unveiled in Beith, Ayrshire, to honour the man many refer to as 'the forgotten Scot'.

Further Reading

Beavan C. *Fingerprints: The Origins of Crime Detection and the Murder Case that Launched Forensic Science*. New York: Hyperion Books; 2003.

Faulds H. *Dactylography: or, The Study of Finger-prints*. London: Halifax, Milner & Company; 1912.

Faulds H. *Nine Years in Nipon: Sketches of Japanese Life and Manners*. Boston, MA: Cupples & Hurd; 1888.

Faulds H, Herschel WJ. *Dactylography and the Origin of Finger-Printing*. Cambridge: Cambridge University Press; 2015.

James SH, Nordby JJ, Bell S (eds.). *Forensic Science: An Introduction to Scientific and Investigative Techniques*. Boca Raton, FL: CRC Press; 2002.

25 JOHN MILSON RHODES (1847–1909)

Freya Doswell

John Milson Rhodes was born in Broughton, Manchester, on 14 September 1847. His mother and father were Ann (née Keith) and Milson Rhodes respectively, with his father employed as a fustian salesman. Together they had three sons of which Rhodes was the youngest. The family lived in Glasgow for part of Rhodes' childhood and his brothers Francis and Thomas Wemyss both graduated from Glasgow Medical School. Rhodes himself began to read medicine at the same medical school but after the family moved back to Manchester, he enrolled at Owen's College and Manchester School of Medicine where he was a major prizewinner. He was awarded Licentiate of the Royal Conservatory of Music (LRCM) and Licentiate of the Royal College of Surgeons (LRCS) in Edinburgh in 1874 before later being awarded MD from Brussels in 1899. He set up as a general practitioner in 1874 in the affluent area of Didsbury, Manchester, where he spent his working life. With a special interest in learning disabilities and epilepsy, he also took on many voluntary roles reforming the provision of health care in Manchester's workhouses.

In 1880, Rhodes was appointed Overseer of the Poor for Chorlton, Manchester. This was a role that was defunct elsewhere in the country following the 1834 Poor Law Amendment Act. It was a voluntary position, which involved gathering epidemiological information rates of poverty in the area, as well as inspecting workhouse standards. This role was further refined for him when he was elected chairman of the Board of Guardian's for Chorlton in 1882. He held this position for 27 years. In this capacity, he inspected Chorlton Union Workhouse in Withington where he pioneered the care of children and the 'feeble minded', including epileptic patients. On inspection, he was very critical of the lack of medical care provided to residents and recommended that nursing care be provided in particular to the feeble minded and insane. In his capacity as guardian, Rhodes established the Northern Workhouse Nursing Association in 1891, of which he was its first executive chair, to ensure the placement of trained nurses in workhouse infirmaries. This was pioneered in London by Florence Nightingale two decades before, and Rhodes made certain these good working practices became common place in Northern England as well. As executive chair of the association, he held to account workhouses in the region who failed to provide professional nursing care, through the publication of annual reports.

By this point in his career, Rhodes was regarded nationally and abroad as an expert in care of the poor. In the first decade of the twentieth century he chaired the central poor-law conference of England and Wales and the Association of Poor Law Unions. He delivered evidence before the Royal Commissions on the care and control of the feeble-minded (1904–1908) and on the poor laws (1905–1909). He also lectured to statistical and scientific societies and a lecture to the BMA entitled *Pauperism Past and Present*, in 1890, was discussed in a leader in *The Times* before being published in French and widely circulated in pamphlet form. He particularly lectured on matters of workhouse treatment, nursing care of special groups and the link between poverty and disease. One such example of this epidemiological observation was when he visited slum areas in New York, noting the higher infant mortality rates compared to affluent New York. He noticed that infant mortality was lower amongst Jewish communities in the slum areas of New York as well as in Cheetham, Manchester, which had a sizable Jewish population at the time. He postulated this was due to the higher rates of breastfeeding in those communities having a protective effect, which correlates with modern beliefs in this subject. On the other end of the epidemiological spectrum, he also noted the higher prevalence of gout and dyspepsia in the wealthier Didsbury residents.

Rhodes also worked specifically in the care of patients with neurological illness. He campaigned to secure funding for a new 'colony' for people with epilepsy in Cheshire, which led to the establishment of the David Lewis Epileptics Colony; the institute still exists in the same building today, although the word 'Colony' has been replaced with 'Centre'. In 1897, in his capacity as poor law guardian, Rhodes was sent by the Chorlton and Manchester Joint Asylum Committee to Europe, in search of better systems of medical care that could be applied in the Chorlton workhouse and further afield. Rhodes observed that in places such as Germany, Austria and Belgium, their patients were separated from the main population of workhouse residents. In 1902, he travelled to the United States to observe how patients with epilepsy were treated there. He returned to the United Kingdom recommending that patients with learning disabilities, or 'imbeciles' as was the term used at the time, and severe epilepsy be removed from the mainstream workhouse setting. These patients were to be treated with, amongst other recommendations, specialised nursing care and fresh open air. In 1904, he began laying the foundation stones for the Langho Colony for Epileptics in Ribble Valley, Lancashire, which opened its doors in 1906 to the people of Manchester suffering with severe epilepsy. Here, residents were treated as per the findings and recommendations that Rhodes and colleagues had published in the *Poor Law Officers' Journal*, including open-air treatment. By 1909, under Rhodes' stewardship, the Board of Guardians ruled that Chorlton Workhouse deliver special dietary provisions to children, the 'feeble minded' and the sick, based on a more scientific basis than prior practice which provided the same rations to all.

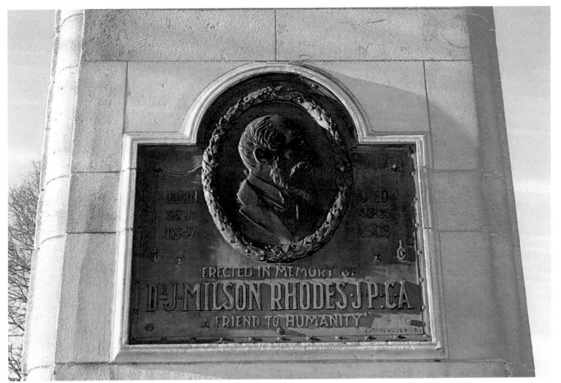

Memorial to Dr J. Milson Rhodes on Didsbury station clock. (Courtesy of Wikicommons/Wikidwitch.)

Throughout his career, Rhodes was also devoted to the plight of children in difficult social circumstances. This may have been through poverty or medical illness, in particular neurological illness. He orchestrated the development of cottage residential homes for children in Styal, Wilmslow. Opened in 1898, the initial 14 cottages housed around 300 children. They were built so that children could be removed from the workhouse to reside in homes specially designed to care for children. These homes had an infirmary, recreational hall, school rooms and a swimming pool. Whilst Rhodes was with the Chorlton Board of Guardians, three further cottages were added in 1903. The cottages housed thousands of children over the 58 years that they were open, finally closing in 1956.

Other notable positions were held by Rhodes. He was appointed Justice of the peace and visiting justice for HM Prison Strangeways in 1906. Furthermore he was one of the founder members and vice-president of the French-based Society for International Public Assistance, recognising his social justice and liberal beliefs. He was a Liberal, being an active member of Didsbury Liberal Club and was a sidesman at Emmanuel (Anglican) Church. He was elected as Liberal Councillor for Lancashire in 1892 representing Withington. He was later Alderman for Lancashire. In terms of other medical roles he was a factory surgeon and a medical referee for an insurance company. He wrote frequently on topics as diverse as infant mortality, the alleged increase in insanity and hospital floors. His article 'The Poor Law and the medical profession' was published posthumously in the *BMJ* in 1910.

It was particularly through his voluntary campaigning and his continued attention to detail to the epidemiology of the poor and their ailments that led to Rhodes being regarded nationally as an expert in poor law. He is noted in history to have been a key public figure in the reformation of the poor law. His interest in the Chorlton Union Workhouse was such that it was mentioned that he knew the name and history of all the patients on the Imbecile Ward as it was then named.

Rhodes never married and left no children when he died on 25 September 1909. His death was recorded as an accidental strychnine overdose. It is reported he medicated himself to treat an unspecified heart condition. On the evening of his death, his heart condition was particularly tiresome but as he was due to deliver a lecture in Europe Rhodes medicated himself to relieve the symptoms. However, dosing using a dangerous medication ultimately meant that too high a dose was used on that particular day. A funeral attended by many was held at Emmanuel Church in Didsbury and he was cremated at Manchester Crematorium. There was had a clock tower named in honour of him posthumously in Didsbury with a commemorative plaque, commissioned by contributions from local residents after his death. The clock is inscribed with the words 'A Friend to Humanity', acknowledging the life work of Rhodes as a campaigner for social justice. He is also one of a select band of doctors to have a public house named in honour of him; the Milson Rhodes Public House is found in Didsbury.

Further Reading

Anon. John Milson Rhodes, M.D., J.P. *British Medical Journal* 1909;2:1104–7.

Anon. Celebrating a visionary doctor. *Manchester Evening News* 2003; 12 January.

Barclay J. Rhodes, John Milson (1847–1909). In: Matthew HCG, Harrison B (eds.). *Oxford Dictionary of National Biography.* Volume 46. Oxford: Oxford University Press; 2004.

Rhodes JM. *Pauperism, Past and Present.* Manchester: Statistical Society; 1891.

26 WILLIAM CLOSE (1775–1813)
Emma L. Vinton and Neil Metcalfe

William Close was born on 25 May 1775 in the rural town of Field Broughton near Cartmel. He was the son of a mole catcher and was educated in Walney by Reverend Samuel Hunter. In 1790, when he was 15 years old, he was apprenticed to Mr Roger Parkinson, a surgeon in Burton-in-Kendal where he lived until completing his indenture in 1796. Over the following year he attended the University of Edinburgh Medical School and was awarded a diploma in Medicine on 18 April 1797. He immediately began work as a general practitioner and opened a practice in Dalton-in-Furness.

In 1803, Close married Isabel Charnock of Newton, near Dalton. They had two children together; John in 1805 and Jane in 1806. Close lived a prudent lifestyle and was respected by his peers. He did not own his home and surviving records of his stocks, books, chemicals and work equipment demonstrate his frugality. His love of horse riding meant that he could travel significant distances that would have otherwise been inaccessible. Locals described him as a slender man who was very clever but changeable.

During his relatively short life Close achieved many things. In 1799, he introduced smallpox vaccination to the Lake District only three years after its discovery by Edward Jenner (1749–1843). He elected the nearby village of Rampside to test his vaccine. He proposed that poorer children were inoculated. Several children had been previously exposed to the infection from peers and all escaped without manifesting symptoms of infection. This very open experiment established the efficacy of the vaccine and for five years the locality remained free of smallpox due to Close's efforts.

As well as being committed to his medical role Close contributed significantly to the fields of engineering and physics. With the advent of the industrial revolution Barrow became an early centre for ship building and the mining of slate, coal, copper, iron ore and saltpetre. Close enjoyed learning about the professions of his patients and spent many hours with local miners and traders. He helped the miners by improving the function of tallow-burning lamps. He devised a new technique for sand-tamping explosive charges and later published a paper with the consent of his colleague who had invented a technique for preventing their premature explosion. This was greatly received by miners who were increasingly concerned about their safety. The Isle of Walney was surrounded by water and Close developed a fascination with fluid mechanics. In 1804, he developed novel double-cased water-filled jackets that would go on to resolve the problem of air leaking into industrial condensers. He published a paper 'Observations on the practicability and expense of recovering land from sea at Walney Channel' and went on to design a hydraulic pump based on Goodwin's engine design. The prototype lifted water at a rate of 20 pints per hour and was well received by locals who had long suffered, trying to make the waterways work for them.

Musical instruments featured heavily in Close's life. In 1797, he opened a workshop in his home in Dalton. He made trumpets, bugles and French horns from brass, occasionally from silver. Sounds at that time were restricted to match the tube lengths of instruments. Experienced players could achieve additional notes by using 'lipping' technique, but this was a challenge for novice players and Close was keen to find a solution. From 1715 onwards, shanks or crooks were used to change the base note of each instrument allowing additional notes to be played. Close worked on several modifications and on 2 September 1811 he applied to patent his invention, this being the drainage spittle-cock. This prevented moisture from accumulating in the tubes, dulling performance. Whilst studying these drainage holes he thought carefully about adding additional holes to allow players to play an octave scale and shortly afterwards he developed his prototype 'the uncoiled trumpet', out of brown soap and paper. Since 1801, Close had been crafting these out of rolled lead and pewter and he achieved the best configuration for achieving the desired variations in sound. He worked on his new 'polyphonian' instruments until the year before his death in 1813.

Examples of Close's instruments were sent to the bands of The Duke of Cumberland and The Duke of Kent, the Bandmaster of the British Army and to Mr Thomas P Musical Instrument maker of 89 St. James St., London. In the same year, Close successfully obtained a patent for his keyed brass trumpets that could be fingered to produce any number of sounds. Though these were replaced in 1818 by German made valves, Close's contributions to music are undoubtedly noteworthy. In 1810, his paper 'Improvements in various brass instruments' was presented to the Society of Arts and Manufacturers. They offered him a silver medal but he modestly turned it down. His musical talents were not well known and only Mr Thomas Percival, musical instrument maker, displayed the phrase 'POLYPHONIAN' on his shop door, sometimes to the bemusement of his customers. Close's persistence led to the creation of the four-octave chromomatically scaled trumpet, played in the brass bands of today.

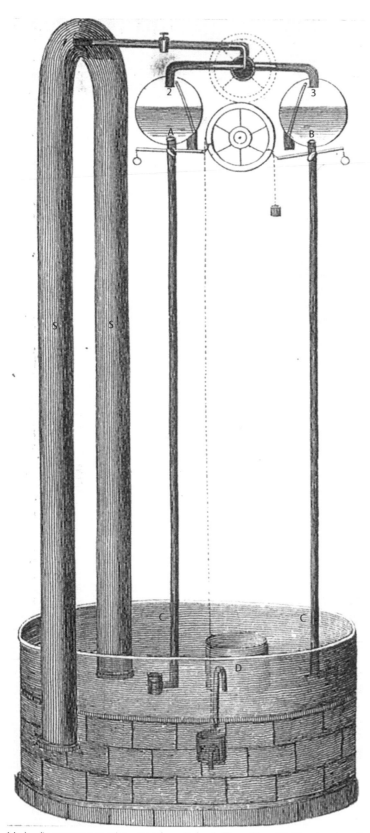

Hydraulic apparatus to raise water above its level. (From Close W. Construction of an hydraulic apparatus, which by means of the syphon raises water above its level, and performs its alterations without attendance. *Nicholson's Journal* 1802;1:27–32.)

Close also had a fascination with ink. He recognised that inks often faded if exposed to humidity and light. The advent of printing reduced the need for stand-alone inks but Close believed that important documents should be preserved where possible so he began experimenting with a range of recipes. His first indelible ink recipe comprised:

"200 grs oil of lavender
25 grs copal in powder (dried crystalline resin from the S. American tree: *Bursera copal*)
2.5 to 3 grs lamp black (for red ink add red sulphuret of mercury)

With the assistance of a gentle heat, dissolve the copal in the lavender in a small glass phial, and then mix the lamp black or red sulphuret with the solution upon a marble slab… put the composition in to a bottle and keep it excluded from the air."

His ink was a success and was used in a range of medical and legal documents as well as his own research. One of these was his analysis of 250 births, deaths and marriages in the Dalton Parish Registers, a technique used by modern public health professionals to map and predict communicable disease patterns. He also spent many hours drawing and mapping his local region and studying items of archaeological and historical significance. When 30 years old he edited, with additions, a previous book by Thomas West about the topography and history of Furness. It was called *Antiquities of Furness* (1805) and his 86-page supplement described various aspects of local archaeology, botany and geology. One further piece of work was not completed. In the last ten years of his life he had been preparing *Itinerary of Furness and the Environs*. It provided brief information about all the towns and villages within 21 miles of Ulverston and had he not died before its completion, is thought to have ultimately become as widely known as Thomas West's *Guide to the Lakes* (1778).

Close died of tuberculosis when 38 years old. On Sunday 17 June 1813 eight bearers carried his coffin to Walney Chapel burial ground and he was laid to rest under his favourite ash tree in a nine-foot-deep unmarked grave. A commemorative plaque marking his many achievements was erected at his former home at 2 Castle Street, Dalton. His obituary in *Gentleman's Magazine* described him as a doctor deservedly esteemed for his candour, sincerity and benevolence. His widow is said to have destroyed most of his writings after his death but many survive in the collection at Barrow library.

Further Reading

Anon. Obituary: With anecdotes of remarkable persons. Mr. Wm. Close, surgeon and apothecary. *Gentleman's Magazine* 1813;83:298.

Close W. On the lamp for tallow, and the combustion of that material. *Nicholson's Journal* 1799;3:547–48.

Close W. Description of an engine for raising water by the lateral motion of a stream of water through a conical tube. *Nicholson's Journal* 1801;4:293–98 and 493–95.

Close W. Construction of a hydraulic apparatus, which by means of the syphon raises water above its level, and performs its alterations without attendance. *Nicholson's Journal* 1802;1:27–32.

Close W. Composition of writing ink, possessing the permanent colour, and other essential properties, of the ink used for printing. *Nicholson's Journal* 1802;11:145–50.

Close W. *Observations on the Defects of the Trumpet, Bugle and French Horn, and the Extensions of their Musical Powers.* Furness; 1812.

Gardner-Thorpe D, Gardner-Thorpe C, Pearn J. William Close (1775–1813): Medicine, music, ink and engines in the Lake District. *Journal of the Royal Society of Medicine* 2004;97(12):599–602.

Gardner-Thorpe D, Pearn J. Tubular branches, additaments, holes and ventiges. William Close (1775–1813), Lake District Apothecary and Surgeon; and his invention of Polyphonian trumpets and French horns. *The Galpin Society Journal* 2005;58:38–45.

Gaythorpe H. William Close: Surgeon, apothecary, historian, musician of Dalton-in-Furness. *Annual Reports, Proceedings, &c., of the Barrow Naturalists' Field Club* 1909;17:166–80.

UK Patent Office. Rolls Chapel Reports. 8th Report. Abridgement of the Specification of Patent No. 3505. [William Close of Dalton] for Improvements on trumpets of different denominations, namely, the treble or common trumpet the French horn or tenor trumpet, and the bugle horn: 92.

27 WILLIAM GILBERT GRACE (1848–1915)
Neil Metcalfe

William Gilbert (WG) Grace was born in Downend, Mangotsfield, near Bristol on 18 July 1848. He was the eighth child of nine of Martha and Henry Grace (1808–1871), the latter a general practitioner and Poor Law parish medical officer. Much of his childhood revolved around cricket. He played with his family in the orchard at Chestnuts, his home in Downend, and played for the West Gloucestershire club as early as 1857, a day after his ninth birthday. The first time he made a substantial score was in July 1860 when he scored 51 for West Gloucestershire against Clifton; he later wrote that none of his great innings gave him more pleasure.

Away from cricket and roaming the surrounding fields, Grace's schooling was first with Miss Trotman in Downend before Mr Curtis of Winterbourne. He subsequently attended Ridgway House where he was a 'steady working lad, accurate at mathematics, with no mischief in him, passionately fond of [collecting] eggs and snakes'. Following an illness with pneumonia he received home tuition from Reverend John Dann between 1862 and 1864.

Grace was an outstanding athlete as a young man. He won the 440 yards hurdling title at the National Olympian Games at Crystal Palace in August 1866. In addition to running, he was an excellent thrower, as evidenced when he threw a cricket ball 122 yards (112 m) during an athletics event at Eastbourne. He also played football for the Wanderers, although he did not feature in any of their FA Cup-winning teams.

However, becoming a first-class cricketer was Grace's aim. Initially many factors were against him, including his not being born in nor having close ties to a first-class county and not being initially eligible to have membership in the Marylebone Cricket Club (MCC), the custodians of the game, as being the son of a provincial doctor was not a high enough ranking position in society for the club. He was also frowned upon for requesting expenses to be paid whilst claiming to play as an amateur or gentleman. This meant only by accruing a huge amount of runs, as well as wickets, was he able to play first-class cricket. A breakthrough inning in 1864 was his 170 at Hove for South Wales. In June 1865, Grace Played for Gentlemen of the South versus Players of the South in his first-class debut. He bowled extremely well and had match figures of 13 for 84. It was this performance that earned him his first selection for the prestigious Gentlemen versus Players fixture that season. His performance in that match at Lord's brought their first success against the Players in 19 matches. In July 1866, Grace confirmed his potential with his debut first-class century with an innings of 224 not out for the All England eleven against Surrey at The Oval. This was a record score at the Oval, a record he would break again there in 1871. In 1868, Grace scored two centuries in a match, only the second time in cricket history that this had occurred. He was awarded MCC membership in 1869.

Grace's cricketing feats were remarkable. In 1871, he became the first ever player to make over 2000 runs in a season and that was also the year he started to captain the new county side Gloucestershire, which he continued until 1899, and saw the press hail him as 'The Champion'. Grace became the first batsman to score a century before lunch in a first-class match when he made 134 for Gentleman of the South at The Oval in 1873. In the same season, he became the first player ever to complete the 'double' of 1000 runs and 100 wickets in a season. He went on to do the double eight times in all. By the time he was 27 years old he had scored 50 first-class centuries, at a time when pitches and protective equipment were poor. His highest score of 344, when playing for MCC against Kent in August 1876, was the first triple century scored in first-class cricket and broke the record for the highest individual score in all classes of cricket.

It took Grace 11 years to qualify as a doctor. Following the 1858 Medical Act it was a requirement to have 30 months of training compared to the previous apprenticeship model. This had been done by his father as well as all of his three older brothers with Henry (1833–1895) practising at Kingswood-Hill, Alfred (1840–1916) being a general practitioner in Chipping Sodbury and Edward Mills (1841–1911), who later became a coroner for the Lower Division of Gloucestershire, all working in medicine by this time. Grace enrolled at Bristol Medical School on 7 October 1868 but he was not known as a great scholar. One example of this is that he was said to have rebuked members of his teams for reading as he believed doing so ruined their eyes for the cricket. He was a rare attender at medical school as sport took up a lot of time, including occasional winter tours such as the six months from October 1873 to play in Australia. Although unsuccessful at a sporting level, Grace had more success personally as he combined the tour with a honeymoon with his wife Agnes Nicholls Day (1853–1930). He and Agnes would go on to have four children. Spells at St Bartholomew's Hospital and Westminster Hospital Medical School culminated in Grace receiving his diploma from the University of Edinburgh in November 1879, having been awarded LRCP (Edinburgh) and qualifying as MRCS (London).

After qualifying Grace took over from William Day (1822–1879) as the Poor Law medical officer for the northern half of the Bristol parish of St. Philip and Jacob, a role his father had previously handed over to Day. As a Poor Law medical Officer, he answered to the Board of Guardians of the Barton Regis Union. The guardians often disapproved of his long absences and requests for locums to cover his playing cricket. Despite being unhappy with the £90 a year salary,

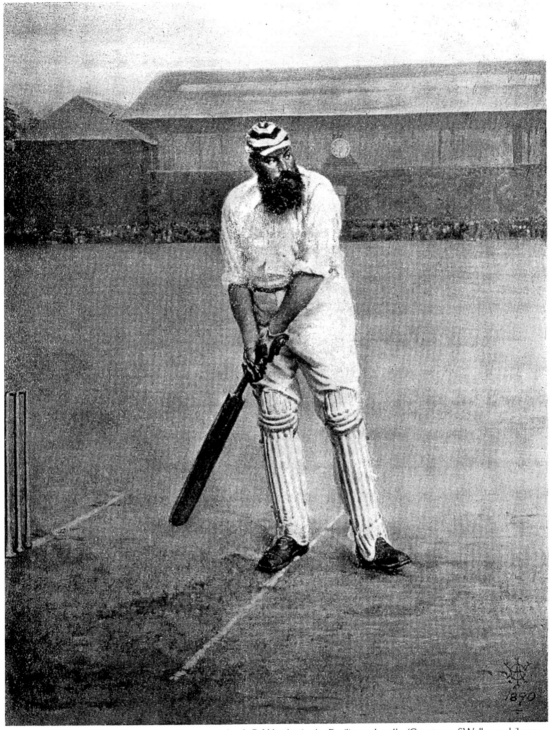

Portrait of William Gilbert Grace, from the portrait by A.S. Wortley in the Pavilion at Lord's. (Courtesy of Wellcome Library, London.)

he was able to top this up with private work from his house at Thrissell House, 61 Stapleton Road in Easton, a relatively poor district of Bristol. He was also surgeon to the Pennywell Colliery and the local public vaccinator about which he was said to have an incredible ability to identify smallpox.

It is believed that Grace tried to be a good doctor though his medical skills were mixed. He provided defensive and vague evidence at inquests but was celebrated following his race to a gas leak explosion in February 1886 where he helped dress and treat wounded miners. He was known to be generous to many and at Christmas would play open house for his poorer neighbours; one year there were over 100 guests. Even during a cricket match he helped save injured Gloucestershire team mate Arthur Croome (1866–1930) by holding a neck wound together for almost half an hour that had been caused by an accident on railings when fielding and doing so prevented what otherwise was believed could have been a fatal haemorrhage. On another occasion, against Kent, he stitched the eye of Richard Palmer (1848–1939), the Kent wicket keeper, only to then be aggravated when he was promptly stumped by him and on leaving the field reported 'After all I've done for you – that's what you do for me!'

By the 1880s, Grace mixed his general practitioner work with Test match cricket. Although the early matches were recognised retrospectively, Test cricket began in 1877. Grace made his debut in 1880 in the first ever Test match in England. In this match he played with his brothers, Edward Mills and George Frederick (1850–1880), the latter of whom was also destined to be a doctor but died from pneumonia when 30 years old just two weeks after this match in which Grace had scored England's first-ever Test century against Australia. He captained England and played in 22 Tests through the 1880s up to 1899, all of them against Australia, and was an automatic selection for England at home. His only Test-playing tour of Australia was that of 1891 to 1892. His highest Test score was 170 in 1886. Regarding his dual careers, during a match against Middlesex in 1985, he was 163 not out at the close of the first day's play. That evening, he recalled, was spent delivering a baby before he completed his double century the next morning.

Grace's later years continued to feature sporting successes. Despite his fondness for good food and drink affecting his physique, he was the sole recipient of the *Wisden* Cricketers of the Year award for 1896, the first of only three times that *Wisden* has restricted the award to a single player. He left general practice in 1899 in order to take up the post of manager of the newly formed London County Cricket Club. He ultimately scored 124 first-class centuries, the last for London County Cricket Club against MCC at Crystal Palace on his 56th birthday in 1904. His last first-class cricket match was in 1908 which was two years after his sons WG Junior and Charles had retired form their own first-class cricket careers. At the end of his first-class career he had amassed 54,211 runs (average 39.45) and taken 2809 wickets (average 18.14), which as of 2018 puts him 5th and 10th in the overall top run scorers and wicket takers in the history of first-class cricket. By then he had founded the English Bowling Association in 1903, becoming its first president as well as captaining England against Scotland in the first bowls international in the same year. He was keen on curling and played to a golf handicap of nine. He played minor cricket and the last match of any kind that Grace played in was when he scored an unbeaten 60 for Eltham versus Northbrook on 8 August 1914, a few days after the outbreak of the First World War (1914–1918). He was reportedly distressed by the war and was known to shake his fist and shout at the German Zeppelins floating over his home in South London. When Sir Henry Leveson-Gower (1873–1954) remonstrated that he had not allowed fast bowlers to unsettle him, Grace retorted: 'I could see those beggars; I can't see these'.

Grace was the first great international sport star and arguably the most famous celebrity in Victorian England. He died at Fairmount, his home in Mottingham, Kent, on 23 October 1915, at 67 years of age, after a stroke. There may have been more famous doctors and general practitioners than Grace but there are few more famous cricketers.

Further Reading

Grace WG. *W.G.: Cricketing Reminiscences and Personal Recollections*. London: J. Bowden; 1899.

Hawke MB, Harris GRC, Gordon H. *The Memorial Biography of Dr. W.G. Grace*. London: Constable; 1919.

Toghill P. Dr WG Grace, LRCP Edinburgh, MRCS England, 1879. *British Medical Journal* 1979;1:1269–70.

Tomlinson R. *Amazing Grace: The Man Who Was W.G.* London: Little Brown; 2015.

PART 2: GENERAL PRACTITIONERS FROM THE FIRST HALF OF THE TWENTIETH CENTURY

The previous section of this book has shown the careers of some of the names that helped establish the role of the general practitioner, as well shown how some general practitioners led other notable careers. All doctors at the beginning of the twentieth century were private. Some waived fees though unemployed patients had to rely on the stigmatised social welfare provisions of the Poor Law. Incomes of the doctors varied, though the average general practitioner was not wealthy.[1] Some worked in hospitals as physicians and surgeons to help their income but did not undertake extra training for such. Medical literature, particularly in the format of journals, was available though not necessarily focused to the general practitioner, and books specifically for the general practitioner were absent. The following section reviews the first 50 years of the twentieth century to exemplify some of the general practitioners who brought about changes to this status quo. It will again include general practitioners that contributed to general society either directly or indirectly.

Medical Politics and Medical Education in the First Half of the Twentieth Century

The major Act of the early twentieth century that affected modern social welfare and the general practitioner was the National Insurance Act (NIA) 1911. This Act introduced National Health Insurance (NHI) and had been proposed by David Lloyd George, the Chancellor of the Exchequer in 1908. It aimed to give the working classes the first contributory system of insurance against illness and unemployment. All male workers who earned under £160 a year had to pay four pence a week to which the employer paid three pence and general taxation paid an extra two pence, leaving Lloyd George to call it 'ninepence for fourpence'.[2] Workers were to gain access to free treatment for tuberculosis and were placed on the 'panel' (or list) of a named general practitioner who received an annual 'capitation' fee to provide for their general medical care.[2] General practitioners thus became responsible for the provision of primary health care within a national system funded by the state. Due to pressure from the Co-operative Women's Guild, the Act also included maternity benefits.

Several factions opposed the NIA.[2] These particularly included a large section of the Conservative Party and there was also opposition from some friendly societies and some trade unions that had their own insurance schemes. The BMA was one such union initially against it and there was much tension between the friendly societies and the doctors regarding the way that the NHI was financed.[2] Considering specialist care was not included, much of the effects of NHI and reform concerned general practitioners, who had to provide general medical services within their poorly equipped surgeries. The man who was the medical trade unionist *par excellence* and who gave the profession the organisational strength to make its demands felt was Alfred Cox.[2] He had been a general practitioner in Gateshead and had done much to fight friendly societies before becoming Deputy Security in 1908 and then Medical Security of the BMA in 1912. His support of NHI and his demonstration to thousands of general practitioners of how they were to actually benefit from the scheme did much to strengthen the BMA's position under the NIA, and Cox lived to see his dreams fulfilled when friendly societies were abolished in 1948.[2]

With regard the social reform leading to NHI and its subsequent implementation, the Highlands and Islands Medical Service (HIMS) justifies mentioning. Its history is intertwined with the work of Alexander Grant, a general practitioner from Ballachulish who had become interested in the rights of workers when working as a medical officer at a quarry company. In 1906, he was passionate for the cause of agricultural workers and in response oversaw the formation of the Highland Crofters and Cotters Association. His overall interest in social reform and such projects led to him providing evidence to a committee tasked with responding to poor provision of medical care in the Highlands.[3] He was able to exemplify and argue that medical and nursing services were either poor or non-existent in many areas within the crofting counties. Crofters did not qualify for services under the NHI, and anyway, the method of money-collecting of NHI contributions was impractical in these rural parts of Scotland. In addition, doctors struggled to make any living in such sparsely populated areas. The ultimate report, the *Dewar Report*,[3,4] led to Grant's pilot suggestion of HIMS being established in 1913 with a Treasury grant of £42,000. Doctors were given a basic income but could continue to treat private patients. Fees were set at minimal levels if they could be paid but medical care was still provided on a non-contributory basis if required. State resources were directed to basic needs, and they provided a house, telephone, car or motor boat to help provide the required care, as well as finances to help further study and provide locum cover for holidays. By 1929, there were 175 nurses and 160 doctors in 150 practices. Care was being delivered to all sections of the community and was of a higher standard than much of the rest of the United Kingdom. This led to working with HIMS becoming an attractive career option for nurses and doctors.

Several decades later, in 1948, the NHS was formed and several general practitioners from this time deserve mention. Considering that HIMS was the nearest matched service example available to the planners of the NHS, one of its general practitioners, Alexander Macleod was able to show how good and equal a service it was possible to provide. His career developing the service and supporting its widespread adoption into the NHS was important. Also, at the BMA between 1944 and 1949, was Harry Guy Dain who, as well as being a general practitioner, was also the chairman overseeing these politically charged and revolutionary times for social and health care. He had to oversee various disagreements with the government as the majority of doctors at this time were opposed to the idea of becoming employees to the state. Doctors were in a powerful position, since without them the NHS could not operate. Several compromises were given by the government to general practitioners especially, whose surgeries remained private businesses that could be bought and sold, and the NHS in effect gave these practices contracts to provide health care.

Towards the end of the 1940s, general practice was seen to be struggling. From an education point of view this had been recognised in 1948 with a BMA report *The Training of a Doctor*,[5] also known as the *First Cohen Report* after the chairman Sir Henry Cohen (1900–1977). The report suggested better education for general practitioners in order to keep their professional knowledge up to date, even if it meant being trained by hospital specialists rather than those from general practice who knew the job and its demands. The same year saw the first general practitioner trainee scheme commence[6,7] and two years later the BMA's *General Practice and the Training of the General Practitioner (the Second Report)*,[8] the *Second Cohen Report*, was published. This recommended specific general practice training for three years from registration and before the assumption of independent general practice. A similar finding of a need to increase general practitioner training was seen by an Australian general practitioner, Joseph Collings, who visited the United Kingdom to undertake a review of general practice in England and Scotland for the Nuffield Trust. He spent a year visiting 104 general practitioners in 55 practices and published his far-reaching report, the *Collings Report* in *The Lancet* in 1950.[9] It was largely condemning, not only of the poor knowledge of many general practitioners who undertook no postgraduate training, but also of their ill-equipped surgeries and the payment structure that did not incentivise general practitioners to improve them.[9] Whether a combination of these reports would lead to change will be addressed in the next part of the book.

General Practice Research in the First Half of the Twentieth Century

A leading researcher from before the Second World War (1939–1945) was William Pickles. He had benefited from the work of James Mackenzie, first of all indirectly by Mackenzie having delivered Pickles' wife into the world in Burnley, but more directly following reading Mackenzie's *The Principles of Diagnosis and Treatment in Heart Affections* (1918).[10] This had convinced him of the possibilities of research within general practice. He started undertaking detailed recordings of his patients at his practice in the Dales, which ultimately led him to describe various infectious diseases. This included being the first to observe the condition that was ultimately to become known as Hepatitis A, as well as documenting an outbreak of epidemic myalgia, now known as Bornholm disease.[11] He wrote numerous papers and was later encouraged to collate his findings, leading to his writing *Epidemiology in Country Practice* (1939).[12]

Although Mackenzie and Pickles were the two most prominent researchers at the time, there were other contributors to the medical literature in this period. Arthur Campbell Stark's most significant contribution was *An Index to General Practice* (1923).[13] This book outlined and defined important concepts of the reality of general practice and how it differed from hospital specialists. More specific advice in helping and advising those entering general practice came from William Sykes who published *A Manual of General Medical Practice* (1927).[14] Ernest Le Fleming published *An Introduction to General Practice*[15] in 1936 in which his views on a more patient-centred approach, compared with the more commonly practised doctor-centred approach, was given to the reader. Later Charlotte Naish, a pioneer of health promotion for children, wrote *Breast Feeding*[16] (1948), the first general practice book written by a woman.

Featured General Practitioners Making Major Contributions to Society in the First Half of the Twentieth Century

There were two female general practitioners who particularly had an influence on society in the first half of the twentieth century. Ethel Williams was the first female doctor in Newcastle and separately also the first woman in the North of England to have a driving licence, which she gained in 1906. However, it was her devotion and energies in the Suffragette movement and social welfare for which her career is generally remembered and she was said to have substantiated women's ability to contribute to society. Similarly, though at a later time, Edith Summerskill played a key role in the formation of the Socialist Health Association as a committed socialist and feminist. She enjoyed a long political career, first being elected MP in 1935 at a time when there was a total of eight female MPs. Her medical career helped influence a number of roles she had within the government, particularly during the Second World War and around the mid-twentieth century; she is remembered for also having written several books.

Again within public life, Chuni Lal Katial exerted some influence. He was a member of Krishna Menon's India League, which campaigned for Indian self-rule. When Mahatma Gandhi visited England for the Second Round Table conference in 1931, it was Katial who assisted him in his wish to stay 'amongst the poor', as well as arranging a visit at his house with Charlie Chaplin. He later proposed and helped develop Britian's first health centre as well as becoming the first mayor in the United Kingdom of South Asian origin in 1938, for Finsbury.

Regarding contributions from general practitioners to English literature in this time period, the largest was perhaps from Archibold 'AJ' Cronin. His medical career came to an end due to ill health, which inadvertently helped him follow a writing career. *Hatter's Castle* (1931)[17] was Cronin's first published novel but his most famous was *The Citadel* (1937),[18] the plot for which was inspired from his time practising in South Wales and working within the mining industry. The novel has been said by some to have helped highlight health inequalities at the time, and ultimately became a Hollywood film success on release in 1938, being nominated for four Oscars. In addition, the aforementioned Sykes also published novels and had some success with a series of detective novels, the best known of these, *The Missing Money Lender* (1936),[19] being published in the Penguin Book series.

Within the music industry, a significant contribution was made by Louis Neel, who conducted amateur groups and was persuaded to form an orchestra of young professionals recruited in 1932 from the Royal Academy of Music and the Royal College of Music. The Boyd Neel London String Orchestra, which later became the Boyd Neel Orchestra and is now the Philomusica of London, made its debut at the Aeolian Hall London on 22 June 1933. Neel ultimately left medicine to devote himself full-time to music and this led to conducting for various operas as well as embarking on world tours with his orchestra and publishing a book about these experiences called *The Story of an Orchestra* (1950).[20]

In terms of sporting achievements, the main success from a general practitioner at this time came from Ran Laurie. He had a glittering rowing career in the 1930s that had led him to successes in the Boat Race and other regattas. Together with his rowing partner he achieved a fourth place in the coxless pairs at the Berlin Olympics in 1936. The Second World War stopped any further chances of rowing for an Olympic medal until the London 1948 Olympic games in which he won gold in the same event.

References

1. Digby A. *The Evolution of British General Practice 1850–1949*. Oxford: Oxford University Press; 1999.

2. Honigsbaum F. *The Division in British Medicine: A History of the Separation of General Practice from Hospital Care 1911–1968*. London: Kogan Page; 1979.

3. Dewar J (Chmn.). *Report to the Lords Commissioners of His Majesty's Treasury*. Highlands and Islands Medical Service Committee (Cd 6559);1912.

4. Sheets JW. Dr Roger McNeill and Public Health in the Highlands and Islands of Scotland. *Journal of the Royal College of Physicians of Edinburgh* 2011;41:354–60.

5. Cohen H (Chmn.). *General Practice and the Training of the General Practitioner*. London: Butterworths; 1948.

6. Ministry of Health and Department of Health for Scotland. *Report of the Interdepartmental Committee on the Remuneration of General Practitioners*. London: HMSO; 1946.

7. Horder JP, Swift G. The history of vocational training for general practice. *The Journal of the Royal College of General Practitioners* 1979;29:24–32.

8. Cohen H (Chmn.). *General Practice and the Training of the General Practitioner*. London: Butterworths; 1950.

9. Collings JS. General practice in England today: A reconnaissance. *The Lancet* 1950;255(6604):555–79.

10. Booth CC. Research and the general practitioner. *British Medical Journal* 1987;295:1614–19.

11. Mackenzie J. *Principles of Diagnosis and Treatment in Heart Affections*. London: Henry Frowde, Hodder & Stoughton; 1918.

12. Pickles W. *Epidemiology in Country Practice*. Bristol: John Wright; 1939.

13. Stark A. *An Index to General Practice*. London: Bailliere, Tindall & Cox; 1923.

14. Sykes WS. *A Manual of General Medical Practice*, London: Lewis; 1927.

15. Le Fleming EK. *An Introduction to General Practice*. London: E Arnold & Co; 1936.

16. Naish FC. *Breast Feeding: A Guide to the Natural Feeding of Infants*. London: Lloyd-Luke Medical Books Ltd; 1956.

17. Cronin AJ. *Hatter's Castle*. London: Gollancz; 1931.

18. Cronin AJ. *The Citadel*. London: Gollancz; 1937.

19. Sykes WS. *The Missing Money Lender*. London: Penguin Books; 1936.

20. Neel B, Finch DJ (eds.). *My Orchestras and Other Adventures: The Memories of Boyd Neel*. Toronto: University of Toronto Press; 1985.

28 ALFRED COX (1866–1954)

Priya J. Shah

Born on 5 May 1866 in Middlesborough, Alfred Cox was the second son of eight children born to Thomas Benjamin Cox and Dinah Sanderson Skilbeck. His parents were a bridgeyard worker and the daughter of a blacksmith respectively. Initially Cox tried to pursue a career in teaching. This was not successful as he did not enjoy the post he had as monitor in Albert Road Board School because he was unable to use it as a step to becoming a pupil teacher. Therefore, when he was 17 years old he began to study for the civil service lower division, during which time he met a doctor who persuaded him to become his dispensing assistant in Carlisle. This provided Cox with a method of entry to the medical profession and he went on to read medicine at Durham University when 21 years old, during which time he continued to work as a dispensing assistant. On graduating in 1891, he became a general practitioner in Gateshead where he would practise for 17 years. In 1894, he married Florence Amelia, daughter of Thomas Cheesman, an iron merchant, in Newcastle with whom he had no children.

Whilst in Gateshead, Cox helped to found the Gateshead Queen Victoria Nursing Association and, in 1898, he also founded the Gateshead Medical Association. He played an active part in local politics, joining forces with the rector in a campaign for slum clearance. He also helped to form various societies for the discussion of medico-political and medico-ethical matters across the North of England, through which the dissatisfaction of doctors with the BMA became evident at the time. This then led to him helping to give the BMA a chance to reform itself by providing them with a motion to change the way that they handled their medico-political practice across England. This was done in order to rectify those abusing practice conduct and it resulted in a new constitution for them. Cox was a member of this constitution committee from 1900 to 1902 and he became the first Honorary Secretary of the Gateshead division, which replaced the Gateshead Medical Association that he had formed. He was also Honorary Secretary of the North of England branch between 1902 and 1908, and its president in 1908.

Cox was a keen member of the parliamentary bills (later medico-politico) committee. This was particularly for the time period between 1899 and 1903 and later in the years 1907 to 1908. In 1908, he gave up general practice and became the Deputy Secretary of the BMA with an initial salary of £500 per year. He then went on to succeed his predecessor, James Smith Whitaker (1866–1936), to be appointed as the medical secretary of the BMA in 1912. It was a difficult beginning for Cox with the previous year having seen the implementation of the NIA combined with Whitaker's decision to leave the BMA at the height of this struggle. The NIA gave the British working classes the first contributory system of insurance against illness and unemployment whereby everyone between the ages of 16 and 70 years old that were earning had to contribute four pennies (d) a week, their employers gave three d and the state would give two d, which meant that they were able to receive free medical treatment and medicine. This new measure caused a bitter struggle between the BMA and the government due to the decrease in medical fees for doctors. However, Cox worked arduously to maintain professional unity by holding numerous meetings and giving speeches in support of the NHI scheme to his colleagues and also managing to convey across a system of professional consultation to show the general practitioners how they would benefit from the scheme with the additional funding in the long-term. In just a month of Cox being appointed as the medical secretary 15,000 general practitioners had signed contracts with insurance committees.

When the First World War (1914–1918) started, Cox acted as joint secretary of the Central Medical War Committee where he helped to organise the supply of doctors to the armed forces, for which he was appointed Officer of the Order of the British Empire (OBE) in 1918. As ambassador for the BMA he was successful in cementing relationships between the organisation of doctors in Canada and South Africa. His visit to Canada was mentioned in both the *Canadian Medical Association Journal* and the *BMJ* editorials. By the time that Cox died both the Canadian Medical Association and the South African Medical Association had become affiliated with the BMA. Cox was also a co-founder of the Association Professionnelle Internationale des Médecins (later merged into the World Medical Association which is still operating today) in 1925, which was a successful attempt to bring together doctors practising in different countries. The Association Professionnelle Internationale des Médecins reached a maximum capacity of 23 countries which provided a platform to discuss problems of medical practice and to compare the conditions of medical service and medical education in their respective countries.

In 1932, Cox retired from the BMA after staying for a year beyond retirement in order to oversee the celebrations for the BMA's centenary. On retirement from the BMA he received a cheque of £1000 as well as a book with the names of 7000 subscribers to his testimonial fund, which went towards a portrait of himself produced by Sir Arthur Cope. The contribution to this fund was published in a letter to the editor of *The Lancet*.

After retiring from the BMA Cox took up several different medico-political positions in a number of different societies. Between 1933 and 1938, he was part-time General Secretary of the British Health Resorts Association,

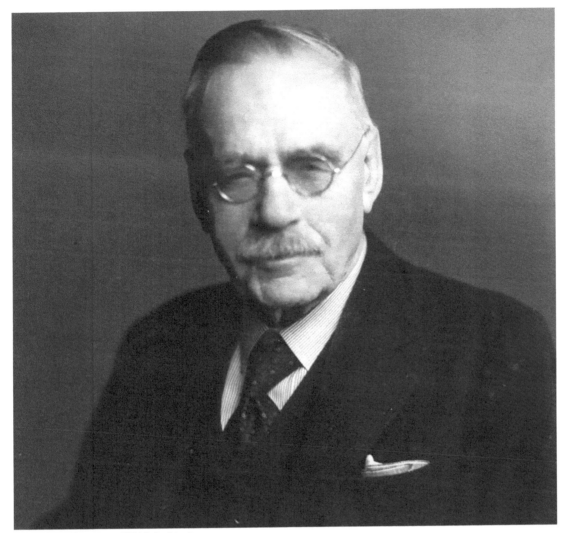

Alfred Cox. (Courtesy of BMA Archive.)

chairman of the advisory council of the medical section in the British Industries House, part-time medical secretary of the London public medical services and medical advisor to the Proprietary Association of Great Britain. Between 1941 and 1946, Cox was also the acting secretary to the National Ophthalmic Treatment Board.

Cox's work was highly commended and acknowledged contemporaneously. He was awarded the honorary degrees of MA from Durham University in 1921 and LLD from the University of Manitoba, Canada in 1930. In 1931, he was awarded the BMA's highest accolade of the gold medal to celebrate all the years of service he had given to them. After several years of poor health, Cox died in a nursing home in Brighton, having outlived his wife, on 31 August 1954 having reached 88 years of age. After his death, Cox was honoured for his caring and selfless work to his community by Gateshead Metropolitan Borough Council who erected a commemorative blue plaque in his honour at his former house in Gateshead on 21 March 2011.

Further Reading

ADB. Editorial comments. *Canadian Medical Association Journal* 1931;25(4):459–60.

Clegg H. Cox, Alfred (1866–1954). In: Matthew HCG, Harrison B (eds.). *Oxford Dictionary of National Biography*. Volume 13. Oxford: Oxford University Press; 2004.

Cox A. *Among the Doctors*. London: Christopher Johnson; 1950.

James T. Dr. Alfred Cox and the South African Medical Association. *South African Medical Journal* 1980;57(11):416–21.

Little EM. *History of the British Medical Association, 1832–1932*. London: British Medical Association; 1932.

Vaughan P. *Doctors' Commons: A Short History of the British Medical Association*. London: Heinemann; 1959.

29 LACHLAN GRANT (1871–1945)
Mason McGlynn and Neil Metcalfe

Lachlan Grant was born in the town in Johnstone, in the west Central Lowlands of Scotland, on 18 April 1871 into an affluent industrial family. Grant's father owned and operated a prosperous cabinet-making business in Johnstone; his mother was a descendent of a distinguished textiles family. This was all to change, however, when in October 1878 the City of Glasgow Bank collapsed. The vast majority of shareholders suffered catastrophic financial losses, including Grant's father, who ultimately lost both his business and the family's savings. For two years succeeding this, the Grant family faced stern financial hardship until a wealthy aunt offered the family employment in her shop in the Highlands, bringing to an end these difficulties.

The family relocated to Ballachulish. Grant was schooled at Ballachulish Public School, and began learning Scottish Gaelic, a language he would soon be fluent in. Gifted at school, he was admitted to the University of Edinburgh to study medicine in 1889. Grant excelled at university, showing a particular talent for ophthalmology, and graduated with distinction in 1894. Unlikely many Highland contemporaries, he was not averse to returning to the Highlands to practise medicine. In 1896, Grant was awarded MD and began a job as an assistant to a general practitioner in Oban the same year. Remaining in Oban only briefly, he soon relocated to Gesto Hospital in North Skye, assuming the role of medical officer.

In the late 1890s, Grant returned to the family home in Ballachulish and began working as a doctor overseeing the health of slate quarry workers. In 1900, he accepted a job as the medical officer for the quarry company. His return to Ballachulish, and subsequent appointments within the company proved to have been pivotal for Grant. He would go on to remain a doctor serving Ballachulish for the next 45 years, working as a general practitioner until his death in 1945. Whilst working at the quarry in 1902, he spoke freely about the quality and quantity of accommodation for the quarry workers, hoping with his criticism to appeal to those within the organisation for change. Displeased with what they viewed as sedition, the quarry company promptly dismissed him from his post. Ultimately, however, the loyalty of the workers to him proved fortuitous for Grant. The quarrymen unwaveringly laid down their tools and went on strike until Grant was reinstated. In late 1903, with a signed agreement from the managers at the quarry, he returned to work, concluding the workers' protest.

By this time highly interested in politics, a revitalised Grant did not cease urging for reform where he viewed it necessary. Between 1905 and 1908, Grant served as the medical officer once more for a hospital in Northern Skye. In 1906, during his time in Skye he became impassioned by the cause of agricultural workers, and in response oversaw the formation of the Highland Crofters and Cotters Association; an entity dedicated to campaigning for fair and just working conditions for farm labourers. From his time at the slate quarry onwards, Grant wrote unremittingly about economics, social reform and the provision of medical care in the Highlands, as well as about the preservation of Gaelic language and culture. In 1911, he was awarded a diploma in Public Health and, in 1912, gave evidence to a committee tasked with responding to poor provision of medical care in the Highlands. The report emerging from this, The *Dewar Report*, after its chair, the businessman and MP Sir John Dewar, was influenced greatly by evidence submitted by Grant, who spoke of the barriers to swift and efficient medical care in the Highlands. He proposed a centrally governed health service, and outlined an infrastructure that bore striking resemblance to what would eventually become the young NHS. Before implementing this service, which he believed could work for the whole of Scotland, Grant proposed a pilot scheme, which took the form of the HIMS, established in 1913. Critically, when a NHS was imagined for the entire United Kingdom 35 years later, only Grant's pilot scheme was considered as a possible model. Further, when the *Beveridge Report*, which laid out the initial plan for the NHS in 1942, was being commissioned, Miss Muriel Ritson (1885–1980) served on the commission and had been the service administrator for the HIMS.

It is worth noting that Grant, in addition to being a general practitioner and journalist, continued to publish medical research throughout his career, erecting a laboratory just adjacent to his rooms. Grant had a particular interest in tuberculosis. From his laboratory he was able to more quickly and accurately diagnose the disease when he encountered it amongst his patients, in addition to performing research on its effects on the body. In 1921, he was awarded FRCP and FRCS of Glasgow. In 1930, drawing upon his extensive experience treating work-related diseases in the slate quarry, he accepted a job as the medical officer for health at the new aluminium plant in Kinlochleven. In this role for British Aluminium he continued to publish as an occupational physician about the effects of working with aluminium. Having written for much of his life about developments in the Highlands, in 1934, he published a pamphlet, entitled *A New Deal for the Highlands*, expounding his vision for the advancement of the Highlands and the surrounding Islands. In it he campaigned against economic migration to Canada and New Zealand, which he felt was pulling skilled young people away from the community. Following the publication of his

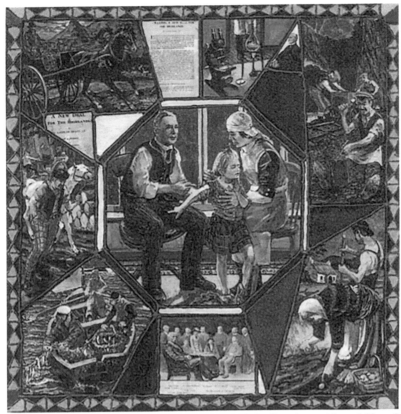

Portrait of the life of Lachlan Grant by Alastair Smyth. Separate panes include: Grant immunising a child; a reference to transport problems for doctors in the Highlands and Islands; his research career; his patients from the Highland crofters, fishermen and forestry workers; slate quarry workers who were his occupational health interest; his participation in the Dewar committee; Ramsay MacDonald M.P. and Prime Minister who became his friend and correspondent. (Courtesy of Dr James Douglas.)

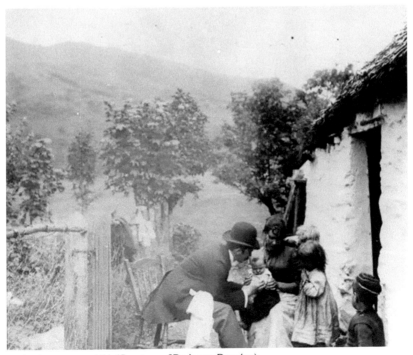

Image of Grant vaccinating a young child. (Courtesy of Dr James Douglas.)

pamphlet, the Highland Development League was formed in 1936, which Grant co-founded. From this entity, the Highland Development Board followed.

Grant died at his home in Ballachulish on 31 May 1945, survived by his wife and family. His legacy lives on today not only as a skilled and dedicated general practitioner but increasingly, with hindsight, as a man ahead of his time in being a truly unsung hero of the NHS. In 2014, a painting by Alastair Smyth and commissioned by James Douglas was presented to the Scottish Headquarters of the RCGP in Edinburgh to recognise and celebrate Grant's life of Grant. Furthermore, in 2011 a monument was erected to his memory in Ballachulish, commemorating his commitment to reform for workers. It is suitably sculpted in slate.

Further Reading

Dewar J (Chmn.). *Highlands and Islands Medical Service Committee. Report to the Lord Commissioners of his Majesty's Treasury.* Edinburgh: H.M. Stationary Office; 1912.

Douglas J, Tindley A, Smyth A. Dr Lachlan Grant (1871–1945). *Occupational Medicine* 2014;64:233–34.

Grant L. Aluminium and health. *British Medical Journal* 1932;9:686.

Grant L. *A New Deal for the Highlands* 1935;4–6.

Grant L. Diagnosis of early pulmonary tuberculosis. *British Medical Journal* 1935;1:446.

Macleod R. *Dr. Lachlan Grant of Ballachulish, His Life and Times.* Argyll: House of Lochar; 2013.

Tindley A, Cameron EA. *Dr Lachlan Grant of Ballachulish, 1871–1945.* Edinburgh: John Donald Publishers; 2015.

30 ALEXANDER JOHN MACLEOD (1894–1979)

Rebecca N. Woollin

Alexander John Macleod was born on 26 July 1894 in Leurbost, on the Isle of Lewis in Scotland. He was educated in the Nicolson Institute of Stornoway and after completing his education, joined the British Army. He served in the Ross Mountain Battery during the First World War (1914–1918) and was wounded at Gallipoli, being mentioned in despatches. From there he returned to the United Kingdom where he worked in the Officers Training Corps unit until the end of the war.

After completing his service in the army, Macleod decided to study medicine and began his medical degree at the University of Glasgow. During his time here he was a regular on the sports field, even losing his right eye during a shinty match at the university.

Following his graduation in 1924, Macleod undertook many locum roles including working in an asylum, an experience which he liked as it allowed him to appreciate a different approach to medicine. In 1928, he joined the crew of a whaling ship, becoming their medical officer for a year long trip to the Antarctic and collecting specimens for the Natural History Museum. In 1929, he began his first job as a general practitioner in Applecross in the Highlands of Scotland.

In 1932, Macleod was offered a job as general practitioner in Lochmaddy, North Uist, which he accepted. This meant that he was the sole general practitioner for a group of 16 islands and was assisted by several nurses. This job was as a part of the HIMS, a group which helped subsidise coverage by a doctor and nurses for each area included and made it possible for people who previously struggled to receive health care to have equal ability to be cared for pre-NHS, at a time when health care fees were private. This service was taken as an example of how a good and equal service could be provided when the idea of the NHS was being conceived and Macleod was passionate that all the best features of this service be included in the future NHS.

Macleod was the ideal person for this position. Firstly, he was fluent in both English and Scottish Gaelic. Secondly, he was passionately committed to providing the services he could. Thirdly, having been raised in the Highlands himself he was more than used to struggling against the elements; he travelled by foot, horse, car, boat and even tractor to reach his patients no matter the weather. In 1933, he became the first doctor in the Western Isles of Scotland to use a helicopter service to transport a patient. This was for Reverend Malcolm Gillies of the parish of North Uist who was in hospital in Glasgow and wished to return to North Uist to receive palliative care and live his last days amongst his family and parishioners. Macleod persuaded a local newspaper, the *Daily Record*, to fund the flight from Glasgow back to North Uist. This flight proved that an air ambulance service for the islands was feasible and led to the formation of the first air ambulance service in the United Kingdom. It was named the Outer Hebrides Air Ambulance.

During his time in North Uist, Macleod helped deliver over 2000 babies and became well respected in the field of obstetrics. One such birth was of John Gillies (1952–), former chairman of the RCGP Scotland (2010–2014), who recalled Macleod being known as 'An dotair Mor' which is 'the big doctor' in Scottish Gaelic. Macleod published a paper, 'Manual dilatation of the pelvis' in the *BMJ* about the techniques which he created to aid difficult births, having no access to emergency obstetric care compared with urban contemporaries. He performed caesareans by himself and was assisted in his obstetrics duties by his wife Julia (1933–1972), also a general practitioner by training. She also helped at his general practice whenever Macleod was predisposed and fully covered his duties when in 1944, he became very ill with pneumonia and took several months to recover. During this time, the community showed their appreciation and raised money to support the family at that difficult moment. Together they had five children, including son John (1935–2009) who followed his father into becoming a general practitioner, starting at the same Lochmaddy practice in 1973.

Macleod was committed to teaching and took on many trainee general practitioners who were keen to learn the ways of rural practice, gaining the nickname of the 'Lochmaddy School of Postgraduate Medicine' for the quality of the teaching and experiences provided.

In 1952, the RCGP was founded and Macleod was a founding member. He represented the Western Isles of Scotland for the BMA for 25 years and fought for incentive payments in 1963 for rural doctors who, at the time, were paid less than their urban counterparts. He was also a member of the Scottish Council (1962–1967) and a member of the Public Health Committee (1962–1964). Public health was an important part of practice for Macleod who was an avid promoter of vaccines, trialling them on his own children before putting them into practice on his patients. The role in which he took most interest in was on the Highlands and Islands Subcommittee of the Scottish General Medical Services Committee (1954–1974).

In 1967, Macleod was appointed OBE in recognition for his services to general practice. He retired in 1974 and died on 27 August 1979 aged 85 years old. In 2012, a memorial was erected in North Uist to celebrate the contribution of the Macleod family to the health of the community and their achievements in general practice.

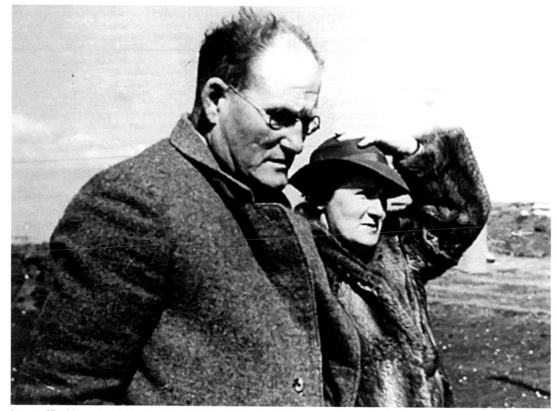

Image of Dr Alexander Macleod and his wife, Dr Julia Macleod. (Courtesy of Lorna Macleod.)

Further Reading

Macleod A.J. Manual dilatation of pelvis. *British Medical Journal* 1943;2(4319):484–85.

MacLeod A.J. Addiction to alcohol. *British Medical Journal* 1960;1:1953.

Macleod A.J. Alternative to salaried service. *British Medical Journal* 1965;1(5438):863–64.

Macleod A.J. Helicopters and medical emergencies. *British Medical Journal* 1968;3(5611):184.

31 HARRY GUY DAIN (1870–1966)

Adam J. Jakes and Harriet Metcalfe

Harry Guy Dain was born on 5 November 1870 in Birmingham. He was the eldest of six children of Major Dain, a draper, and his wife, Diana Weaver. He was educated at King Edward's Grammar School in Five Ways and Aston from 1883 to 1887. Thereafter he attended Mason College, which later became the medical department of Queen's College, Birmingham, and qualified with MRCS LRCP in 1893 and passed the MBBS a year later.

In terms of family and home life, Sir Harry married his first wife Flora Elizabeth Lewis (d. 1933), a nurse, on 17 July 1897. They had four children together, with one of his sons, Basil Guy Dain (1902–1976), following in his father's footsteps and practising medicine in Birmingham. He wed his second wife, Alice Muriel Hague, a dispenser, on 1 February 1939. His leisure interests included gardening and playing bridge.

Sir Harry spent his entire medical career in Birmingham. His first appointments were as Resident Medical Officer (RMO) at the children's hospital and assistant House Surgeon at the general hospital before becoming a general practitioner. He ultimately became a partner at a medical practice in Selly Oak, Birmingham, where he remained for the rest of his medical career.

It was the introduction of the NHI Act in 1911 that developed Sir Harry's interest in medical politics and enabled him to act as a key player in medico-political affairs for over 50 years. He was an active member of the first Insurance Committee and the first Panel Committee in Birmingham before becoming chairman. Later, in 1917, he became a member of the Insurance Acts Committee in London. For six years he chaired the annual conference of Local Medical and Panel Committees (1919–1924) and for 12 years (1924–1936) he was chairman of the Insurance Acts Committee. During this period it was said that his name was suggested for every sub-committee or deputation to the government.

Sir Harry also held other roles in medical politics. He was a direct representative of general practitioners in England and Wales at the GMC from 1934 to 1961. This was the longest period of service of any medical practitioner. Between 1937 and 1942 he was chairman of the BMA's representative body, his membership of which spanned the period 1919 to 1957. He was a member of the BMA Council from 1921 to 1960, serving as chairman between 1943 and 1949. Even whilst serving on the Council, he continued to work at his practice in Birmingham where he was popular with patients.

Sir Harry's involvement with the BMA coincided with the creation of the NHS. As BMA chairman for much of the 1940s, he became one of the chief spokesmen for general practitioners. Initially, he was opposed to the idea of the profession entering the NHS, deeply suspicious of government involvement in medicine. He feared doctors would become salaried civil servants and that patients would lose their right to choose their own doctors. He fought against the prospect, real or imagined, of state control of the medical profession. He felt that an extension of the NHI scheme with the preservation of private practice on a large scale would be more beneficial to the profession. With the incoming Labour government and Aneurin Bevan as Minister of Health, Sir Harry's fears grew. 'The Act', he told a BMA meeting in Exeter, 'is part of the nationalisation programme which is being steadily pursued by the government. What the Minister appears to have done is to have taken the Bill which we had partly fashioned and to have inserted into it the Socialist principles of State ownership of hospitals, direction of doctors, basic salary for doctors, and abolition of buying and selling of practices'.

In a speech in 1948, Sir Harry urged the profession to refuse service under the Act. However, the BMA's vote went against this advice and he accepted this outcome, pledging that the profession would 'do its utmost to make the new Service a resounding success'. The widespread respect and admiration for him and his powers of persuasion and prestige within the profession persuaded many general practitioners to join the NHS in 1948. It was said one of his greatest achievements was to keep the profession united in the face of the most severe pressures.

Sir Harry was skilled in clear thinking and persuasive speech, able to present facts clearly and identify the root of a problem. He was 'better known as a steady negotiator than a forceful leader'. He was described as a 'smart, dapper little man with blue eyes, a kindly face and a brisk manner'. He was 'terse and lucid where others were flatulent and foggy'. In an interview with the *Sunday Express* following his appointment as BMA chairman the then 73-year-old Sir Harry joked, 'I think they hesitated about approaching me to the job last September because they didn't think I'd last the year out, but they are finding there is plenty of life in me yet'. Away from medicine his leisure interests included gardening and playing bridge.

Several honours were bestowed on Sir Harry. In 1936, the Dain Testimonial Fund was established to honour his work on behalf of Insurance Practitioners. This was used, at his request, to help finance the education of the children of medical practitioners who had fallen on hard times. From the BMA he was awarded gold medal in 1936. In recognition of his services to his profession Sir Harry received the honorary degrees of LLD from the University of Aberdeen in 1939, and MD from the University of Birmingham in 1944. For his service to the RCS and a member for more than 20 years standing he was elected FRCS in 1945 having also served for some years on the council. In 1957, he became the first recipient of the Claire Wand Award for outstanding services to general practice. He was knighted

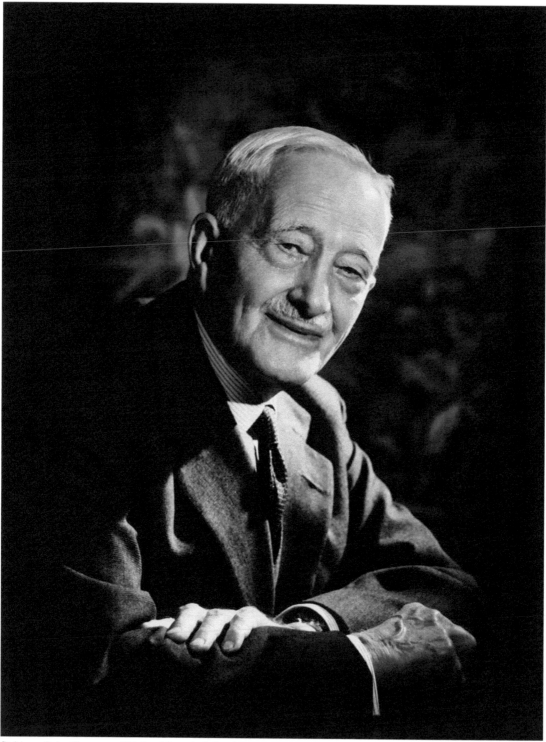

Sir Harry Dain. (Courtesy of National Portrait Gallery.)

in 1961, a year after he retired, at 90 years old. He was quoted at the time to reveal: 'I'm not retiring. I think retire is an ugly word and I shall continue to serve the profession in an advisory capacity'. He died on 26 February 1966.

Sir Harry's house and surgery survive as private residences called Bournbrook House on the corner of Bristol Road and Alton Road in Selly Oak. It was used as a surgery until 2009, when Bournbrook Varsity Medical Practice moved into adjacent larger premises. As a tribute to its original founder, the consulting rooms on the third floor of the new premises have been named the 'Dain Consulting Suite' and the residences in the adjacent converted technical college have been renamed Dain Court.

Further Reading

Anon. At 73, family doctor gets the biggest job of his life. *Sunday Express* 1944; 20 February.

Anon. Sir Guy Dain, F.R.C.S., Hon. M.D., Hon. L.L.D. (1870–1966). *Annals of the Royal College of Surgeons of England* 1966;38(6):391–2.

Croton L. Sir Harry Guy Dain MD, LLD, FRCS (1870–1966). *Aesculapius* 2012;1:82.

Stevenson D. Dain, Sir (Harry) Guy (1870–1966). In: Matthew HCG, Harrison B (eds.). *Oxford Dictionary of National Biography.* Volume 14. Oxford: Oxford University Press; 2004.

32 JOSEPH SILVER COLLINGS (1918–1971)
Stuart Pinder and Neil Metcalfe

Joseph Collings was born on 26 June 1918 in Sydney, Australia. Following an interruption in his studies by the outbreak of the Second World War (1939–1945), during which he worked for the Scientific Liaison Bureau and an Army Intelligence unit, he graduated from the University of Sydney in 1946 with degrees in agricultural science and medicine, before practising as a locum doctor in New Zealand between 1946 and 1947.

Collings later moved to the United States and became a Research Fellow at the Harvard School of Public Health. Whilst at Harvard in 1948, he conducted studies in general practice in the Canadian province of Manitoba for the provincial government and later on regions of the United States on a grant from the Rockefeller Foundation.

Following this, Collings then travelled to the United Kingdom on a grant from the Nuffield Trust. This was to undertake a review on the state of general practice in the United Kingdom and Scotland and its ability to provide primary care under the newly formed NHS. He spent a year in the United Kingdom, during which he visited 104 general practitioners in 55 practices, covering a range of urban and rural areas.

In 1950, Collings published his findings in *The Lancet*. His report, entitled 'General practice in England today: a reconnaissance', took up nearly half the issue of the journal. His critical view on the failings of general practice was controversial and drew unfavourable comment. However, this report, which became known as *The Collings Report*, produced a sharp professional debate and then reaction.

Two years after the start of the NHS, *The Collings Report* highlighted the failings in general practice. It revealed the broad disparity in the quality of service provided. Collings observed several practices of an excellent standard but described others as dingy and ill-equipped with a deplorable standard of medicine. His writing style spoke plainly and painted vivid images of his observations and opinions: 'Few skilled craftsman, be they plumbers, butchers or motor mechanics, would be prepared to work under such conditions or with equipment so bad'. One practice he visited was one with four partners and two assistants, which had a patient list of 20,000. He described it as consisting of:

> A small dilapidated waiting room, three equally small and untidy consulting rooms, and a kind of cupboard that served as a dispensary... The consulting rooms were dirty and ill-equipped. There were no examination couches... apart from a few rusty and dusty antique instruments, there was no sign of any sort of equipment... The desk and floor were littered with papers. Only one of the consulting rooms was equipped with a hand-basin and hot and cold water.

Contrary to popular opinion at the time, Collings described rural practices as generally providing superior health care than those in urban areas. Policy makers contemporaneously believed city-based doctors benefitted from collaborations with academic medical centres and greater access to continuing medical education. However, he described these relationships as more adversarial than collaborative, and reserved his highest praise for the doctors in HIMS in Scotland, identifying that general practice standards in Scotland were higher than England as a whole.

Collings primarily blamed the state of general practice on its leadership, in addition to policy makers and specialty societies. He described the medical knowledge of many general practitioners as out of date, and the overall state of general practice as 'bad and still deteriorating'. There was no real postgraduate training in general practice at that time, and the NHS payment system failed to encourage a high standard of care, by penalising general practitioners who spent money on their practices and equipment.

The BMA was hostile to the report and quickly commissioned another survey by Stephen Hadfield (1908–2007), the then assistant secretary of the BMA. Published in 1953, Hadfield's *A Field Survey of General Practice 1951–1952* was more positive than *The Collings Report* but confirmed many of Collings' concerns including that there was significant scope for improvement both of conditions and of attitudes and standards.

The main analytical criticism of *The Collings Report* was in regards to the unique ethnographic techniques that Collings employed producing it. The report was the only article published by *The Lancet* between 1946 and 1955 that used a qualitative method of data collection. With the exception of mass observation, qualitative research was under developed in the United Kingdom whilst gaining popularity in the United States. His research method was both innovative and pioneering, as it was the first time ethnographic techniques had been applied to the profession in the United Kingdom, having previously only been employed in studies on manual workers.

A separate criticism of the *Collings Report* cited the method of how the 55 general practices were chosen. The selection criteria that Collings had used consisted of three regions he was advised 'would present the general picture' by regional officers of health, medical officers of health and consultants, based on their judgements. London was excluded from the report due to 'it's aggregation of teaching hospitals and many other complicating factors peculiar to a city of this size'. The report also provided no information on the refusal rate of practices asked to participate in the study, and

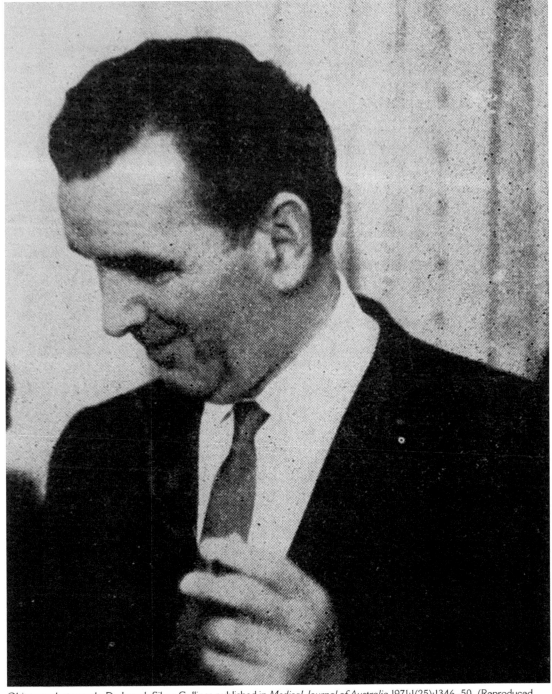

Obituary photograph: Dr Joseph Silver Collings published in *Medical Journal of Australia* 1971;1(25):1346–50. (Reproduced with permission from *The Medical Journal of Australia*.)

the levels of cooperation provided, which brought criticism about the accuracy of generalising beyond the practices studied.

Despite these criticisms, Collings' frank and devastating condemnation of several of the practices visited made the report 'the single most effective factor in mobilising opinion in favour of constructive change' according to the official NHS historian, Charles Webster. *The Collings Report* galvanised the establishment of the College in 1952. The following year, committees on undergraduate and postgraduate education were established, and guidelines for medical student and postgraduate training were developed over the ensuing decade.

After publishing his report in 1950, Collings returned to the United States as a Research Fellow at the Harvard School of Public Health, before returning to New Zealand in 1951 to work in general practice. In 1952, he returned to the United States where he became Assistant Medical Director of the Health Insurance Plan of Greater New York, in charge of professional practices. That same year he was also appointed as a consultant to President Harry Truman's commission on the Health Needs of the Nation.

Collings later returned to Australia and set up his own practice in an industrial part of Melbourne. Although under the Australian payment system this type of practice was poorly remunerated. He endeavoured to provide a wide range of services for his patients, including physiotherapy and minor surgeries. Having played a major role in catalysing the establishment of the College, in 1958, he became one of the founding members of the Australian College of General Practitioners. In 1961, he moved from general practice to hospital medicine and accepted an invitation to become Head of the Department of Physical Medicine at Royal Melbourne Hospital, where he worked for the last decade of his life, and developed a special interest in spinal injuries.

Collings died in 1971, and was survived by his wife and their three children. He is fondly remembered by those who knew him for his warmth of character and good humour, as an exceptional teacher and as a doctor who cared greatly for his patients. His impact on the structure of primary care in the United Kingdom was formidable and long lasting. He had a crusading zeal for identifying and correcting deficiencies in health care provision. His obituary in the *Medical Journal of Australia* stated that 'in many ways he was too far ahead of his time; and many regarded his visions of better medical centres, better medical training, and a position for the general practitioner at the top, rather than the bottom of the hierarchy as merely visionary', a vision he worked upon to try and make a reality.

Further Reading

Collings JS. General practice in England today: A reconnaissance. *The Lancet* 1950;255(6604):555–79.

Crock HV. Obituary: Joseph Silver Collings. *Medical Journal of Australia* 1971;1(25):1346–50.

Loudon I, Horder J, Webster C. *General Practice under the National Health Service 1948–1997*. Oxford: Oxford University Press; 1998.

Petchey R. Collings report on general practice in England in 1950: Unrecognised, pioneering piece of British social research? *British Medical Journal* 1995;311:40.

Sturmberg JP. *The Foundations of Primary Care: Daring to Be Different*. Milton Keynes: Radcliffe Publishing; 2007.

Sydney MB. Obituary: Joseph Silver Collings. *The Lancet* 1971;297(7704):867–68.

33 WILLIAM NORMAN PICKLES (1885–1969)

Christopher Goode

William Pickles was born in Camp Road, Leeds, on 6 March 1885. He was the second son of six for Leeds general practitioner John Jagger Pickles (1851–1925). All but the youngest son entered the medical profession. He attended Leeds Grammar School and was awarded a Leeds Infirmary Scholarship. When he was 17 years old, he entered the Medical School of Yorkshire, which later merged with the University of Leeds, in 1902. He worked as Lord Berkeley Moynihan's (1865–1936) surgical dresser for six months from whom he learnt a great deal. Whilst still a student he also worked as dispenser for a general practice often covering if the general practitioner was called away.

Pickles failed his first attempt at the London MB in October 1908. He was awarded LSA in March 1909. He worked as a locum general practitioner in various practices for a number of months but then returned to Leeds General Infirmary as a resident obstetric officer. Not satisfied with his qualification Pickles retook his examination and was awarded London MB in 1910. He then returned to a variety of general practice locum posts, including one in Bedale in the North Riding of Yorkshire where he assisted Drs Horsfall and Eddison. This is when Pickles' first interest in epidemiology arose. He studied an outbreak of typhoid in Bedale and traced it back to a water pump that had been contaminated by a gypsy woman. He ordered the pump to be closed to help limit the spread.

In 1913, Pickles joined the general practitioner partnership in Aysgarth in Wensleydale, where he would eventually work until his retirement. The practice included eight villages and at the time the district had a population of 4267. At the outbreak of the First World War (1914–1918) Pickles was assigned to the Royal Naval Reserves on *HMS Albion*, patrolling the South Atlantic and sailing to Cape Verde. This experience led him to write to the *Journal of the Royal Naval Medical Service* about Vincent's disease, with this becoming his first publication when it was published in 1919. Vincent's disease caused malodorous ulceration of the gums, now known to be caused by fusospirochaetal organisms. It was widespread amongst sailors due to poor dental hygiene. This gave Pickles many cases to document. During this period he became engaged to Gertrude Tunstill (1891–1969) and married her in Aysgarth Church in 1917. The next year he was awarded MD from London and returned to work at his Aysgarth practice, where he worked with Dean Dunbar (1884–1934) who was a friend from medical school days.

Pickles had an investigative nature and believed that general practitioners had unique opportunities to make valuable observations which other medical practitioners did not. It was James Mackenzie's (1853–1925) book *The Principles of Diagnosis and Treatment in Heart Affections* (1918) which convinced Pickles that is was possible for a general practitioner to make important and original observations. In 1927, he attended a correspondence course in London, as he wanted to learn the latest methods of diagnosis and treatments from consultants. He would continue to take refresher courses to help keep his knowledge up to date. This proved useful in October 1928 when an epidemic of jaundice occurred in the Yorkshire Dales. Pickles kept records of all the 118 cases that he and Dunbar saw. By careful documentation and enquiry they were able to find 132 additional sufferers. In many cases, they were able to find the source of the infection and from this information Pickles accurately calculated the incubation period of the disease. Gertrude maintained and organised all of his charts and notes. His findings were published in the *BMJ* in 1930. Today the disease Pickles and Dunbar had been investigating is known as hepatitis A which is spread via the faecal–oral route. In 1933, Pickles documented an outbreak of epidemic myalgia, also known as Bornholm disease, in Wensleydale. The condition was practically unknown in the United Kingdom until his description of it. It is known today to be caused by Coxsackie B virus. Pickles also wrote important epidemiological descriptions of measles and farmer's lung, the latter being a hypersensitivity pneumonitis caused by repeated inhaling of dust from mouldy hay.

In 1954, Pickles met Professor Major Greenwood (1880–1949) in London. Greenwood was an epidemiologist and statistician. He knew of Pickles' various articles and encouraged him to write a book on all of his findings. This would lead to Pickles publishing *Epidemiology in Country Practice* in May 1939. It was well received but the outbreak of the Second World War (1939–1945) prevented it from achieving worldwide reputation sooner, as the remaining stock of the book was destroyed at the publishers John Wright of Bristol due to a direct hit from an air raid in April 1941. During this time he was invited to lecture in Australia, South Africa and the United States. He also lectured at nearly every medical school in the United Kingdom.

In the 1950s, Pickles' advice was much sought after. He became a member of many different committees including the Medical Advisory Committee of the Central Health Services and the Nuffield Provincial Hospitals Trust Medical Advisory Council. He was also a prominent member of the BMA and became a founding member of the Society for Social Medicine and the International Epidemiological Association. He received the Steward Prize for 'His researches in the field of epidemiology' and was awarded an honorary DSc from the University of Leeds on 19 May 1950. When the College was created, the Foundation Council proceeded to unanimously nominate him the first president of the College and he gave the first James Mackenzie Lecture in 1954. He was appointed Commander of the Order of the British Empire

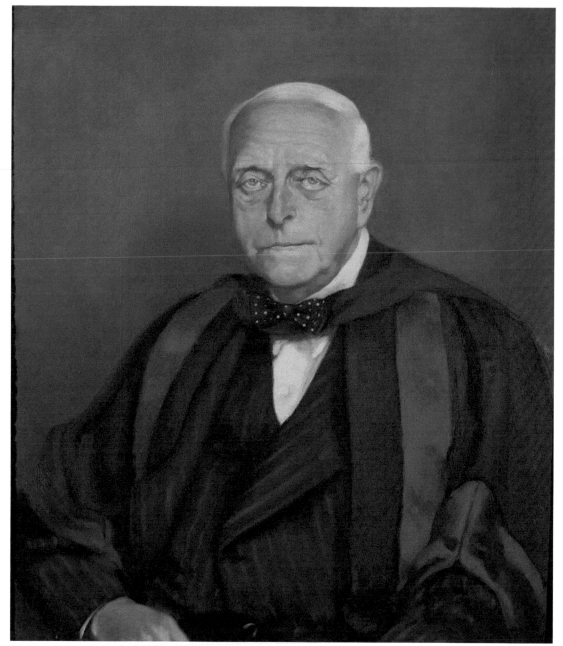

RCGP presidential portrait of William Normal Pickles CBE (1885–1969). Artist: Christopher Sanders. (Courtesy of RCGP Archives, London.)

(CBE) in 1957, Honorary Fellow of the College in 1958, became the second ever recipient of the Foundation Council Award in 1961 and was awarded FRCP (London) in 1963.

In 1965, Pickles suffered a partial tibial artery occlusion in his right leg, which ultimately required a leg amputation. Despite this he reportedly remained in good spirits. Shortly after a prostatic operation he contracted pneumonia and died on 1 March 1969 aged 83 years old. His wife outlived him by six months.

Pickles had been offered the post of epidemiologist for the Ministry of Health in 1931, as well as many other opportunities; however, he never wanted to leave his patients in Aysgarth and only retired in October 1964 when 79 years old. Consequently, his obituary in the *BMJ* stated: 'As well as being a great field epidemiologist Will was a great family doctor of our time. Scrupulously careful in recording and visiting, never underrating a patient or his symptoms, he was courteous and kind to all, even the most awkward patients'.

Further Reading

Moorhead R. Pickles of Wensleydale. *Journal of the Royal Society of Medicine* 2001;94:536–40.

Pemberton J. *Will Pickles of Wensleydale. The Life of a Country Doctor.* London: Geoffrey Bles; 1970.

Pickles WN. Vincent's disease. *Journal of the Royal Naval Medical Service* 1919;5:87.

Pickles W. Epidemic catarrhal jaundice: An outbreak in Yorkshire. *British Medical Journal* 1930;1:944–46.

Pickles W. *Epidemiology in Country Practice*. Bristol: John Wright; 1939.

Pickles WN. The country doctor and public health. *Public Health* 1944;58:2.

Pickles WN. Epidemiology in country practice. *The Practitioner* 1955;17:76–87.

34 ARTHUR CAMPBELL STARK (1864–1928)
William Mark Stevens

Arthur Campbell Stark was born in Norwich on 17 October 1864. In his early teenage years, he left his family home to live with and train as an apprentice to the chemist James Robinson (1838–1901). Following this apprenticeship, Stark went on to obtain the qualification of a pharmaceutical chemist and began being able to dispense medication to the public.

In the 1890s, Stark was dispensing in London's St George Hanover Square, and demonstrating materia medica and pharmacy at St George's Hospital. Under his teaching, the students learnt about the therapeutic qualities of different compounds and medicines. He also aspired to further his own education and to become more directly involved with the treatment of patients. For this reason, he studied for a LSA which he was awarded in 1903. He was also awarded MBBS in 1904 by the University of London. During these years he won the gold medal of the University of London, a medal still awarded annually to the strongest final year London-based medical student. He also won the gold medal of the Society of Apothecaries.

The 1911 census describes that, after qualifying, Stark was working as a general practitioner near Wanstead Park, Essex. In the First World War (1914–1918) he worked at Wanstead Park Military Hospital. This hospital had 50 beds in 12 wards, which increased to 75 by 1917. It also had a fully equipped operating theatre, in which he was responsible for treating wounded soldiers. Along with working at the hospital, Stark also furthered his surgical expertise by working as a district surgeon for the St. John Ambulance Association.

Despite his notable achievements and qualifications, Stark's true legacy and his impact on practice came through his teaching and his research. Whilst demonstrating materia medica and pharmacy at St George's Hospital in 1893, he published *Practical Pharmacy for Medical Students*, a text designed to help students who were undergoing the examinations of the Conjoint Board in Practical Pharmacy. The book outlined the mode, character, incompatibilities and production of many drugs used at the time. This text was received sufficiently well to warrant publication of a revised edition, published in 1900, which was adapted to include drugs added in the *British Pharmacopoeia* of 1898.

Stark later became a lecturer of Biology at Westminster Hospital Medical School. He was also a vocal member of the academic community from 1905 to 1927, and his correspondence regarding many different topics featured regularly in the *BMJ*. His contributions focussed particularly on puerperal sepsis, glandular fever, acidosis of the blood as well as an analysis of the state of obstetrics at the time. Regarding this latter topic he wrote in the *BMJ* in September 1919, that infant mortality rates were unacceptably high. In an effort to improve this, he identified that practical midwifery teaching of the time was of a low standard and advocated its improvement. He also recommended more extensive involvement of general practitioners at childbirth.

Perhaps Stark's most significant work, however, came in 1923. This was when his book entitled *An Index to General Practice* was published. This book outlined and defined important concepts of general practice for the first time. Today, it also acts as a useful historical text on the life of a general practitioner at the time.

There were several important principles that Stark identified in general practice in his *An Index to General Practice*. Firstly, he noted that 'Many of the disorders, the treatment of which makes up a large proportion of the general practitioner's work, are scarcely seen at hospitals', thereby differentiating doctors who practised general practice from those in hospitals based on experience with different conditions. In many conditions, he mentioned, treatments were effective before ever requiring a patient to go to hospital. Conversely, a clinician at hospital was likely to have specialised in a particular branch of medicine and, therefore, tended to have experience of rarer diseases, limited to their specific field of interest.

Stark's second point was to note that: 'To the hospital physician, or surgeon, a patient is a more or less interesting example of a disease, and what he is concerned with is the treatment and pathology of that disease, as he sees it. He never sees the beginning of the disease, and not often the end of it, and the individuality of the patient, and his fate, are of minor importance. In general practice, on the contrary, the individuality of the patient is the first consideration'. This was an early documentation of the principle and benefit of a general practitioner building a strong rapport and relationship with patients.

Stark went on to highlight the importance of social histories and patient-centred care in a third point, in which he stated: '[the patients] temperament, his surroundings, and the routine of his ordinary life, must always be considered, and a practitioner who fails to take these into account will not be very successful'.

Finally, Stark wrote that the general practitioner will encounter 'a large number of human beings, diverse and interesting', and that they can expect to 'have to listen gravely to nonsense and to bear patiently with prejudices, yet…must understand and sympathise with the patient's point of view'. This showed understanding of the necessity of empathy in the career of a general practitioner, and appreciation of the varied nature of patients in general practice.

AN INDEX

TO

GENERAL PRACTICE

BY

A. CAMPBELL STARK

M.B. AND B.S. (LOND.), L.S.A. (ENG.), PH.C.

EXHIBITIONER AND GOLD MEDALLIST OF THE UNIVERSITY OF LONDON ; GOLD
MEDALLIST OF THE SOCIETY OF APOTHECARIES ; LATE LECTURER ON
BIOLOGY AT WESTMINSTER HOSPITAL MEDICAL SCHOOL ; LATE DEMON-
STRATOR ON MATERIA MEDICA AT ST. GEORGE'S HOSPITAL MEDICAL
SCHOOL ; LATE DISTRICT SURGEON ST. JOHN AMBULANCE
ASSOCIATION ; LATE SURGEON TO THE WANSTEAD PARK
MILITARY HOSPITAL ; AUTHOR OF "PRACTICAL PHAR-
MACY FOR MEDICAL STUDENTS," ETC., ETC.

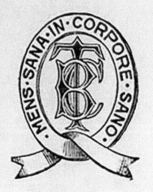

LONDON

BAILLIÈRE, TINDALL AND COX

8, HENRIETTA STREET, COVENT GARDEN, W.C. 2

1923

All rights reserved

Book cover of *An Index to General Practice*. (Courtesy of RCGP Archives, London.)

On 20 June 1923, The *BMJ* published that Stark's work was 'admirable and all too short'. The article highlighted that it is curious 'that although a large majority of medical students go into general practice, no attempt is made during their curriculum to train them for their special work', and that 'those who are setting out on the same journey will avoid many a wrong turning by having his little guide-book with them'.

Stark's death was registered in West Ham, Essex, on 18 March 1928, and was announced in the *BMJ* on 14 April 1928. He was succeeded by his wife, Ellen Bailey. The couple were married in 1891, when Stark was 27 years old. They ultimately had two children, and their son Michael Cecil Stark (1892–1974) followed his father into general practice.

Further Reading

Anon. A useful guide. *British Medical Journal* 1923;1(3261):1097–98.

Stark A. *Practical Pharmacy for Medical Students*. London: Bailliere, Tindall and Cox; 1893.

Stark A. *Aids to Practical Pharmacy for Medical Students*. London: Bailliere, Tindall and Cox; 1900.

Stark A. *An Index to General Practice*. London: Bailliere, Tindall and Cox; 1923.

35 WILLIAM STANLEY SYKES (1894–1961)
Duncan Blues

William Stanley Sykes, son of Arthur Stanley Sykes, was born on 5 August 1894 and grew up in the small market town of Morley, West Yorkshire. Upon finishing secondary education at Rossall School, he went on to begin his medical training in 1912 at Emmanuel College, University of Cambridge.

The outbreak of the First World War (1914–1918) interrupted Sykes' studies at Cambridge. He briefly joined the Royal Navy, before being sent back to finish his studies. As a student he was awarded MRCS and LRCP in 1919. In 1921, he graduated with a Bachelor of Medicine, Bachelor of Surgery (MBBChir) and completed a diploma in Public Health.

Sykes started his working career with a move to London to work at St Bartholomew's Hospital, first as house surgeon and extern midwifery assistant, and then house anaesthetist. This job in anaesthetics sparked a lifelong interest in the subject, which ultimately became his passion. He soon returned to his hometown of Morley, taking up a job in general practice and being appointed honorary anaesthetist at Leeds General Infirmary, Leeds Dental Hospital, Dewsbury Infirmary and St. James's Hospital, Leeds. He also achieved a Diploma in Anaesthetics in 1935.

At the commencement of the Second World War (1939–1945), Sykes immediately volunteered for service in the Royal Army Medical Corps (RAMC). He worked as an anaesthetist under the rank of Major. His troops were captured in Greece, where they became prisoners of war for four and a half years. Undeterred, he continued to practise anaesthesia in very basic and testing conditions and was said to run the hospital and inspire his junior and senior colleagues alike. Upon returning to the United Kingdom, he was appointed Member of the Order of the British Empire (MBE) in recognition of his work during the war.

Sykes gave up administering anaesthesia immediately after the war, following a heated dispute with the hospital authorities. He had threatened to quit unless hospital conditions were improved, particularly relating to hygiene standards. He was well known for his bullish attitude of accepting nothing but the best.

Following this dispute, Sykes returned to work as a general practitioner in Morley. It was in this role that he worked until his retirement in 1959. A year before his death, he started to suffer from ill-health, though nevertheless was reported to have remained cheery and determined. He died suddenly in 1961, leaving behind a widow and stepdaughter.

Sykes enjoyed writing in any free time he had. His first publication, *A Manual of General Medical Practice* (1927), was written to help and advise those contemplating or having recently started working in general practice. It offered an insight into the profession, with varied chapter headings such as 'Starting a practice', 'The diseases of general practice' and 'Strange and unusual symptoms and happenings in practice', to name but a few. A review was published in the 1927 *Canadian Medical Association Journal* stating that 'this manual of practice is filled with instruction in both the art and science of medicine as applied in general practice, and many of the diseases met within general practice are dealt with in a practical way both in diagnosis and treatment'. The review concludes that 'a book of this type should be in the hands of every young student, while any physician may read it with pleasure and profit', indicating its practicality and trans-Atlantic appeal at the time.

However, Sykes' greatest passion was anaesthetics and it is in this field that his publications soared. He contributed an article about ethyl chloride to the thirteenth edition of *Encyclopædia Britannica* (1926), and, in 1931, published his first book about anaesthetics, entitled *Modern Treatment: Anaesthesia*. He then spent the majority of his post-Second World War career investigating the history of anaesthesia. His tenacious approach to research ultimately led to the publication of *Essays on the First Hundred Years of Anaesthesia* (1960), which garnered enormous praise. He explained in the foreword of the book how the death of his father and grandfather during surgery inspired him to write it; in one chapter he asked, 'is there any device in the whole of anaesthesia that has not killed somebody?' The book offered new insights into the historical development of anaesthesia and challenged some widely believed perceptions, including the coining of the word anaesthesia and the date on which chloroform was first used as an anaesthetic. His research proved to be akin to that of a historian, and he used original documentation to present his arguments. Medical historians today continue to use it as a key reference. The second volume was published posthumously in 1962.

Sykes also enjoyed writing fiction as a hobby. He published a series of detective novels, using his medical background for inspiration in the narrative. The best known of these, *The Missing Money Lender*, was first published by John Lane (London) in 1931 before becoming part of the Penguin Book series in 1936. It sold well in the United Kingdom and North America. The story revolves around the mysterious murder of a young Jewish man. Reviews at the time praised its intelligent and gripping plot, though modern commentators heavily criticise certain elements within the book. It has been noted to contain some anti-Semitic undertones in relation to the murder victim. Additionally, one reviewer complained of Sykes and his apparently snobbish attitude towards what he considers to be menial professions. These characters are described in a particularly negative light on numerous occasions. Similar prejudices were not uncommon contemporaneously. Despite some of these comments, Sykes was remembered by friends as a dear and loyal friend. Those who knew him spoke of his quiet disposition and brilliant mind.

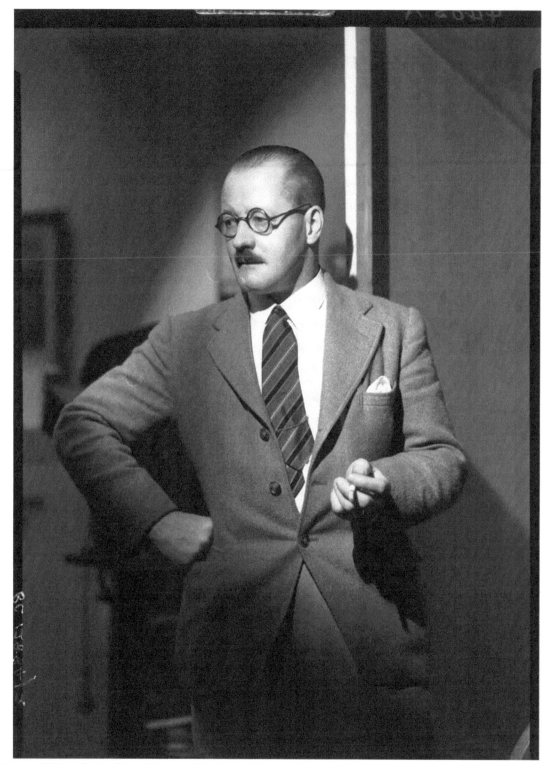

Image of William Stanley Sykes. (Courtesy of the National Portrait Gallery, London.)

Further Reading

Sykes WS. *A Manual of General Medical Practice*. London: Lewis; 1927.

Sykes WS. *The Missing Money Lender*. London: Penguin Books; 1936.

Sykes WS. *Essays on the First Hundred Years of Anaesthesia*. Edinburgh: E. & S. Livingstone Ltd; 1960.

36 SIR ERNEST KAYE LE FLEMING (1872–1946)

Rhea Nicholson

Ernest Kaye Le Fleming was born in July 1872 in Tonbridge, Kent, the fourth of seven children to Reverend John and Harriet Mary Neville. His father was an army tutor, who was known far and wide as 'The Preceptor', with the 1881 census showing that several of his students were living with the Le Flemings in the family home. Reverend Neville's career clearly influenced his sons with Sir Ernest's brothers all going on to have either esteemed military or athletic careers. Sir Ernest, however, seems to have been more influenced by his maternal family; his grandfather, William Henry Neville (LSA 1816), was a surgeon and appointed apothecary extraordinary to Queen Victoria in June 1840.

In regards to his education, Sir Ernest was educated, as were his brothers, at the Tonbridge School from 1885 to 1891. He matriculated on 9 October 1891 at Clare College, University of Cambridge and was awarded BA in 1894. During his time at the University of Cambridge, he competed in the Oxford-Cambridge golf varsity, a sport that he retained a lifelong passion for and was once noted as having said, 'It is wonderful what a game of golf will do to reconcile bitter opponents!' After graduating, he decided upon a life in the medical profession and began his training at St George's Hospital, London, qualifying in 1898. He was awarded MB and Bachelor of Surgery (BChir) at Clare College in 1900 and MA in 1928. In July 1901, he married Florence Murton Beeching (1873–1957), with whom he would have two sons.

Sir Ernest began his medical career as a house surgeon and physician at St George's in 1898, progressing to become an assistant surgical registrar. He was also the editor of the *St George's Hospital Gazette* during his years there. Finding hospital medicine to be lacking something, he moved to Wimborne, Dorset, to set up a general practice and it was here that he found his true passion, being once quoted as saying he was 'constantly refreshed by the bond of sympathy, loyalty and affection that should exist between the doctor and his patient'. When the First World War (1914–1918) broke, he joined the RAMC, where he was given the honorary rank of Lieutenant. He was employed at the Royal Victoria Hospital, Netley, from 1914 to 1919, which treated some 50,000 wounded soldiers during the course of the war. He returned to general practice after the war and continued to have an esteemed and gratifying career as a family practitioner until his death.

Such was his passion for general practice, Sir Ernest published a book entitled *An Introduction to General Practice* in 1936 in which he set forth advice to students. In the book, he revealed a preference for a patient-centred approach to general practice consultations rather than the paternalistic approach to them, stating that in his view 'doctors… often adopt an air of mystery about their art and… treat their patients as if they were little children' and that 'every adult patient will have quite definite ideas of his or her own anatomy… and, absurd and erroneous as these opinions may be, they must be treated with all respect'. He also revealed 'it is unthinkable that lack of means to pay should deprive any individual of his most pressing need in time of sickness', showing his support for a universal free-to-all health care system, years before the formation of the NHS. It was this opinion that led him to become a member of the Ministry of Health Advisory Committee on NHI. *An Introduction to General Practice* was well received and a review in the *BMJ* described it as a 'high level of excellence of a book from which patients as well as doctors will derive lasting benefit'.

Sir Ernest believed that all medical professionals should play an active role in societies to help form lasting relationships with fellow practitioners so to continue learning from each other long after qualifying. He held positions on various committees, advisory panels and councils throughout his life. He was elected the direct representative for England and Wales of the GMC in 1928, 1933, 1938 and also in 1946, the year of his death. His election in 1938 saw him receive the highest number of votes for one candidate.

However, it was Sir Ernest's work within the BMA that had the furthest reach. Locally, he was president of the Dorset and West Hants branch, and Honorary Secretary of the Bournemouth branch. Nationally, he was the chairman of the Representative Body between 1931 and 1934, before becoming the chairman of the Council between 1934 and 1939. In this role he truly excelled, and his qualities of a 'gifted leader' were discovered. He was described in his obituary in the *BMJ* as being a 'master in getting through a long and complicated agenda without any sense of hurry or injustice'; he was able to control both large meetings and intimate gatherings, shape policy and conduct routine business with ease. His interest in preventative medicine and the role lifestyle had upon health led him to be selected to chair the BMA Report of the Committee on Nutrition in 1933, and the Report of the Physical Education Committee in 1936. In time, Sir Ernest would be named vice-chairman of the BMA.

Sir Ernest's role as vice-president of the Medical Officers of Schools Association, and his position as medical officer of Canford School, Wimborne, allowed him to influence the health of the next generation. In a speech at his former school's speech day in 1938, he said he wanted 'to see boys and girls taught in schools, in a clear and simple language, the functions of their own bodies' in order to raise awareness of the differences between the well and unwell state of the body from an early age.

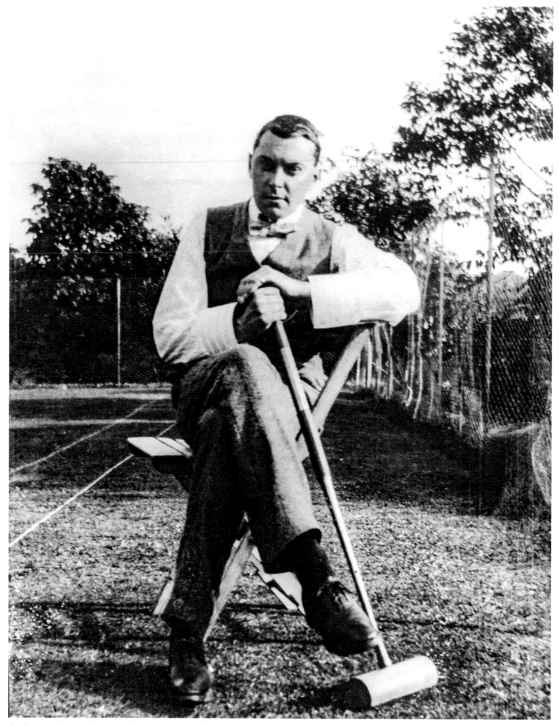

Sir Ernest Kaye Le Fleming. (Courtesy of the Priest's House Museum, Wimborne.)

Such was Sir Ernest's standing, he was awarded numerous awards throughout his career including an honorary MD from both Trinity College, Dublin, in 1932, and the University of Melbourne in 1935. He was honoured with a knighthood in the New Year's Honours list of 1937, one of the few general practitioners compared with their hospital specialists, to receive this distinction at the time. The BMA bestowed the honour of a gold medal on him in 1941, but due to rationing in the Second World War (1939–1945) he never received the medal in person which was instead presented to his widow in 1947.

Sir Ernest suffered from ill health during 1945 but had appeared to make a full recovery. His death on 16 July 1946, aged 72 years old, was sudden and a surprise to all who knew him. His outstanding service to the profession did not go unrecognised and over the following months numerous glittering obituaries were written. The *BMJ* wrote 'his commanding figure and resonant voice were the outward expression of personal qualities above those of the ordinary man'. At the GMC's annual meeting that year the presidential address, from Sir Herbert Eason (1874–1949), praised his 'sound common sense and his peculiar faculty of... putting his finger unerringly on the vital point of discussion'. Sir Henry Souttar (1875–1964), the president of the BMA in the year of his death, said 'contact with him was in itself an education in new fields of medical thought'.

Further Reading

Anon. Obituary: Sir E. Kaye Le Fleming. *British Medical Journal* 1946;2(4464):141–42.

Anon. Obituary: Ernest Kaye Le Fleming. *The Lancet* 1946;248(6413):145.

British Medical Association. Physical Education Committee Report. *British Medical Journal* 1936;1(3928):149–78.

Le Fleming EK. Overcrowding in schools. *British Medical Journal* 1934;2(3860):1204.

Le Fleming EK. *An Introduction to General Practice.* London: E Arnold and Co; 1936.

Le Fleming EK. The threshold of general practice – Sir Kaye Le Fleming's advice to newly qualified practitioners and medical students. *British Medical Journal* 1938;1(4028):141–42.

37 CHARLOTTE NAISH (1908–1959)

Jeannine D. Lemon and Neil Metcalfe

Frances Charlotte Naish was born on 17 January 1908 and was one of eight children. Her father Albert Ernest Naish (1871–1964) was a professor of medicine and her mother Lucy Naish (1876–1967) a lecturer in osteology, both at the University of Sheffield. Her family were distinguished Quakers. She grew up in Sheffield and was educated at Sheffield High School and eventually became head girl at Girton College, University of Cambridge. She was one of the first women to sit on College Council and to have a book published on general practice.

Naish undertook her medical studies at the Royal Free School of Medicine where she won an Owen Roberts scholarship and Grant Medal for surgery. Qualifying in 1933, she was awarded MBBCh in 1936 and MD in 1948. In 1935, she married Paul Weston Edwards, who was later to give her valuable help, including statistical advice, for her research in general practice. After qualifying in 1936, she worked as a house surgeon at the Royal Free Hospital London, then proceeded to house physician at the Devon and East Cornwall Hospital in Plymouth. She returned to the Royal Free Hospital as an obstetric assistant. Throughout this period, she received the Mabel Webb and A.M. Bird postgraduate scholarship. She started her own general practice in Islington in 1936 and was also medical officer at three child welfare centres. It was here where she first developed her passion for infant welfare work. Her efforts were dependent upon personal contact and the continuity with mothers and children all in one service. However, with the outbreak of the Second World War (1939–1945) her general practice and clinics were dispersed. After assistantships in South Wales and Leicestershire she settled in York, soon succeeding to senior partner. Her practice has been reported to have had the first general practice children's clinic. Still deep set on advocating and promoting children's health through her own observations and clinical acuity she became an expert on breastfeeding. As a result, her book entitled *Breast Feeding* won her the Sir Charles Hastings Clinical Prize in 1947. This was the first general practice book written by a woman.

In 1948, Naish started what she called her 'experiment in family practice'. She held weekly clinics for mothers and babies only, encouraging the attendance of babies. Naish was a pioneer in combining preventative and curative medicine, which was then later adopted by many. Throughout her time as a general practitioner, she was continuously publishing her work in a number of journals through which her research and experimental style developed. Her article in *Medical Press*, in 1951, on successful breastfeeding highlighted the undue influence doctors' experiences within their own family affected breast feeding mothers. She suggested that male doctors tend to make sweeping generalised assumptions based on flimsy evidence. For an example, she described men whose children are breastfed with ease tended to attribute breastfeeding difficulty with the mother's psychology. Consequently, it was felt that these male doctors did not supervise the progress of those babies; thus the less fortunate women than the wives of doctor's were left to cope with underfed infants. Naish was one of the very first general practitioners to start taking into consideration the socio-economic factors that affect their patients. She started treating her patients holistically, mother and child as one and their health intertwined.

To encourage preventative medicine and health education in the practice Naish started a mother's club where she and other partners in the surgery gave talks. In addition to this she also held father's clubs which discussed family problems. Through these clinics she was able to conduct numerous experiments using her patients. In 1954, an article was published in *The Lancet*, which detailed the positive results she noted on increasing breast milk production when giving small amounts of iodine to mothers who previously had been producing only small amounts of milk. Iodine is required by the body to make thyroxine in the thyroid gland and if low in amount can be one of the causes of an underactive thyroid condition also called hypothyroidism. Common symptoms of hypothyroidism include, depression, dry skin, loss of hair, tiredness and weight gain. These are symptoms, which Naish noticed in many of her multiparous patients, including herself. During a short space of time she was able to identify groups of women that were suffering from subclinical hypothyroidism, which was impacting on their ability to breastfeed their children. Although her findings were significant, she always highlighted that her results were not statistically valid. As her research and experiments continued, her research style became geared toward randomly controlled trails, which would validate her discoveries.

As a medical officer to a mother and baby home and a member of the local medical committee of city health, hospital management and the chairman of the advisory panel on child health to Leeds Regional Hospital Board, she was able to advocate the needs of mothers and their babies. She was able to incorporate health services by getting health visitors who were funded by the local authority to attend one general clinic that would treat mother and child. Naish had a keen interest in training students in the organisation and scope of good general practice. She recognised the family doctor has a vital part to play and thought, therefore, that undergraduate medical training should become directed more towards preparing students for family practice. As a result, medical students from the University of

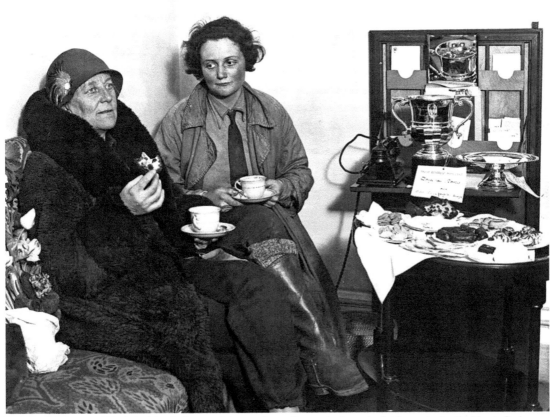

Drs Vaughan (left) and Naish (right) enjoying a well deserved cup of tea and cake at the finish on winning the Monte Carlo Rally Ladies' Cup on 28 January 1932. They won in their Triumph, No 229, despite a prolonged stop whilst treating a Danish competitor seriously injured on the road. (Courtesy of Jean-François Bouzanquet from the Veloce book *Fast Ladies – Female Racing Drivers*, 2009.)

Leeds attended her clinics as part of their paediatric placement. She lectured students, nurses and midwives in medical gatherings. She also had the opportunity to take part in leading child health conferences. She spoke twice at the annual meetings of the BMA where many described her as an excellent speaker who created a lively interest in her subject.

Her achievements led to Naish becoming one of the only two women on the first College Council (1954–1955) and was re-elected in 1959. In 1954, she retired from general practice and begun a new venture in Cumberland with her husband. They opened a special school for disabled children with psychosomatic disorders. Naish was mother, housekeeper and RMO to each of the children. Her understanding and patience brought tremendous improvements and happiness to children whose prognosis was hopeless. Her work filled an obvious need though time dedicated to this role meant that she did not have other time to be able to publish about it.

Away from medicine Naish had a variety of interests. She was a faithful Quaker and spoke at many gatherings of the Society of Friends. She enjoyed motor racing and she was second driver and mechanic to Janet Vaughan (1899–1993), a doctor, when they were the first British women to win the Monte Coupe des Dames. This was in spite of a lengthy stop close to the end of the rally, when they stopped to help another crew. They set a broken leg and gave extensive medical assistance, giving up any chance of a good final time but still hanging on to The Ladies Prize. The following year she herself drove to win a Royal Automobile Club rally. An excellent swimmer, she won the Yorkshire junior championship in her youth. She was an avid walker, sailor and painter. She was a mother to three daughters and two adopted sons whom she looked after often with little help. During the last 10 years of her life she had a number of serious illnesses, from which she rebounded with character and spirit. A year after a pancreatectomy in March 1958, Naish died when 51 years old. She was remembered by many with gratitude for the help she gave them, for her unselfish giving but mainly for her love of all children.

Further Reading

Dyhouse C. Driving ambitions: Women in pursuit of a medical education, 1890–1939. *Women's History Review* 1998;7(3):321–43.

LJL. F. Charlotte Naish. M.D. *British Medical Journal* 1959;1:977–78.

Naish FC. Morbidity and feeding in infancy. *The Lancet* 1949;1(6543):146.

Naish FC. Some everyday problems in infant care in general practice. *Medical Press* 1951;225(14):332–36.

Naish FC. Successful breast-feeding. *British Medical Journal* 1951;1(4707):607–10.

Naish FC. Thyroid for laction. *The Lancet* 1954;267(6847):1077–78.

Naish FC. *Breast Feeding*: A *Guide to the Natural Feeding of Infants*. London: Lloyd-Luke Medical Books; 1956.

38 ETHEL MARY NUCELLA WILLIAMS (1863–1948)

Geraldine M. Hayes

Ethel Mary Nucella Williams was born to Charles and Mary Ketton Williams on 8 July 1863 at Cromer in Norfolk. Williams' father was a country squire and close personal friend of the famous author Lewis Carroll. As a young girl Williams developed a keen interest in gardening, walking and literature and later went on to join Newcastle's Literary and Philosophical Society.

Williams attended Norwich High School and despite women being unable to obtain degrees from the University of Cambridge at the time, she attended lectures at Newnham College between 1882 and 1885, developing an interest in medicine. She studied at the London School of Medicine for Women and was awarded MB in 1891 and MD in 1895. Finding that women were unable to gain clinical training in England, she completed her hospital training in Europe, for the most part in Vienna and Paris but also gaining knowledge of public health methodology in Switzerland and Italy. In 1889, she returned to Cambridge to undertake a diploma in Public Health. In the same year, she signed her name on the Declaration in Favour of Woman's Suffrage organised by the Central Committee of the National Society. Her medical career began shortly after this pivotal moment as a RMO at Clapham Maternity Hospital followed by being medical officer at the Blackfriars Dispensary for Women and Children.

With this new experience Williams left London and became Newcastle's first female doctor. She selected Newcastle as she believed that only cities with a population exceeding 250,000 people would tolerate a female general practitioner. At the time, Newcastle had the fewest doctors per capita of cities in the United Kingdom of this scale. In 1896, she founded a general practitioner practice with her friend Ethel Bentham (1861–1931). A few years later Williams was elected president of the Newcastle Women's Suffrage Society. At this time she was shirked by her male peers and was struggling to prove herself in the wider community with few patients accessing the practice's services.

Williams was the first woman in the North of England to drive a car, gaining her driving licence in 1906. This was highly unusual for the times and what was thought to be even more unusual was the fact that she serviced it herself. Her car is thought to have been fundamental to the suffragist movement. Williams and her colleague Bentham led the Newcastle division of an organisation called the National Union. They worked closely with the local Labour movement despite Williams' largely Liberal views. A British socialist newspaper called *The Labour Leader* stated that the suffragist movement 'was deep reason to be grateful to woman's suffragists for their help in canvassing and lending motor cars'.

The challenges Williams faced in gaining her medical education, coupled with her belief that social reform was integral to improving care, inspired her to become increasingly involved with the suffragist movement over the next few years. The Mud March of February 1907 was the first publicly organised rally by the National Union of Women's Suffrage Societies (NUWSS). Adverse weather conditions on the day, coupled with the police steering the 3000 protesters in their long skirts into gutters, coined the iconic name 'The Mud March'. Williams reported that 'the feeling of the society was entirely for Adult Suffrage' explaining that the Northern branch of NUWSS wanted votes for adult men and women irrespective of property ownership. After this, she frequented many such protests in the local area. In the same year, her concern and involvement with social welfare led her to become the director of research on the commission into the Working of the Poor Law. Over the next three decades, she became more deeply involved in public affairs despite the increasing workload of her practice, which was rapidly gaining respect from the local community. Williams used her status as a general practitioner to influence the city council and imposed upon them a debate over women's suffrage. In 1912, she refused to pay her taxes until the results of the third Conciliation Bill, proposing votes for property-owning women were publicised. On discovering that the Bill had been unsuccessful, Williams continued to withhold her taxes and as a result had goods seized by the government.

With the start of the First World War (1914–1918) Williams' political activity became decidedly more radical. She left the Liberal Party due to their non-acceptance of women's suffrage, working closely with the Independent Labour Party. A firm pacifist, she became involved with the Women's International League for Peace and Freedom, the Women's Executive of the Patriots League of Honour and the Union of Democratic Control. She was deeply involved with the local community in these troubled times, supporting female workers, women and children in detention and lecturing on sex education. She became a tutor for the Workers' Educational Association and established many women's health courses in the North East.

Eight years after the NUWSS organised the Mud March, Williams became chairman of the North Eastern NUWSS. Besides cofounding the Northern Women's Hospital in 1917, she also became secretary of the Newcastle Workers and Soldiers Council. In this role she arranged anti-war events in support of the Russian revolution. Her passion for the women's peace movement continued after the war. In 1919, Williams was a founding member of the British Delegation of the Women's International League for Peace and Freedom. In addition, she played a large role

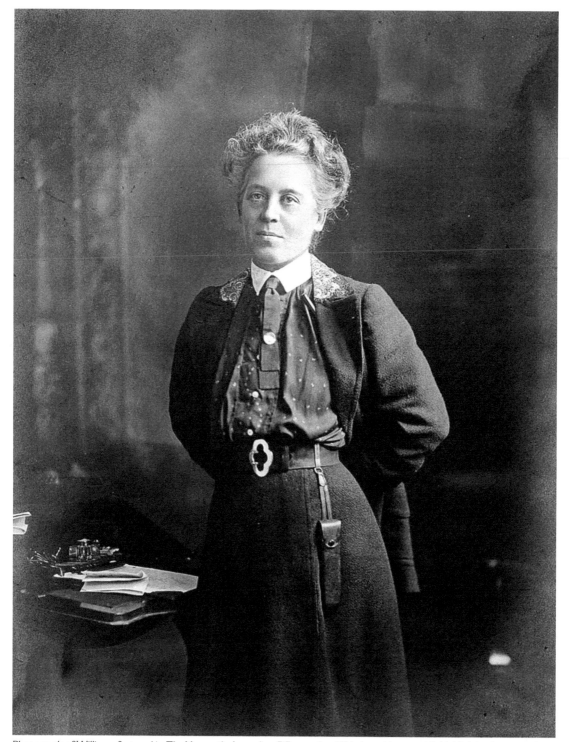

Photograph of Williams featured in *The Newcastle Journal* on 7 September 1914 alongside an article highlighting her contributions to local society and a 'large share of the public life'. (Reproduced with kind permission from Avenue Medical Practice, Jesmond, Newcastle and the Wellcome Library, London.)

in caring for European refugees between the two World Wars and was integral in implementing residential care to improve the quality of the mentally ill.

Williams retired from her work as a general practitioner in 1924 but was still highly involved in education and contributing to the local community. She went on to become a magistrate for Northumberland, was appointed a member of the Senate of Durham University, a Justice of the Peace in 1931 and a member of the University of Newcastle Education Committee. In 1934, Williams became secretary of the Newcastle division of the British Delegation of the Women's International League for Peace. As the Second World War (1939–1945) broke out she relinquished her retirement and left her countryside home to return to Newcastle to aid casualties from the war. As a respected member of the medical community, and an inspiration to female doctors everywhere, she went on to become president of the Federation of Medical Women and Honorary Secretary of the North East Association of Medical Women.

In commemoration of her 'long and valuable public service to her fellow men and women in this district' the local division of the National Council of Women presented Williams' with a portrait of her along with a cheque, which Williams donated the entirety of to the hospital she had founded. On 29 January 1948, Williams died in her home and was laid to rest in Hindley churchyard, Northumberland. In 1950, the University of Newcastle founded the Williams Halls of Residence for the female students in honour of her contributions both to the university and the city.

Williams was a fearless general practitioner, suffragist, pacifist and educator founding her own general practice and hospital despite the constraints women faced in gaining clinical experience at the time. Her focus on the holistic treatment of patients and their social welfare made her an unique clinician. She overcame stereotypes and broke taboos by becoming the first woman to drive a car in the North of England and a lecturer on sex education. As a magistrate, a Justice of the Peace and a member of the Durham University Senate she substantiated women's ability to contribute to society and hence right to vote enabling her to invigorate the suffragist movement.

Further Reading

Crawford E. *The Women's Suffrage Movement: A Reference Guide 1866–1928*. London: Routledge; 2003.

Crawford E. *The Women's Suffrage Movement in Britain and Ireland: A Regional Survey*. London: Routledge; 2013.

Haines CMC. *International Women in Science: A Biographical Dictionary to 1950*. Oxford: ABC-CLIO; 2001.

Law C. *Women: A Modern Political Dictionary*. London: I. B. Tauris; 2000.

39 BARONESS EDITH CLARA SUMMERSKILL (1901–1980)

Clare McGenity and Neil Metcalfe

Edith Clara Summerskill was born 19 April 1901 in London, the youngest child of medical doctor William Summerskill (1866–1947) and his wife Edith Clara Wilde. Baroness Edith was educated at Eltham Hill Grammar School. As a young girl, she accompanied her father to visit patients. This early exposure to illness, suffering and poverty would influence Baroness Edith in later life. Inspired by her father's approach to patients and their hardships, his socialist beliefs and his approval of women's suffrage, Baroness Edith decided to read medicine and attended King's College, University of London and Charing Cross Hospital Medical School from 1918 to 1924.

Baroness Edith graduated from medical school in 1924. At university, she met Edward Jeffrey Samuel (1895–1983) whom she married in August 1925 and they later had two children together, Michael and Shirley. In an unconventional move at the time, she chose to keep her maiden name and to continue her career despite her marriage to Samuel. Working together as general practitioners, the couple formed a medical practice in North London in 1928, where she continued to practise until the latter parts of the Second World War (1939–1945). As a young doctor, she was again exposed to the sufferings and inequalities amongst patients, which strengthened her existing socialist beliefs and directed her career towards politics.

The Socialist Medical Association (SMA, now the Socialist Health Association) was an organisation associated with the Labour Party and founded in 1930. Baroness Edith played a key role in the formation of the SMA and remained a member for many years. By this time a committed socialist and feminist, she also became an early member of the Married Women's Association (established in 1938), which called for an equal relationship between a man and a woman in marriage.

Political movement was the only way that Baroness Edith felt she could make the changes she envisaged to the practice of medicine and public health and thus she pursued a career in politics. She was outspoken in her views of social and political issues relating to women and was quoted on a number of occasions stating 'I am astounded that so many [women] have distinguished themselves despite the conditions which society has imposed on them'. During a Party Political Broadcast on the BBC Home Service on 3 April 1948, which described advantages for voters of the new NHS, she recounted an early experience as a young doctor and reflected, 'It was the suffering of a woman which finally drew me into the political world'. Furthermore, she campaigned for women's birth control, improvements in maternity services, equal rights in marriage and women's rights. She was highly critical of the maternal mortality rates in the United Kingdom and was vocal in identifying negligence from doctors as a cause for many avoidable but fatal infections. Unsuccessful at her first attempts to become an MP in both 1934 and 1935, at a by-election in 1938, she succeeded in becoming an MP for West Fulham. In the 1935 general election, only eight women won parliamentary seats. She was re-elected as MP in 1945, 1950 and 1951 in West Fulham. Following the reorganisation of constituency boundaries she became MP for Warrington between 1955 and 1961. During her time in politics, she supported reforms to laws relating to homosexuality and legalisation of abortions. Her medical background gave her an insight into health risks and gave her direction in many of her campaigns. She fought for a ban on professional boxing due to concerns of associated brain damage and she pushed determinedly for a ban on smoking.

After the start of the Blitz in 1940, Baroness Edith announced in parliament that within the last few weeks 'tremendous change has taken place in the medical service'. She emphasised that the current health service was compromising the treatment and diagnosis of patients and, therefore, proposed that a salaried service would benefit both patients and doctors. She suggested that a state medical service was the best way to achieve this. After the war, the SMA continued to campaign for the introduction of a socialist medical service. At a SMA meeting, Baroness Edith spoke to members, praising the work of the association and the growth of its followers. She reminisced 'half a dozen of us used to sit in a very small room at a time when a socialist doctor was looked upon as an eccentric and an untouchable'. In 1946, the NHS Act created the NHS in England and was implemented by the Minister for Health at the time, Aneurin Bevan.

Baroness Edith joined the National Executive Committee in 1944 and in 1945. She was also made parliamentary secretary for the Ministry of Food. Her role put her in a position of great responsibility for public welfare throughout United Kingdom post-war as food rationing continued after the war. She was most notably involved in the Clean Milk Act 1949, ensuring that contamination of milk by tuberculosis bacilli was avoided. She was made privy councillor in 1949. She briefly held a role as a minister of National Insurance prior to Labour losing the general election in 1951 and she became chair of the Labour Party in 1954.

Fearless in voicing her opinions, Baroness Edith commanded both respect and resentment from colleagues. She had several political enemies including Bevan whom she criticised for taking credit for the creation of the NHS since she felt that those who had worked since the 1930s on a long campaign for a socialist medical service should be

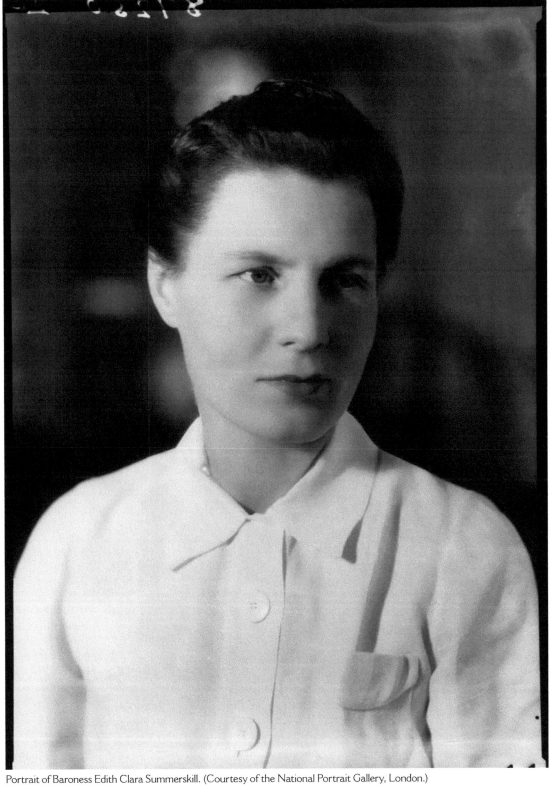

Portrait of Baroness Edith Clara Summerskill. (Courtesy of the National Portrait Gallery, London.)

acknowledged. She later called for his removal from the Labour Party. Some of her colleagues found her fiery character and strong opinions to be overbearing. However, in the context of mid-twentieth-century United Kingdom and as a married woman involved in politics, it is not surprising that she should attract some criticism.

In 1961, she was made a life peeress as Baroness Summerskill of Kenwood and continued her career in the House of Lords. Her long-term campaign for marital gender equality contributed to the Married Women's Property Act of 1964 and the Matrimonial Homes Act of 1967. She was awarded Order of the Companions of Honour (CH) in 1966. She published five books during her lifetime. In 1957, *Letters to My Daughter* was published, a collection of letters written to her daughter Shirley. Shirley followed a similar career path to her mother and became Labour MP for Halifax. Baroness Edith also published *Babies without Tears* (1941), *Wanted – Babies: A Trenchant Examination of a Grave National Problem* (1943) and *The Ignoble Art* (1957). Her last book *A Woman's World: Memoirs* was published in 1967.

Baroness Edith was a general practitioner, politician, socialist and mother. Her passion and determination helped her make a difference to the population throughout the United Kingdom and fuelled her long and successful career. She died suddenly of a heart attack on 4 February 1980, aged 78 years old in her home in Highgate, London. In an obituary in the *BMJ*, she was described by an ex-colleague: 'She was indeed honest, direct, and outspoken… but she was also endlessly compassionate, always ready to champion those in misfortune, especially women and children'.

Further Reading

Merrick J. Vignette: GP and political activist. Baroness Edith Clara Summerskill (1901–1980). *MDDUS Summons* 2014;4:23.

Stewart J. *'The Battle for Health'. A Political History of the Socialist Medical Association. 1930–51*. Hants, UK: Ashgate Publishing; 1999.

Stewart J. Summerskill, Edith Clara, Baroness Summerskill (1901–1980). In: Matthew HCG, Harrison B (eds.). *Oxford Dictionary of National Biography*. Volume 53. Oxford: Oxford University Press; 2004.

Summerskill EC. *Letters to My Daughter*. London: Heinemann; 1957.

Summerskill EC. *A Woman's World*. London: Heinemann; 1967.

40 CHUNI LAL KATIAL (1898–1978)

Camille Gajria

Chuni Lal Katial was born in the Punjab region of India in January 1898. After graduating with honours in medicine and surgery from Lahore University in 1922, he spent five years as a captain with the Indian Medical Service attached to the British Royal Air Force (RAF) in Iraq.

In 1927, Katial moved to the United Kingdom. His first work led to him obtaining the Liverpool diploma in Public Health and Tropical Medicine in the same year as his arrival. The University of Dublin granted him a licence in medicine, enabling him to be a general practitioner. He set up his practice with Satish Chandra Sen (1910–1979) in Canning Town, where the London Docks were situated. In the 1930s, he moved to the practice at 4 Spencer Street in Finsbury in North London, then a densely populated area plagued by endemic disease. He was well known locally, and highly respected by his working-class patients; it was said that at his practice 'the difference between East and West did not exist'.

Katial was a member of Krishna Menon's India League, which campaigned for Indian self-rule. So when Mahatma Gandhi visited England for the Second Round Table conference and stipulated that he wanted to stay 'amongst the poor', Katial assisted him. At the same time, Charlie Chaplin was promoting his latest film in London, and was keen to meet Gandhi due to their shared interests in the struggles of the working classes. Katial arranged the historic meeting at his home in Beckton Road, in Canning Town, on 22 September 1931.

At the BMA Congress in November 1932, Katial heard about plans for a tuberculosis (TB) clinic in East Ham, designed by the architect Berthold Lubetkin. Lubetkin had a reputation for rational responses to social needs. Traditional general practice waiting rooms were generally damp, cold and dark; the proposed building would be well ventilated and able to adapt to medical advances. Although it was never built, it would inspire Katial. At the same time, Harold Riley, an Alderman of Finsbury, had another dream called the 'Finsbury Plan'. This was a comprehensive programme for health and housing that was later abandoned. In 1934, Katial entered public life by election to the Finsbury Borough Council for St. John's ward. He became chair of the Public Health Committee of Finsbury Council in 1935. As a general practitioner, he observed that the average life expectancy for his working-class male patients was under 60 years of age, and noted how health services were haphazard and difficult to access. Building on the Finsbury Plan, he introduced a then new concept of free at the point of access, joined-up health care. He proposed a health centre that would provide a range of facilities including a TB clinic, paediatric services, immunisations and podiatry. There would be dentistry, which was not previously available to most people, and it would be the first to establish a menopause clinic nationally. Case records would be kept in the same building to improve administrative coordination. There were cleaning services in the basement and a lecture theatre.

Katial commissioned Lubetkin to design the Finsbury Health Centre on Pine Street, which opened in October 1938. The reception area was open plan and consulting rooms were all on the ground floor for accessibility. Murals with public health messages decorated the walls. English Heritage described it as 'the finest monument to nascent clinical provision in Great Britain and a brilliant piece of planning; it is very important for its break with the tradition of municipal architecture... It was viewed as the prototype on a national level for modern construction and communal architecture such as NHS clinics'. This radical approach to both health care and architecture predated the 1948 NHS reforms by 10 years.

Meanwhile, Katial had become deputy mayor of Finsbury in 1936 and when he was unanimously elected mayor for the term 1938 to 1939, he became the first mayor of South Asian origin in the United Kingdom. During the Second World War (1939–1945), Katial was a civil defence medical officer, chairman of the air raid precautions medical service and food control committee. He trained St. John Ambulance members in first aid and was a member of the City division medical emergency committee.

After the war, Katial was elected to the London County Council, as one of the two representatives from the Borough of Finsbury. He made a speech when Aneurin Bevan, Minister of Health, laid the foundation stone of the Spa Green housing estate in 1946. He continued medical practice as an examining surgeon for factories in the City of London district. He was later appointed as an executive committee member of the BMA. He also became an FRS of Tropical Medicine. He retired in 1948 and in recognition of his services to health, housing and social welfare, he was the third person to be made a freeman of Finsbury. He asked for the ceremonial casket to be made by local carpenters from wood rather than the customary precious metals.

Katial then travelled to Delhi to become the director-general of the Employees' State Insurance Corporation of India, steering the first statutory social security scheme for workers in India. In the 1970s, he returned to live in London. He died of prostate cancer at Putney Hospital on 14 November 1978.

Inspired by Gandhi's ideal of selfless service, Katial was a pioneer of contemporary public health who had the energy and passion to make things happen.

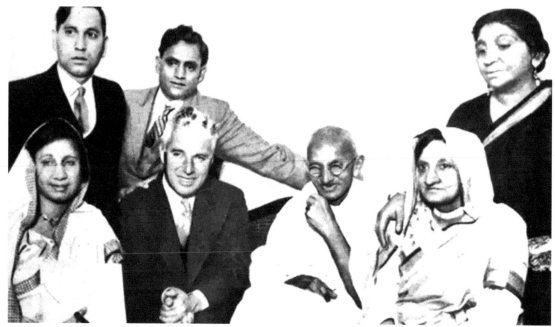

Katial (pictured top left) when hosting Mahatma Gandhi (seated third from right) and Charlie Chaplin (seated fourth from left) at his home in 1931. (Courtesy of Wikimedia Commons.)

Further Reading

Esmail A. Asian doctors in the NHS: Service and betrayal. *British Journal of General Practice* 2007;57(543):827–34.

Gaw A. Vignette: GP and Britain's first Asian mayor Chuni Lal Katial (1898–1978). *MDDUS Summons* 2015;3:23.

Heath I. Observations: Life and Death 'Nothing is too good for ordinary people'. *British Medical Journal* 2009;338:b683.

Historic England. Finsbury Health Centre: List Number: 1297993. *The National Heritage List for England*. London: Historic England; 1972.

Visram R. *Asians in Britain: 400 Years of History*. London: Pluto Press; 2002.

41 ARCHIBALD JOSEPH CRONIN (1896–1981)

Rebecca Jane Helliwell and Neil Metcalfe

Archibald Joseph Cronin, better known as the author A.J. Cronin of *The Citadel* (1937) amongst numerous other pieces of work, was born to Jessie Cronin (née Montgomerie) on 19 July 1896 at Cardross, Dumbartonshire in Scotland. Cronin's father Patrick Cronin worked as a commercial traveller but died when Cronin was seven years old. Jessie moved the family to her parents' home upon the death of her husband and began work as the first female health inspector in Glasgow. Cronin was raised as a Roman Catholic; his mother in particular was of strong faith.

Cronin attended Dumbarton Academy where he obtained a scholarship to study medicine at the University of Glasgow in 1914. His studies were interrupted by the First World War (1914–1918), in which Cronin served in the Royal Navy as a surgeon sublieutenant. He then returned to his studies at Glasgow where he received a commendation prize in clinical surgery amongst other awards. He graduated in 1919 with Bachelor of Medicine, Bachelor of Surgery (MBChB) with honours and he was placed in the top three of his year. He met his future wife Agnes Gibson (1898–1981) at Glasgow Medical School and they later married in 1921.

Once graduated Cronin worked as a general practitioner in South Wales for three years. During this time he was awarded his diploma in Public Health in 1923. From 1924 to 1926, he was appointed medical inspector of the mines for Great Britain. During his time at this post he wrote two reports: the first focused on the effects of dust inhalation, and the second concentrated on delivering first aid in mines. During this time he was awarded MRCP in 1924 and then, in 1925, MD for his thesis titled 'The History of Aneurysm. Being a contribution to the study of the origins, growth and progress of the ideas in medicine' from the University of Glasgow. After two years as a medical inspector, Cronin and Agnes moved to London, where he set up a private practice on Harley Street. Later the two moved the practice to Westbourne Grove in Notting Hill, London.

In 1930, Cronin's medical career came to an abrupt end due to ill health and he moved to the West Highlands in Scotland. With his newfound time he decided to embark on a career in writing, another passion of his. *Hatter's Castle* (1931) was Cronin's first published book and was the first to ever retell the events of the Taybridge disaster on 28 December 1879. The tragedy occurred when the central navigation of the two-mile bridge collapsed, sending a six-carriage train plummeting into the Firth of Tay, causing 75 deaths. The book was later turned into a feature film in 1942.

Cronin went on to write numerous very successful novels. *The Stars Looked Down* (1935) is a novel about a northern mining town, highlighting the poverty and occupational illnesses faced by the nation's mining population, through the eyes of the Fenwick family. *The Citadel* draws inspiration from Cronin's time practising in South Wales and working with the mining industry, and follows the story of a newly qualified doctor starting his career and the obstacles he faced. The novel highlights the gross health inequality across the country and has been reported to have been one of the influences in creating the *Beveridge Report* (1942) and the subsequent creation of the NHS. He described the state of health care pre-1948 as 'guinea-snatching and the bamboozling of patients'.

Many of Cronin's novels were made into Hollywood blockbuster films. This includes *The Stars Looked Down* (1940) starring Michael Redgrave and Margaret Lockwood and *The Keys of the Kingdom* (book published 1941, film premiered 1944) starring Gregory Peck. *The Citadel* (1938) starring Robert Donat and Rosalind Russell, was highly successful and is found in *The New York Times Guide to the Best 1,000 Movies Ever Made* (2004); the film was also nominated for four Oscars, including Best-Adapted Screenplay.

Cronin wrote a series of short stories entitled *Country Doctor*, which gave the inspiration for the BBC's very popular TV series *Dr Finlay's Casebook* (1962–1971). The series focused on a Scottish doctor in the town of Tannochbrae. Later, the stories were created into a BBC Radio 4 show, which received estimated weekly audiences of 12 million.

In 1939, Cronin and his family moved to the United States where he wrote more novels. These proved highly popular and total sales of his books in the United States reached seven million in 1958. In honour of his contribution to literature, he was awarded a Doctor Litterarum (D.Litt) from Bowdoin and Lafayette College in the United States. Cronin continued his life travelling between Switzerland and the United States and died of bronchitis on the 6 January 1981 in Glion, Switzerland.

Despite leaving the profession after a little over 10 years, Cronin influenced medicine in the United Kingdom immensely through his literary work. Drawing from his experience and background allowed him to accurately highlight the struggles miners faced on a daily basis. Similarly, through his work Cronin emphasises the gross health inequality in the United Kingdom in the 1930s prior to the establishment of the NHS in 1948 and his work was one of the many catalysts of this change. The RCGP commemorated the work of Cronin on 27 March 2015 with a plaque placed on 152 Westbourne Grove, West London, the third plaque to be laid by the RCGP.

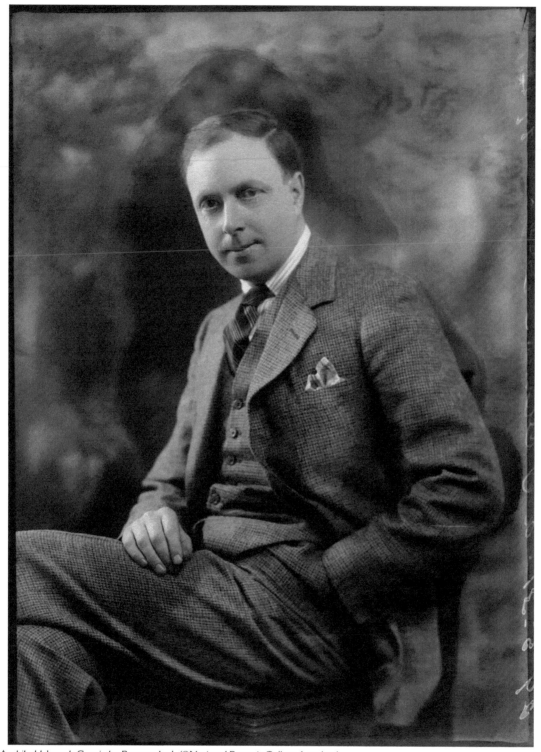

Archibald Joseph Cronin by Bassano Ltd. (©National Portrait Gallery, London.)

In ways that could symbolise his own life, Cronin once stated 'Life is no straight and easy corridor along which we travel free and unhampered, but a maze of passages, through which we must seek our way, lost and confused, now and again checked in a blind alley. But always, if we have faith, a door will open for us, not perhaps one that we ourselves would ever have thought of, but one that will ultimately prove good for us'.

Further Reading

Cronin AJ. *The Citadel*. London: Gollancz; 1937.

Helman C. *Doctors and Patients: An Anthology*. Boca Raton, FL: CRC Press; 2002.

Hodges S. Cronin, Archibald Joseph (1896–1981). In: Matthew HCG, Harrison B (eds.). *Oxford Dictionary of National Biography*. Volume 18. Oxford: Oxford University Press; 2004.

Mahony S. AJ Cronin and The Citadel: Did a work of fiction contribute to the foundation of the NHS? *Journal of the Royal College of Physicians Edinburgh* 2012;42(2):172–78.

42 LOUIS BOYD NEEL (1905–1981)
Daniel James and Neil Metcalfe

Louis Boyd Neel was born into a musical family in Blackheath, South London on 19 July 1905. He was the only child of Louis Anthoine Neel, a paint manufacturer who would later go on to supply water purification equipment to British forces in France and to Buckingham Palace, and Ruby Le Couter, a noted accompanist. His mother would often bring famous musicians of the day back to the family home and the family attended the ballet and the opera together.

In 1918, Neel attended the Royal Naval Academy at Dartmouth to become a naval officer. His maths master at Dartmouth was a music lover and fostered Neel's love of the arts and music but when the 'Geddes axe' saw the armed forces drastically cut in the early 1920s, Neel turned to medicine. He attended Caius College, University of Cambridge, but returned to his native South London for his clinical studies. Neel found time to indulge his love for music by holidaying in the great European cities of culture, particularly spending time in Bavaria where he developed a love of Wagner and saw Mozart's *Così fan tutte* in intimate surroundings in a Munich theatre. He later referred to this experience as formative in his regard for smaller orchestras and his development of the chamber orchestra as a performance genre.

Neel qualified in 1930. He started his medical career as a house physician at St George's Hospital, London, and later worked at King Edward VII's Hospital for Officers near Harley Street. His career would soon take him out of hospital medicine when he became a general practitioner in Elephant and Castle, Southwark. Before it was damaged heavily in the Blitz during the Second World War (1939–1945) this area was thriving and it was for a time considered as 'Piccadilly Circus of South London' with thriving cinemas and nightclubs.

As well as absorbing the local culture and tending to his patients by day and night, Neel continued to devote himself to music and in his spare time studied theory, singing and orchestration at the Guildhall School of Music. He started to gain a reputation as a skilled conductor of amateur orchestras and friends suggested he form his own. The young general practitioner had little money for such an endeavour but inspired by his earlier exposure to baroque and classical music performed on a smaller scale, he formed the first 'modern' chamber orchestra. It has just 17 players, most of whom were recruited by advertising amongst London's music students. He called his group the Boyd Neel London String Orchestra. Professional orchestras at this point usually had up to 100 musicians and a professional ensemble of this scale was virtually unheard of.

The date of the orchestra's first concert, a British premiere of the works of Respighi at the Aeolian Hall, London in June 1933, was set by Neel's day off from surgery, and after the performance he had to rush back for a night on call to deliver a baby. For several years Neel's fame, and that of his orchestra, continued to grow. This part-time general practitioner, part-time conductor continued to straddle the worlds of medicine and music until he turned full-time to the latter when the orchestra was offered its first record deal with Decca Records a few years later. Pieces suitable for such a scale were rarely performed prior to this and Neel uncovered and rediscovered baroque and classical works worthy of his orchestra and also commissioned, championed and popularised new works.

The orchestra's noted releases from this time included the first recording of Vaughan Williams' *Fantasia on a Theme* by Thomas Tallis and Benjamin Britten's *Simple Symphony*. They were the first orchestra to perform in the new Glynebourne opera house and, in 1937, they were invited to the Salzburg Festival where Neel commissioned Britten's *Variations on a Theme of Frank Bridge*. The orchestra toured Europe and came to greater prominence through regular performances on the BBC. In 1939, due to the war Neel return to the Royal Navy as a medical officer where he was thrust by his conscience and the national interest. He still performed when his war work and medical practice allowed and was invited as guest conductor to perform with the Royal Philharmonic and London Symphony orchestras. He also undertook a lecture tour of the Mediterranean and conducted hundreds of concerts for British troops.

After the war, Neel returned to conducting. This was for his own orchestra, the D'Oyly Carte Opera Company and the Sadler's Wells Opera. In 1947, with the Boyd Neel Orchestra, he embarked on a series of world tours playing in Australia, New Zealand, the United States and Canada where, in 1952, he would settle as Dean of the Royal Conservatory of Music in Toronto. He was appointed CBE in 1953. In 1954, Neel founded the Hart House Orchestra, a chamber group similar to his London one. He realised that in Canada there were more trained performers than could be employed, and that a professional orchestra based at the university would stimulate the community. He himself needed active music making. The resulting Hart House Orchestra toured widely over North America and visited the Brussels World Fair in 1958 and Aldeburgh, at Britten's invitation, in 1966. Neel was also in demand as a guest conductor, particularly after he retired in 1971 from his academic post, where his work had substantially raised the prestige of music at the university.

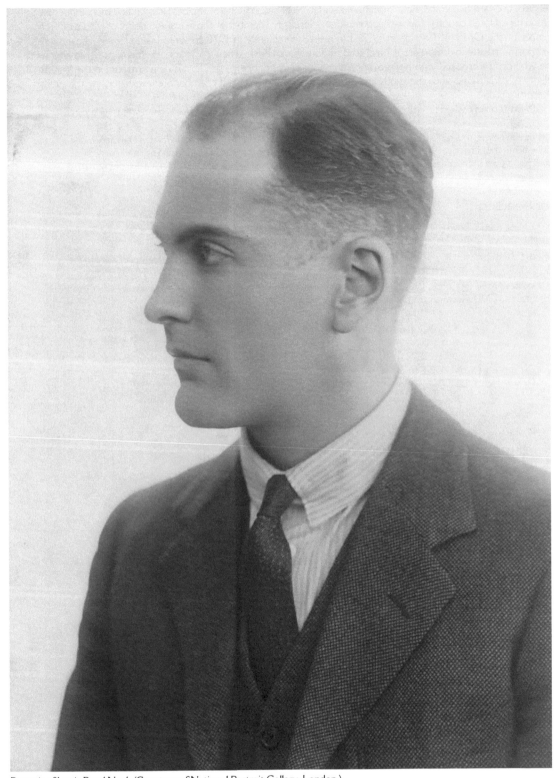

Portrait of Louis Boyd Neel. (Courtesy of National Portrait Gallery, London.)

A relaxed, buoyant figure and a convivial homosexual. Neel became one of the best known and most influential musicians in his adopted country. He was appointed an Honorary Member of the Royal Academy of Music in 1965 and Member of the Order of Canada in 1973. He retired completely in 1978 to write his memoirs. These were published posthumously in 1985 before Neel died in Toronto in 1981, when 76 years old. His legacy remains as someone who can be credited with rediscovering an entire performance genre. This is demonstrated in the growth in popularity of early music since the 1960s and a plethora of small string and chamber orchestras touring the world to great acclaim today.

In 1950, Britten was asked to write an introduction to Neel's book *The Story of an Orchestra*. In it he wrote:

> Let us composers, too, remember what Boyd Neel has done for us. Not only has he asked for and used new music but – here's the difference – he has used it many times. If Boyd Neel and his orchestra like and believe in new music they play it over and over again until the audience gets used to it and begins to like it too; not for it a first performance and then the dusty shelf.

Further Reading

McVeagh D. Neel, (Louis) Boyd (1905–1981). In: Matthew HCG, Harrison B (eds.). *Oxford Dictionary of National Biography*. Volume 40. Oxford: Oxford University Press; 2004.

Neel B, Finch DJ (eds.). *My Orchestras and Other Adventures: The Memories of Boyd Neel*. Toronto: University of Toronto Press; 1985.

Warren CPW. Boyd Neel. In: Cooper DKC (ed.). *Doctors of Another Calling: Physicians Who Are Best Known in Fields Other than Medicine*. Lanham, MD: Rowman and Littlefield; 2013.

13 RAN LAURIE (1915–1998)
Mason McGlynn and Neil Metcalfe

William George Ranald Mundell Laurie was born on 4 June 1915, in Grantchester, Cambridgeshire, to parents Margaret and William Laurie. Of Scottish descent, Laurie, known in his youth as Stan, was educated first at Monkton Combe School, then Selwyn College, University of Cambridge, distinguishing himself early in life as a formidable oarsman. Beginning to row first as a hobby whilst at Monkton, Laurie's rowing abilities quickened whilst at Cambridge. Admitted in 1933 as a science undergraduate, he quickly garnered a reputation as a formidable stroke. This position, the rower at the stern of the boat, bears responsibility for establishing the rate and rhythm for the whole crew. The stroke must strike a delicate balance, pushing the rowers to their very limits, but no further. In setting a demanding pace, it is the stroke who can least afford to tire; the crew is lost without their pacemaker.

In 1934, Laurie delivered one of the strongest performances of his career, stroking the Leander Club to victory in the Grand Challenge Cup at Henley-on-Thames. In doing so, the boat established a record time for the course that would not be broken until 1952. In the same year, he began what would become a three-year streak, rowing in the winning eights against Oxford in the Boat Race. In the boat for the Cambridge Blues with him each and every year was Jack Wilson (1914–1997), lifelong friend, fellow colonial servant and his future Olympic coxless pairs partner. The 1934 crew set a Boat Race record and Laurie, by this time an admirable stroke, occupied this position in the 1935 and 1936 races.

After graduating from Selwyn, Laurie was selected to stroke for the Great Britain team in the Berlin 1936 Olympics. Spectated by Adolf Hitler, the team finished in fourth place. Wilson, who had by this time entered the Political Service in Sudan, was not available to compete; Laurie maintained it was his absence from the crew that had cost Great Britain the gold medal shortly afterwards, Laurie himself joined the government service in Sudan, where he would be stationed until the early 1950s. In 1938, Laurie and Wilson were able to take leave to compete in the Henley Royal Regatta, winning the Silver Goblets for the Leander Club. The advent of the Second World War (1939–1945), however, thwarted the pair's hopes of competing in the Olympics that would have been due for 1940 and 1944, and brought about a lengthy pause to their respective rowing careers.

In 1948, Wilson and Laurie made an anticlimactic post-war return at the Marlow Regatta. This followed a decade in the Sudan, during which time neither had enjoyed much opportunity to row. They struck both banks of the river in the same race. Despite this, the two, now known as 'The Desert Rats', won the Silver Goblets at the Henley Royal Regatta of the same year, just as they had done a decade previously. An easy victory here qualified them for the Olympic squad for the London 1948 Games, the two given to compete only a month later.

Trained at the Leander Club by 1908 silver medalist Alexander McCulloch (1887–1951), and drawing upon much needed extra rations, the pair secured a narrow victory over the Italian boat in the semi-final, progressing to the three-lane final at the familiar Henley-on-Thames course. The two secured gold following a difficult race against the Swiss and Italian pairs; Laurie described it as 'the best row we ever had'. Not only had he just won Olympic gold but his wife, Patricia Laidlaw, whom he had met in Sudan and married in 1944, had also just given birth to their second daughter. In 1951, he was elected a Steward of the Henley Royal Regatta, and he would continue to periodically umpire at Henley for much of the rest of his life. Concluding his colonial service, having risen to the appointment of District Commissioner of Nyala, Laurie eventually returned to the United Kingdom, and in a surprising about-face, applied to medical school at the age of 40 years old.

Despite the incumbent responsibilities of a young family, Laurie qualified as a doctor in 1954. He then worked as a general practitioner in Blackbird Leys, Oxford, for the next 30 years of his life. In this time he served as chairman of the Oxford Duke of Edinburgh's awards committee from 1959 to 1969, and at Save the Children between 1986 and 1989. Laurie continued to remain active at Henley; in addition to umpiring, he sat on the course's management committee between 1975 and 1986. Despite his best efforts in nursing her, Patricia passed away in 1989, having suffered from motor neurone disease. The two, both members of the Presbyterian Church, raised four children in all. In 1990, Laurie married Mary Arbuthnot in Norfolk, where he would remain for the rest of his life, enjoying gardening. On 19 September 1998, Laurie passed away at his home, Hethersett Hall, in Norfolk, having suffered from Parkinson's disease.

Laurie is remembered not only as half of the finest British rowing pair of the generation but as a skilled and firmly principled physician, who was self-effacing to a fault. His son Hugh, an actor, comedian and writer, recalled finding himself in a boat with his father when he was 12 years old, and with his father having taken the oars, nervously wondering whether he knew how to row. On another occasion, the young Hugh was shocked to discover his father's Olympic gold medal when exploring the attic, secreted in a sock. Rowing, it seems, is in the Lauries' blood. Hugh rowed for Selwyn College as a Blue himself in 1980, and Laurie's brother Alan rowed for the Cambridge Blues during the war and served as President of the University of Cambridge Boat Club. Nonetheless it is Laurie, who was described

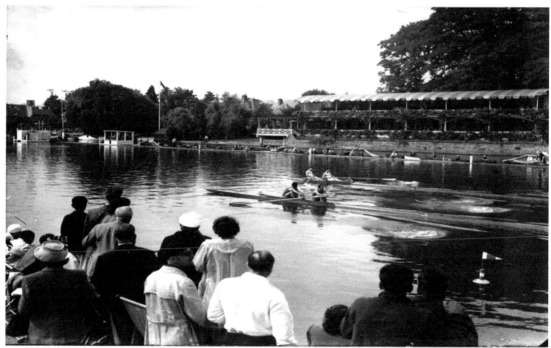

Ran Laurie (seated at the back of the boat at top of picture) with Jack Wilson at the London 1948 Olympic Regatta. (Courtesy of River & Rowing Museum, Henley-on-Thames.)

by A.P. McEldowney, chronicler of Selwyn rowing, as 'not only the most famous oarsmen Selwyn ever had, but also one of the most famous Great Britain ever had'. For this reason, the boat in which Laurie and Wilson secured Olympic gold is on display at the River and Rowing Museum at Henley, a place beholden to Laurie throughout most of his life.

Further Reading

Beasley I. *Before the Wind Changed: People, Places and Education in the Sudan*. Oxford: British Academy/Oxford University Press; 1992.

Brown DJ. *The Boys in the Boat*. London: Penguin Books; 2014.

Dodd C. Laurie, William George Ranald Laurie (1915–1998). In: Matthew HCG, Harrison B (eds.). *Oxford Dictionary of National Biography*. Volume 32. Oxford: Oxford University Press; 2004.

PART 3: CONTRIBUTIONS FROM GENERAL PRACTITIONERS 1950–1967

The Collings Report in 1950 had highlighted that general practice needed to change. The average general practitioner had qualified with MRCS LRCP though this was the lowest ranking qualification of each college that awarded them and the general practitioners had no voting rights.[1] Postgraduate study was lacking as general practice was seen by many to be a small branch of medicine, without its own academic requirements or need to develop further. Similarly, it had no footing in the undergraduate curriculum. Spurts of research and literature activity were not organised collectively and were mainly individually based rather than from research groups. A huge social change had occurred with the formation of the NHS; although the BMA could claim it represented general practitioners, from 1832 there was no representative body speaking for general practitioners academically when such change was occurring. It was over 100 years since attempts at forming a college had been made. This section looks at the development of the College and its early contributors as well as that of others, to the medical landscape for general practitioners from 1950 to 1967 to help transform the field into a respected academic discipline.

The Formation of the College

A number of private meetings and letters helped create a steering committee to try and form a college. John Hunt, later Lord Hunt of Fawley, had been appointed a member of the Committee on General Practice of the RCP on 26 April 1951.[2] He was a private general practitioner working in London. He had mentioned the possibility of forming a college at this committee but his suggestion was neither well supported nor minuted.[2] A letter to the *BMJ* in June 1951 suggesting the same from George MacFeat (1872–1960), a general practitioner from Douglas in Lanarkshire, led to private correspondence amongst a number of doctors that ultimately led to Hunt being invited to submit a memorandum to the General Practice Review Committee of the General Medical Services Committee (GMSC) of the BMA.[2] Around the same time, Fraser Rose, a general practitioner from Preston who had various roles within the BMA, had previously approached the chairman of that same committee about a possible college and he was also invited to submit a memorandum, which he did dated 23 June 1951. Hunt telephoned Rose the day before the meeting of 3 October 1951, the date when they first met each other.[2] Following discussions at the meeting about the two memoranda, Hunt and Rose signed the letter that was sent to both the *BMJ* and *The Lancet* and published on 13 October 1951 (see Figure S3.1).[2] Favourable support came from the BMA and the Worshipful Society of Apothecaries, the latter offering their Great Hall for meetings, and led to a steering committee of 16 members, including five specialists sympathetic to the College being created.[3] They were chaired by the Right Honorable Henry Willink, Q.C. who had been a minister of health between 1943 and 1945.

The steering committee achieved their objective of forming the College. It met eight times and at the final meeting on 19 November 1952 its report was signed, the College was legally constituted, a Foundation Council formed and the report was published in the *BMJ* on 20 December 1952.[2] In the report it was mentioned: 'there is taking place now a world-wide reorientation of ideas about his [a general practitioner] capabilities and correct responsibilities with a steadily growing conviction that general practice is fundamentally as important as the specialities'.[3] Amongst the 23 Council members (see Figure S3.2) was George Abercrombie, who was selected chairman, Rose as vice-chairman and Hunt as secretary. Within three weeks, over 1000 general practitioners had joined the College and over 2000 within six months.[3,4] It was this Foundation Council that created regional faculties to ensure that all views and interests of general practitioners in the United Kingdom and Eire were to be included as well as to organise the finance and general purposes, undergraduate, postgraduate and research committees. These sections were to prepare a report, drafted as a constitution that was presented at the first annual general meeting of the College in 14 November 1953.[1] In the report the Foundation Council mentioned that 'A golden opportunity now presents itself for general practitioners to found an organisation of their own, to watch over their academic interests and their education'. The Foundation Council retired and was elected as the first College Council, with William Pickles elected as its first president (1953–1956).

Research and Academia by General Practitioners

The creation of the College gave fresh impetus to general practice research. Robin Pinsent had served as a member of the steering committee and he was the first chair of the research committee from 1953 to 1964. Within the first year of the committee being formed over 300 member names had been added to the research register, which generated a number of collaborative research projects. Robin Pinsent became research advisor to the College, helping many

College of General Practice

SIR,—There is a College of Physicians, a College of Surgeons, a College of Obstetricians and Gynaecologists, a College of Nursing, a College of Midwives, and a College of Veterinary Surgeons, all of them Royal Colleges; there is a College of Speech Therapists and a College of Physical Education, but there is no college or academic body to represent primarily the interests of the largest group of medical personnel in this country—the 20,000 general practitioners. Many practitioners sadly felt the lack of such a body when negotiations about the National Health Service were taking place.

Preliminary discussions are now being held in the General Practice Review Committee of the British Medical Association about the possible development of such a College of General Practice, to help practitioners in the same ways that the Royal Colleges have helped their own Fellows. Such a proposal must not interfere at all with the present qualifying examinations or with the many other activities of the Royal Colleges. It should be able to help practitioners in a great many ways—by supervising their education and postgraduate work, by improving the standard and status of general practice, and by acting as a repository for its traditions—all at little or no cost to the taxpayer.

We are anxious to collect evidence upon this subject of a possible College of General Practice. If any of your readers have suggestions or comments to make, for or against this proposal, will they please communicate with us?—We are, etc.,

F. M. ROSE,
99, Fylde Road, Preston, Lancs.
J. H. HUNT,
54, Sloane Street, London, S.W.1

Figure S3.1 Letter by Fraser Rose and John Hunt published in October 1951 explaining the plan to start the College. (Courtesy of RCGP Archives, London.)

Figure S3.2 The first meeting of College Council. (Courtesy of RCGP Archives, London.)

researchers over the years but also helping establish local research committees. Over the years these were formed at Birmingham, Dundee, Guildford, Leigh, Manchester and Swansea with the most significant one from this period being the one Pinsent founded in Birmingham with its first Director, Donald Crombie, in 1957. This was initially called the Statistics and Records Unit when formed in 1957, although it became a unit of the College in 1961 and is now known as the RCGP Research and Surveillance Centre. The aim of this unit was to establish and develop a recording system for epidemiological research in general practice. Importantly, it led to general practitioners being able to analyse and use information within their own practices. They publicised the use of the age-sex register[5] and later disease registers.[6,7] Furthermore, it has been involved with the national morbidity surveys, the first of which was being discussed in the research committee as early as 1953.[1] The surveys were then linked with the Birmingham Research Unit, the Registrar General and the Ministry of Health and are now in partnership with the Office of Population Censuses and Surveys and the Department of Health.[4]

A further local unit of note was the Epidemic Observation Unit founded by Ian Watson in 1953. This unit aimed to collate, analyse and led groups of general practitioners who reported syndromes and shared information, mainly about infectious diseases. It was based at Peaslake, Surrey. Watson himself exemplified the new aims of research at the College when at the first meeting of the research committee in Bath in 1953, he suggested researching whether the relatively new medication penicillin would be of use in treating measles that was prevalent at the time.[8] Three years later, the study showed that it did not and hence new collective studies had definitely started.[8] The same unit later made important contributions to understanding respiratory tract diseases.[9]

Single, valuable general practitioner based research still continued and two names particularly feature in this regard. The first was John Fry, who undertook meticulous descriptions of common diseases by recording their content, natural history and outcome seen in every patient from his own practice in Beckenham, Kent. Much of his interest was on childhood illnesses as well as both cardiovascular and respiratory diseases. The other was Robert Hope-Simpson, who moved to Cirencester, Gloucestershire, after the Second World War (1939–1945) to set up practice there. He turned his practice into the Cirencester Research Unit with funds provided by the Public Health Laboratory Service between 1947 and 1973 and then until 1981 by the Department of Health and Social Security. He researched and published particularly on infectious diseases such as herpes zoster and chickenpox. His main important discovery was proving that shingles and chickenpox were caused by the same virus,[10] with his theory initially being aided by studying the isolated community of Yell, one of the north isles of Shetland, Scotland.

Recognition of general practice becoming a discipline was seen with the career of Richard Scott at the University of Edinburgh. Both Scott and the university provided principal dates in the history of general practice, particularly within the undergraduate setting. Firstly, this was because it was Scott who provided the first funded courses of teaching from general practice. He did this with the help of a medical assistant, an almoner, a nurse and a dentist when setting up a NHS practice within the Royal Public Dispensary in West Richmond Street, in July 1948.[11] Within three years, 30 medical students were being provided with three-month courses from this community setting. Then, in 1952, the Rockefeller Foundation offered financial support to further aid the development of general practice as an academic discipline in Edinburgh.[11] Following a merger, by 1956 Scott's dispensary had developed into a department of general practice. In 1963, the University of Edinburgh established a chair in general practice. Considering that the creation and appointment of a chair is the highest ranking academic position at a university, the appointment of Scott to the first chair of general practice anywhere in the world provided the high-ranking academic recognition needed by general practice as a speciality from an external body.[1]

General Practice Literature on the Rise

Born out of the College Research Committee ultimately came the world's first internationally recognised scientific journal of general practice. Pinsent and his colleagues in the research committee soon realised that they needed to communicate with other general practitioners and to 'encourage the publication by general medical practitioners of original work on medical and scientific subjects connected with general practice'.[2] Consequently, a newsletter entitled *Between Ourselves* was first published in September 1953. The three foolscap sheets of duplicated typescript was sent to members of the research register and after three further editions Richard McConaghey, a Foundation Council member, was invited to take over from Pinsent.[1] This he did in 1954. The name of the publication changed to *Research Newsletter* in 1955, ultimately being sent to all members of the College. In 1957, John Burdon, who subsequently edited many issues of the College's *Annual Report* as well as doing much to help in the formation of the MRCGP, joined as assistant editor and a year later its name changed again to the *Journal of the College of General Practitioners* (*Journal*). These early years required time and patience for quality general practice research was still in its infancy in quality and quantity. McConaghey often spent hours rewriting papers and providing references himself to help raise the standard as much as possible.[1] He was later vindicated when, in 1961, the *Journal* was the first general practice journal to be indexed in the *Index medicus*, the hallmark of acceptance of a scientific journal.[1,12,13] This was just seven years into his eventual 17 years of editorship.

Numerous books appeared in this time period. Arthur Watts, who had an active interest in psychiatry, published his first book *Psychiatry in General Practice* in 1952.[14] Pinsent, again, contributed with his *Approach to General Practice* (1953),[15] a book that helped to describe good general practice at the time. The most prolific writer was probably the aforementioned Fry, whose *The Catarrhal Child* (1961)[16] was not only the first clinical book about general practitioner patients but also the first of his over 50 book career. Much of his writing challenged the view of specialists and helped promote the acceptance of a generalist's view. Keith Hodgkin provided the first book to define the presentation of common conditions in general practice, called *Towards Earlier Diagnosis* (1963),[17] which highlighted how hospital-based training ill-equipped many to the actual pathologies seen in general practice. This was similarly discussed in David Morrell's *The Art of General Practice*[18] in 1967, which was the same year that Abercrombie, together with McConaghey, published in eight volumes *The Encyclopaedia of General Practice*,[19] the first comprehensive textbook of general practice.

General Practitioners Involved in Major Medical Politics between 1950 and 1967

There was gloom surrounding general practice at this time for which a lack of financial reward was an important cause. Some initial improvement came about from the work of Solomon Wand, a general practitioner who had initially opposed the NHS's '100% free principle'. Whilst he was BMA chairman (1948–1952) and with the help of others he negotiated remuneration of general practitioners. The BMA and the government reached deadlock over pay but after going to independent arbitration it was decided that because of the altered value of money and changed earnings of professionals from 1939 to that after the Second World War a 'betterment' earnings of 100 per cent would be awarded to general practitioners. This doubling of income was known as the Danckwerts Award and started in 1952.

However, the 1950s and 1960s continued to see low morale within the general practice workforce. General practitioners felt they were second-class citizens and undervalued. Furthermore, finances were not provided for administrative support. In addition, general practitioners were rewarded under a 'pool' system of pay and expenses that penalised those who provided good services to their patients and rewarded those who had large lists of patients, often more than 3000 patients per general practitioner. Many general practitioners emigrated. The work of Annis Gillie did much to alter things. During a distinguished career she was appointed, between 1961 and 1963, as chairwoman of a sub-committee set up by the Standing Medical Advisory Committee of the Central Health Services Council to advise on the future field of work of the general practitioner.[20] During her time on the committee *The Porritt Report* (1962) had been released by the Medical Services Review Committee and was an early review of the new NHS; Burdon had been one of its members.[21] *The Porritt Report* criticised the separation of NHS services into hospital, general practices and local authorities and called for them to be reorganised.[21] *The Gillie Report*, formally known as *The Field of Work of the Family Doctor* (1963),[20] however, concluded against the *Porritt Report* by suggesting it was not necessary to unify the NHS, something of a relief to Ministry of Health Officials at the time.

The work of Gillie and others helped stabilise general practice and made it a wanted career choice. Considering that in 1964, over 18,000 general practitioners had signed undated resignation letters from the NHS, *The Gillie Report*, by profoundly influencing the Family Doctor's Charter, agreed between the BMA and the Minister of Health in 1964, helped reduce this eventuality. James Cameron, chairman of the GMSC (1964–1974) and later chairman of BMA Council (1976–1979) oversaw the negotiations of this contract that did much to improve morale in general practice. This contract provided a basic practice allowance, new allowances for support staff, improvement grants, generous loans for group practice premises and a pay rise. Importantly, *The Gillie Report* also stressed the value of training and education at all stages and the need for a formal, structured postgraduate training pathway for general practice trainees, something that, as discussed in the next part of the book, later became a reality. This time saw tense battles between the government, BMA and the College regarding policies and the future of general practice. Other selected general practitioners who held high-ranking positions and are mentioned in this section also include Ian Grant, who was the second president of the College (1956–1959) as well as vice-chairman of the BMA (1958–1961), and Ronald Gibson who was appointed chair of BMA Council (1966–1971).

Societal Approval of General Practice

This time period does not include general practitioners famed for contributions to society. Of course some contributions from names mentioned previously and in other parts of the book had part of their careers overlap with this time period but instead this time period witnessed when the recognition of general practice being an independent scholarly discipline occurred. The other medical colleges had all received their Royal Charters previously but to get parity from an acceptance point of view with these colleges a defining year was 1967. This was the year that the College was given the prefix 'Royal'. It was presented with its Royal Charter in 1972 when HRH Prince Philip, Duke of Edinburgh was appointed an Honorary Fellow and became President of the College. Since relinquishing the post, he has been the College's patron. Later HRH Prince Charles, the Prince of Wales was Honorary President of the RCGP in 1992.

References

1. Pereira Gray D. The emergence of the discipline of general practice, its literature, and the contribution of the College *Journal*. *The Journal of the Royal College of General Practitioners* 1989;39:228–33.

2. Fry J, Hunt Lord of Fawley, Pinsent RJF (eds.). *A History of the Royal College of General Practitioners: The First 25 Years*. Lancaster: MTP Press; 1983.

3. College of General Practitioners. *First Annual Report 1953*. London: College of General Practitioners; 1953.

4. Pereira Gray D. History of the Royal College of General Practitioners: The first 40 years. *British Journal of General Practice* 1992;42:29–35.

5. Pinsent RFJH. The evolving age-sex register. *The Journal of the Royal College of General Practitioners* 1968;16:127–34.

6. Birmingham Research Unit. Practice activity analysis: Punctuality of appointments. *The Journal of the Royal College of General Practitioners* 1977;27:634–35.

7. Crombie DL, Fleming DM. *Practice Activity Analysis*. Occasional paper 41. London: Royal College of General Practitioners; 1988.

8. College of General Practitioners, Study Group. The complications of measles. *Research Newsletter* 1956;4:51–68.

9. Watson GI. *Epidemiology and Research in a General Practice*. London: Royal College of General Practitioners; 1982.

10. Hope-Simpson RE. The nature of herpes zoster: A long-term study and a new hypothesis. *Proceedings of the Royal Society of Medicine* 1965;58(1):9–20.

11. Howie J, Weller D. The University of Edinburgh. In: Howie J, Whitfield M (eds.). *Academic General Practice in the UK Medical Schools 1948–2000: A Short History*. Edinburgh: Edinburgh University Press; 2011.

12. Anon. Mac. *The Journal of the Royal College of General Practitioners* 1975;25:627–29.

13. Jones R, Pereira Gray D, Barley S, Buckley G, Wright AF, Jewell D. Fifty years of the Journal. *British Journal of General Practice* 2010;60(581):934–37.

14. Watts CAH, Watts BM. *Psychiatry in General Practice*. London: J & A Churchill Ltd; 1952.

15. Pinsent RJFH. *An Approach to General Practice*. Edinburgh: E. & S. Livingstone; 1953.

16. Fry J. *The Catarrhal Child*. London: Butterworth; 1961.

17. Hodgkin K. *Towards Earlier Diagnosis: A Family Doctors Approach*. London: E & S Livingstone Ltd; 1963.

18. Morrell D. *The Art of General Practice*. London: Faber; 1967.

19. Abercrombie GF, McConaghey RMS (eds.). *The Encyclopaedia of General Practice*. London: Butterworth; 1963–67.

20. Central Health Services Council, Standing Medical Advisory Committee (Chmn. Gillie AC). *The Field of Work of the Family Doctor: Report of the Sub-Committee*. London: HMSO; 1963.

21. Medical Services Review Committee (Chmn. Porritt A). *A Review of the Medical Services in Great Britain*. London: Social Assay; 1962.

44 LORD JOHN HENDERSON HUNT (1905–1987)

Olivia Macnamara

John Henderson Hunt was born in Secunderabad, India, on 3 July 1905, to Edmund Henderson Hunt (1874–1952), a surgeon and chief medical officer of the Railway Hospital in Secunderabad, and Laura Mary Hunt, the daughter of a tea plantation owner. At an early age, Lord Hunt moved to England with his mother whilst his father remained in India. During his early childhood, he was exposed to the medical world not only through the work of his father but also through his own experiences. Following his move to England he fell ill with diphtheria, requiring him to have his tonsils removed. This was a procedure which contemporaneously was carried out by painting the tonsils with cocaine and the using a tonsil guillotine. Lord Hunt reportedly said that he thought 'it must have been the last time the procedure was ever performed in Great Britain'.

After attending Charterhouse School, Lord Hunt received the scholarship to attend Balliol College, University of Oxford in 1923. His academic excellence did not go unnoted; Lord Hunt was awarded the Theodore Williams Scholarship in Physiology in 1926 and he graduated with a 2:1 with honours in Physiology in 1927. He completed his medical training at St Bartholomew's Hospital Medical School and qualified in 1931. It was here that he undertook his first post as a house surgeon.

Lord Hunt's career quickly advanced. In 1934, he was awarded a doctorate from the University of Oxford for his work on Raynaud's syndrome. During the same year he was awarded MRCP. He had intended to work primarily in neurology and general medicine and his prior success had prepared him well for a consultant role. However, after attaining a job as the chief assistant to the Consultative Neurological Clinic at St Bartholomew's Hospital in 1935, he became disillusioned at this time he felt that the treatment options in Neurology were limited. A colleague of Lord Hunt, John Horder (1919–2012), wrote that 'Diagnosis fascinated him, but it was not enough. In the then neurology of 1935, effective treatments were few'.

In 1937, Lord Hunt made the decision to enter general practice, joining George Cregan as a partner in his practice at 83 Sloane Street, London. Horder wrote that this decision to become a general practitioner had been considered by Lord Hunt's other colleagues to be 'professional suicide'. At this time there were many differences between the pay and status of hospital specialitities and general practitioners.

Second World War (1939–1945), Lord Hunt served as a neurologist with the rank of Wing Commander in the RAF from 1940 to 1945. When the NHS was formed in 1948, he made the decision not to enter it but to set up his own practice, also on Sloane Street. This private practice had its own laboratory and radiography facilities on site, allowing him to provide a high level of care. The excellence of the services he provided, in addition to the dedicated and wealthy clientele he had established during his time in general practice, meant that his practice thrived.

Despite not joining the NHS, Lord Hunt became increasingly aware of the uncertain position of general practitioners in the early stages of its organisation. A report published in 1950 by Joseph Collins (1918–1971) in *The Lancet* detailed the limitations of the early NHS which summarised it as having overworked and demoralised doctors providing low standards of patient care. Seeing the discrepancy between the care described in this report and that provided in his own practice convinced Lord Hunt of the need for an academic body to represent and support general practitioners, as well as to standardise education and postgraduate training, ultimately improving patient care.

Lord Hunt was not alone in this view. Fraser Rose (1897–1972), a general practitioner from Preston, had previously approached the chairman of the GMSC regarding a possible college. Both Rose and Lord Hunt had been invited to each submit a memorandum to the Review Committee. Seeing Rose as a potential supporter of a new college, Lord Hunt spoke to Rose for the first time by telephone on 2 October 1951. The very next day, during the General Practice Review Committee meeting, Rose co-signed letters drafted by Lord Hunt proposing a new college for general practitioners, which were delivered to the *BMJ* and *The Lancet* the same day. In the letter they wrote:

> There is a College of Physicians, a College of Surgeons, a College of Obstetricians and Gynaecologists, a College of Nursing, a College of Midwives, and a College of Veterinary Surgeons… but there is no College or academic body to represent primarily the interests of the largest group of medical personnel in this country – the 20,000 General Practitioners.

These letters provoked a strong response, with vocal responses of both support and opposition. Some members of the RCP and RCS feared that by fragmenting the members of the Royal Colleges, their power and influence would be diluted.

However, Lord Hunt persevered, gathering a group of influential figures to form a committee investigating the aims and requirements of the proposed college. This steering committee, with George Abercrombie (1896–1978) as chairman, Rose as vice-chairman and Lord Hunt as secretary, prevailed and on the 19 November 1952 the College was formed.

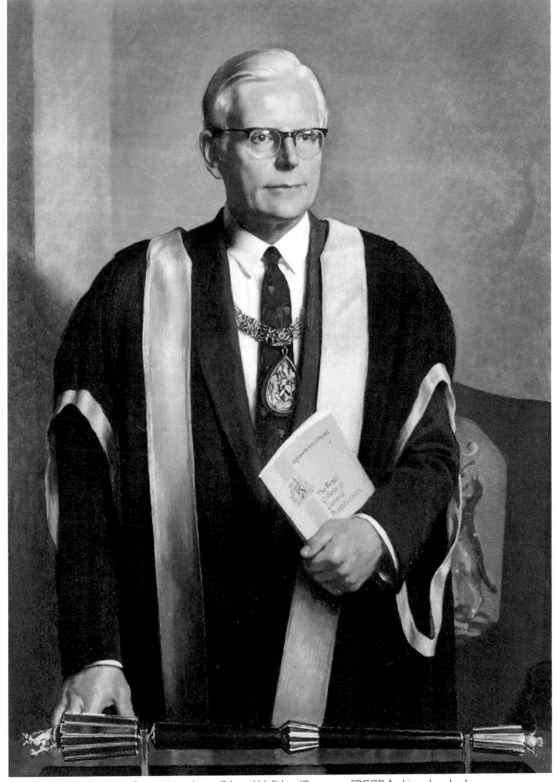

RCGP presidential portrait of Lord Hunt. Artist: Edward Halliday. (Courtesy of RCGP Archives, London.)

In January 1953 and for the first time a foundation membership was offered to general practitioners who met designated criteria. Within six months, 2000 doctors had joined and this number steadily increased. Lord Hunt served as the first Honorary Secretary of College Council until 1967, the year that the College was granted the 'Royal' prefix. Lord Hunt's key role in the formation of the College did not go unnoticed. In the first annual report it was stated that *'the measure of success so far achieved by the College would not have been possible without [John Hunt]'* .

Unsurprisingly, Lord Hunt received multiple national and international honours. He was president of the following: the Hunterian Society (1953), the General Practice Section of the Royal Society of Medicine (1956), the Medical Society of London (1964–1965), the RCGP (1967–1970), the Harveian Society (1970) the Chelsea Clinical Society (1971) and the Society of Chiropodists (1974). He was a consultant in general practice to the RAF. He was awarded FRCP (1964) and FRCS (1966) as well as honorary fellowships of the American Academy of Family Physicians and the Royal Australian College of General Practitioners. He was made an Honorary Member of the College of Family Physicians of Canada, which also awarded him the Victor Johnston Medal. He received the Baron Dr Ver Heyden de Lancey memorial Award in 1978 and was made a gold medallist and Fellow of the BMA in 1980. He gave the Lloyd Roberts Lecture (1956), the 19th James Mackenzie Lecture on 'The foundation of a college' (1972), the Albert Wander Lecture (1968) and the Paul Hopkins Oration (1969).

Lord Hunt was appointed CBE in 1970 and was made a life peer in 1973. He became Lord Hunt of Fawley but also became the first general practitioner to be honoured in this way. In this latter capacity he frequently attended debates and took his parliamentary duties seriously. He spoke effectively on several different issues and made a particularly notable contribution to the debate on the 1978 Medical Act which materially revised the status of the GMC.

He wrote on various subjects. This included peripheral vascular disease, accident prevention and early diagnosis. With his detailed knowledge of the creation of the College he provided valuable contributions as co-editor of *A History of the College of General Practitioners: The First 25 Years* (1983).

During his life, Lord Hunt was supported by his wife Elisabeth (née Evill), whom he married in 1941. They had five children: two daughters and three sons of which two sons became general practitioners. He was a big man who, in spite of a hip problem, walked prodigiously, including on one occasion from Lands End to John o'Groats. He played tennis and croquet at his country house near Henley-on-Thames. He suffered from poor eyesight throughout his life and lost the sight in one eye in 1967, which greatly taxed his patience and that of his family. He later suffered from Parkinson's disease and died on 28 December 1987 at his home, Seven Steep, in Fawley, Buckinghamshire.

In his James Mackenzie Lecture, Lord Hunt stated that his successors had achieved all that the steering committee had initially set out to do. However, he was still looking to the future, stating 'The welfare of this College during the years to come will depend entirely on the younger members. You must continually be looking ahead...' This was a perspective that could be viewed as still being relevant today.

Further Reading

Drury VWM. Hunt, John Henderson, Baron Hunt of Fawley (1905–1987). In: Matthew HCG, Harrison B (eds.). *Oxford Dictionary of National Biography*, Volume 28, Oxford: Oxford University Press; 2004.

Fry J, Hunt Lord of Fawley, Pinsent RJF (eds.). *A History of the Royal College of General Practitioners: The First 25 Years.* Lancaster: MTP Press; 1983.

Horder J. *The Writings of John Hunt.* London: RCGP; 1992.

Hunt JH. The foundation of a College. The conception, birth, and early days of the College of General Practitioners. *The Journal of the Royal College of General Practitioners* 1973;23(126):5–20.

Linnet M. John Henderson, Lord Hunt of Fawley. Hunt. *Royal College of Physicians Heritage: Lives of the Fellows* 1988;8:234.

Pereira Gray DJ. Lord Hunt of Fawley CBE, DM, FRCP, FRCS, FRCGP *British Medical Journal* 1988;296:218–19.

45 FRASER MACINTOSH ROSE (1897–1972)

Priyana Sen and Neil Metcalfe

Born in South Side River Denys in Nova Scotia, Canada, on 3 February 1897, Fraser Rose was the youngest son and eighth child of the Reverend John Rose (1849–1922). It was Fraser McAulay (1872–1943) who came to deliver him into the world and to whom his parents acknowledged with appreciation when naming their child after him. His parents were originally from Inverness; they later moved to Canada but returned to Scotland to reside in the Outer Hebrides when Rose was 12 years old. He was educated at the Nicolson Institute in Stornoway in the Western Isles, Scotland. He is arguably most well known for his key role founding the College, along with John Hunt (1905–1987). He lived a life of numerous achievements within the medical field and beyond.

Rose was 17 years old at the start of the First World War (1914–1918). He was already part of the Ross Mountain Battery of the Highland Territorial Division when war broke out and so went straight into the war. His main post was as a driver, which meant caring for the horses and much of his time was spent in Gallipoli. He took part in the first landing at Cape Helles on 25 April 1915, two months after which he was wounded on 28 June 1915. He was later evacuated to England with dysentery in November 1915. On 6 August 1916, he returned to serve with the same unit at the Struma Front in Macedonia but, in summer 1918, he suffered from sciatica and returned to England. He was discharged a week before Armistice as a result of this injury.

Rose began his medical training in 1919 at the University of Edinburgh and qualified five years later in 1924. During his student years both his interest and talent for administration led to his election as secretary, then president of the Student Representative Council. He then went on to work as a house surgeon at Bradford Royal Infirmary (1925) followed by being an RMO at the Queen Alexander Hospital for Sick Children, Brighton (1925–1926). Following his training he was short listed along with the future president of the Royal College of Gynaecologists, Charles Read (1902–1957), for the post of resident surgical officer at Preston Royal Infirmary where Rose was successful in obtaining the post (1926–1927).

After completion of his medical and surgical training Rose entered general practice in July 1927. This was at his house on Fylde Road, Preston, the building which is now the Guild Pub that has, since 2009, a blue plaque commemorating that he had lived and worked in the building. He worked there until his retirement in 1968. He initially worked with AT Gibb (b.1892) before then working with Ronald B Guyer (1899–1962). The partner he worked longest with was Callum M. MacKenzie (1914–1990), who joined the practice in 1946, and they worked together for 22 years. He also worked with RE Gibson towards the end of his career. Hunt, when writing Rose's obituary, mentioned that Rose 'often admitted his indebtedness to his partners, without whose help and forbearance much of his other work would have been impossible'.

Rose held various positions. He was Honorary Secretary of the Preston division of the BMA for 16 years (1936–1952), later being chairman of it (1954–1955), and was the first president of the North Lancashire and Westmorland branch of the BMA (1950–1951). Furthermore he served as an active member of the BMA Council from 1942 to 1962 save for the post-war years up to 1950 and he was a member of at least 10 BMA committees, ultimately leading to him being awarded a BMA Fellowship in 1959. Locally, he became a member of 14 committees in Lancashire. Nationally, he served on the Insurance Acts Committee (1941–1948) and, in 1953, he was appointed as a member of the NHS Appeals Tribunal, Central Health Services Council and NHS Standing Medical Advisory Committee. His influence shaped the formation of the health service, BMA service provision and, as described below, the formation of the College. Regarding these committee works he admitted that 'evenings, half days and weekends are all submerged into one thing or another'.

As alluded to, Rose's work in helping found the College that he is best remembered. Several attempts at forming a college of general practitioners had taken place before 1950 but were without serious longstanding commitment. Following the formation of the NHS in 1948, general practitioners felt an ever increasing need for a college in order to prevent professional isolation and to also improve both the consistency and quality standards of general practice. With many other specialists having a college of their own Hunt wrote 'GP's had muddled along, and time and time again they had found themselves left behind'. Between 1951 and 1952 other doctors and general practitioners had suggested the formation of a college in both letter and spoken format. Rose had approached the chairman of the General Practice Review Committee of the GMSC of the BMA about the possibility of forming a college. He was then invited by the same committee to submit a memorandum (dated 23 June 1951) to their meeting on 3 October that year. Hunt believed this was the first time an active response was taken to help form a college of general practitioners. It was the day before Rose submitted his memorandum that Hunt first spoke to Rose, having been appointed as a member of the Committee on General Practice of the RCP.

Collaborative work with Hunt soon moved college proposals forward. The meeting commenced at 1500 on 3 October 1951. During the meeting Hunt mentioned he had previously drafted a letter proposing the formation of a

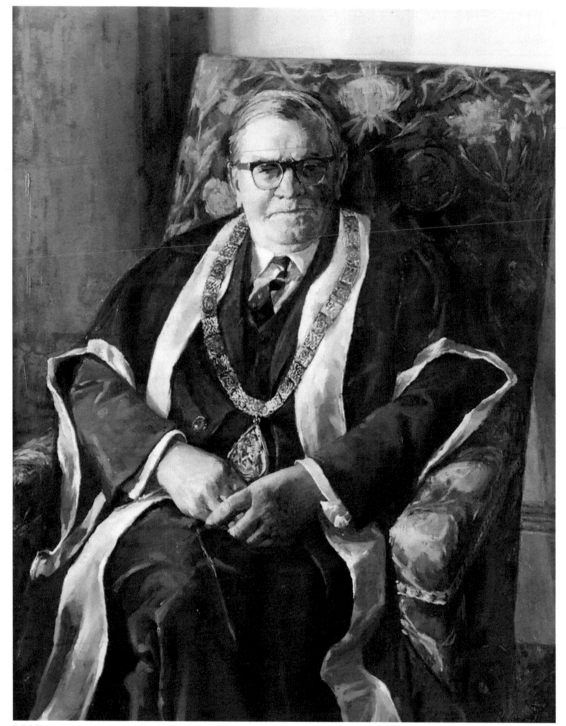

RCGP presidential portrait of Fraser Rose. Artist: Roy Kearsley. (Courtesy of RCGP Archives, London.)

college, some of which was identical to the third paragraph of Rose's memorandum. It was this letter that Rose and Hunt co-signed and submitted to the *BMJ* and *The Lancet*. In doing so they opened a forum via which comments for and against the proposition could be discussed. Rose was later described by Hunt to have played an 'immeasurably important part at this time...in the formation of the college with his friendship and wisdom, his generosity and unselfishness, his influence on the Council of the BMA, his readiness to always help and advise, his quiet humour and good sense and his judgment of character'.

Rose and Hunt co-signed another letter to the journals announcing the formation of a steering committee of which Rose was one of the first general practitioner members. Rose also served time as the vice-chairman of the Provisional Foundation Council (1951–1952) and Foundation Council (1952–1953). The Provisional Foundation Council served to lay the foundations of the college under the recommendations of the steering committee and to build up membership before the first annual general meeting took place. At the first annual general meeting of the College Rose said that doctors had joined 'not because we think we are good practitioners but because we want to be better ones'. At the College he later became Chairman of Council (1956–1959) and president (1962–1964).

Rose was appointed OBE in 1962. In the same year he was awarded Honorary Fellowship of the College. The Fraser Rose Medal was established by the College in honour of his contribution to general practice for which candidates who perform outstandingly in their membership examination and are nominated annually. In his latter years he had two operations for cataracts, and complications of other illnesses such as type 2 diabetes sometimes made regular travelling from Preston to London for BMA meetings difficult, yet he attended most.

Rose often stayed at the Caledonian Club, Belgravia, before travelling back to Preston. He was an avid reader and owned a collection of wide literary works with a particular interest in poetry and history. He completed *The Guardian* crossword every morning at breakfast and, during his student years, wrote a privately circulated autobiography of his early life. He also took an interest in photography and had his own dark room, was a talented debater and was widely rehearsed in literature and travel. He held firm views, yet was always willing to try and understand other viewpoints. Following retirement in 1968, he became an avid gardener and spent his holidays where his parents settled upon their return to Scotland in 1909, the Outer Hebrides.

Rose devoted much time in his later years to genealogical research of his family tree, tracing his ancestors in Canada and Scotland. In 1927, he married his first wife Margaret Jean Howe (1900–1937) and they had two sons, one of whom, Lewis, became a professor of general practice in North America, and a daughter. In 1940, he married his second wife Catherine H Dickinson (1904–1977) and together they had two sons. Two of his sons followed their father's footsteps into general practice. One of his other sons became a radiologist and the other a surveyor whilst his daughter trained as a nurse.

Rose's various talents interests and achievements were plentiful. Despite all his works he cared not for a man's social status in life and was said by Hunt to be 'quite oblivious to social class', and was an incredibly hard working, determined and committed man. Rose died on 2 October 1972, aged 75 years old.

Further Reading

Fry J, Hunt Lord of Fawley, Pinsent RJF (eds.). *A History of the Royal College of General Practitioners: The First 25 Years*. Lancaster: MTP Press; 1983.

Hunt JH. Obituary Fraser Mackintosh Rose. *British Journal of General Practice* 1972;64(622):845–47.

Hunt JH. Obituary F.M. Rose. *British Medical Journal* 1972;4(5832):119.

Hunt JH. Fraser Macintosh Rose O.B.E., M.B.Edin., F.R.C.G.P. *The Lancet* 1972;2(7781):831–32.

JHH. Dr F.M. Rose: Founding of GP College. *The Times* 1972; October 11:18.

RCGP. RCGP Archive. Reference Box Numbers: B/HUN/A2-2, B/HUN/A2-4, B/ROS/A/1-2, B/ROS/A/3-1, B/ROS/1-1, B/ROS/B2-2.

46 GEORGE ABERCROMBIE (1896–1978)

Anizatul Ahmad and Neil Metcalfe

George Francis Abercrombie was born on 25 June 1896 in Kensington, London. He was the only son to George Kennedy Abercrombie, a solicitor from London, and Margaret Jane Forbes. He was educated at Charterhouse School, Ganville, and later graduated and qualified from Caius College, University of Cambridge, in 1922. However, during his time as a medical student with only three months experience at Addenbrooke's Hospital (1917–1918), he joined the Royal Naval Volunteer Reserve (RNVR) as a surgeon probationer in the First World War (1914–1918) he served on *HMS Warwick*. In the Second World War (1939–1945) he served again in the navy on four further destroyers including on *HMS Sheffield*, *HMS Birmingham*, *HMS Lochinvar* and *HMS Anson*, the latter a King George V class battleship. He earned the rank of surgeon captain and, in 1950, was appointed as Honorary Physician to HM King George VI.

Upon qualifying as a doctor, Abercrombie undertook his house appointments at St Bartholomew's Hospital, London. During his time there, he worked as a resident midwifery assistant before working as a house physician at the Hospital for Sick Children, Great Ormond Street. His career in general practice began in 1924 at a practice in Hampstead.

Apart from his clinical work, Abercrombie took a leadership role at various organisations and had a keen interest in academia. He was president of the Hampstead Medical Society, assistant in the antenatal department and lecturer in general practice at St Bartholomew's Hospital. In 1948, he was nominated to the Committee of the Emergency Bed Service and was invited to succeed the chairman, Geoffrey Evans (1886–1951). He contributed a vast amount of effort and time to the King's Fund and was the chairman for the committee for 15 years. In 1950, the Royal Society of Medicine formed a new section, the Section of General Practice. Due to his passion and dedication to general practice, he was appointed as the first president for the newly formed section. It became one of the strongest sections in the society. His 20 years of contribution for the new section led to him, in 1970, being awarded an honorary fellowship by the Royal Society of Medicine.

Driven by a strong determination to improve the quality of general practitioner training, Abercrombie joined and contributed a valuable role in the steering committee to establish the College. He was appointed as the chairman of the Provisional Foundation Council on 19 November 1952 when the College was founded and became the chairman of the Foundation Council until 1956. He mentioned in a paper that at this time he had concerns about the quality of the newly qualified general practitioner and stated his desire to provide better training in the specialty. He later became the third president of the College (1959–1962). John Hunt (1905–1987), a colleague and co-founder of the College, praised Abercrombie for his excellent work and described him as the best chairman that the College ever had. Abercrombie was awarded Honorary Fellowship of the College in 1962.

Abercrombie was heavily involved in writing. He was co-editor with Richard McConaghey (1906–1974) of the eight volumes of *The British Encyclopaedia of General Practices* (1963–1967). In terms of his papers, his presentation of 'The art of consultation' at the fifth James Mackenzie Lecture in 1958 was commented to have been outstanding in the College's Seventh Annual Report. During this paper he remarked: 'As a family doctor, I am not concerned with percentages, but only with people, with men, women and children, individuals, one at a time. The average expectation of life without operation may be so and so, the mortality of the operation such and such, but that is not the point. The point is what will happen to this, to my patient. How one's heart still warms to the surgeon who won't operate!'

Apart from his time serving in the Second World War, Abercrombie worked as a general practitioner until his retirement in 1966. After he retired, he wrote for *Medical Digest* about aspects of his varied career and interests such as his involvement in the RNVR, his participation in the establishment of the College and his writing. His column, entitled 'Musing on the Past', was published monthly. In one of the articles, he shared about how his initial thought of becoming a surgeon changed as he progressed through his medical training as he wanted to have the first contact with patients as a general practitioner. He valued good quality English writing and the College named an award for special meritorious literary work in general practice after him.

As a person, Abercrombie was described as a great and popular figure. He enjoyed much that he did in life. Mountain climbing was one of his favourite activities and he climbed the Matterhorn three times and went climbing in Lofoten Island. He also played chess to a high standard, which included beating former world champion José Raúl Capablanca whilst Capablanca played in simulatenous exhibition games. He enjoyed being a member of the Sherlock Holmes Society and wrote a celebrated paper about Dr Watson. Hunt depicted Abercrombie as an all-rounder which was supported by George Sarum, the Right Reverend, the Lord Bishop of Salisbury, who remarked on their previous time together on *HMS Birmingham* that 'As a doctor, he treated everyone from the Captain to the youngest Boy Seaman with the same skill, compassion, humour, and total lack of sentimentality... As a shipmate he might be playing chess with four officers or ratings simultaneously; acting as compere on a ship's radio programme; making a fourth at

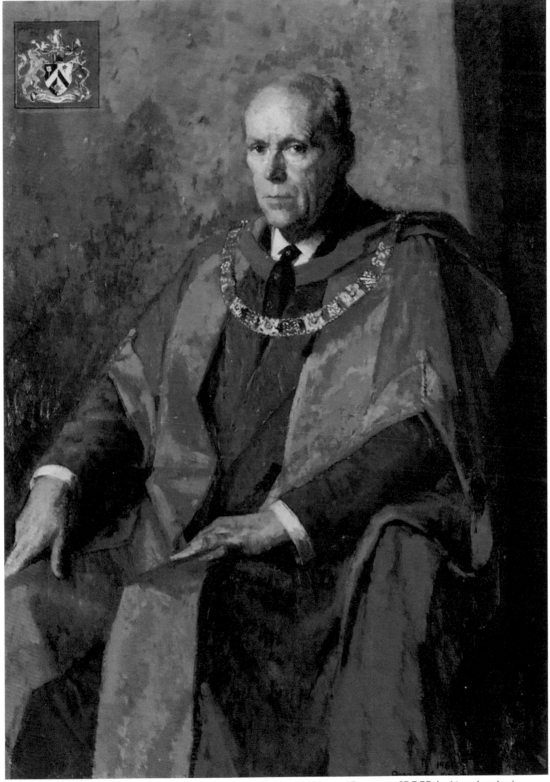

RCGP presidential portrait of George Abercrombie. Artist: Rodney Wilkinson. (Courtesy of RCGP Archives, London.)

bridge; recounting a story with brilliantly dry humour; displaying his considerable skill on the dance floor; or contributing to a serious discussion in cabin or Ward Room'.

Abercrombie died on 26 September 1978 at 82 years of age. He left a widow, Marie, whom he married in 1932. He had a son, George Forbes (1935–), he became a urologist, two married daughters and nine grandchildren. He was an influential general practitioner, a brave royal officer, an astute leader and successful writer.

Further Reading

Abercrombie GF. The art of consultation. *The Journal of the College of General Practitioners* 1959;2(1):5–21.

Abercrombie GF, McConaghey RMS (eds.). *The Encyclopaedia of General Practice*. London: Butterworth; 1963–67.

Gray DP. History of the Royal College of General Practitioners – The First 40 Years. *British Journal of General Practice* 1992;42(354):29–35.

Lord Fawley. George Francis Abercrombie, VRD, MA, MD, HON. FRCGP. *The Journal of the Royal College of General Practitioners* 1978;28(197):765–66.

Sarum G. George Francis Abercrombie, VRD, MA, MD, HON. FRCGP. *The Journal of the Royal College of General Practitioners* 1978;28(197):766.

47 ROBIN PINSENT (1916–1987)

Umair Shahid and Neil Metcalfe

Robert John Francis Homfray Pinsent was born on 4 October 1916 in the village of Horrabridge in Devon. He received his medical education and training at Selwyn College, University of Cambridge, and the Charing Cross Medical School, completing his studies in 1941. At Charing Cross he showed his ability to galvanise others as he organised his fellow students in preparing the Charing Cross Hospital against the potential damage and destruction from the Blitz. As well as completing his medical education in 1941, he married Ruth Morrison in the same year, with whom he would have one son and three daughters.

After serving in the RAMC during the Second World War (1939–1945), Pinsent entered into practice in Handsworth, Birmingham, in 1946. At first, he undertook this role alone but subsequently formed a partnership with Laurie Pike (1925–1998), in 1956, in which he worked until his retirement in 1978. Much effort was put into the practice and a favourable reputation was gained for the quality of the clinical work. The practice became a teaching practice used by the University of Birmingham for some of its undergraduate medical students.

Pinsent served as a member of the steering committee which set up the College in 1952 and he would go on to play a crucial part in the research activity of the College. On 20 January 1952, he wrote a proposal for a research organisation within the College and the College's Research Committee was formed by Pinsent in 1953. This resulted in the research register of the College gaining 300 names within a year and led to a number of research projects. Pinsent served as the committee's first chairman (1953–1964), and his choice of an alcohol-free hotel in Bath for the inaugural meeting was later revealed by George Watson (1909–1979), in 1977, to have been Pinsent's only mistake since 1952. Furthermore, Pinsent's skill and enthusiasm for research also led him to be named research advisor to the College in 1963, a position he held for 20 years. His vision and initiative in realising the importance of research in general practice not only had an impact in the United Kingdom, but also around the world, such as in North America and in Australia, the latter being exemplified when he became an Honorary Member of the Royal Australian College of General Practitioners and North America. His enthusiasm for stimulating research did not cease upon retirement, as he corresponded with Canadian colleagues to encourage them in their endeavours.

Pinsent's influence could be seen in literature as well. He published *An Approach to General Practice* in 1953, and this preceded a flurry of publications on this subject by others. His strength was not simply in publishing material himself, although Pinsent did write many publications, but rather in encouraging and coordinating others. Thus his name does not appear in many studies, that owe a great deal to his work. For example, he played a key role in the first National Morbidity Survey (1956–1958), along with Donald Crombie (1922–2000), with whom he had a long and productive working relationship. Pinsent also started to send out the newsletter *Between Ourselves* in 1953 to a group of research enthusiasts. This newsletter evolved into the *Research Newsletter* in September of the same year, with its first paragraph from Pinsent stating:

> The White Paper on Clinical Research in relation to the National Health Service is a milestone in the history of man's inquiry into sickness and disease; for the definition of research laid down by the joint committee expressly includes field studies in epidemiology and in social medicine, and observations in general practice. It is clearly implied that research in the field of medicine seen by the general practitioner is potentially as valuable as that carried out in a hospital ward or a university department. This is a challenge to those in general practice, who see the beginnings of disease, to make a fuller contribution to its study by investigating more fully the problems they handle.

This far-sighted statement of the need for a research evidence base for general practice set the tone for the early observational studies of disease in the community by a number of general practitioners.

The importance of Pinsent's work in the research activity of the College can be shown by his collaboration with Crombie at the internationally renowned Birmingham Research Unit, with its roots in the early 1960s and set up in its current form in 1967. This unit was involved in development of the age-sex and diagnostic registers, as well as the National Morbidity Studies. The unit also obtained a grant from the National Institutes of Health in the United States to fund a study of diabetes. This led to a survey of 19,412 patients over 10 practices between 1960 and 1961 in order to find out the prevalence of diabetes in a general population as well as the use of glycosuria testing paper and relevance and use of the oral glucose tolerance test in certain sub-groups. It was published in the *BMJ* in 1962 and this paper was not only useful for the data it gathered on the subject but also highlighted the quality of work that was being produced at the Birmingham Research Unit. This in turn led to a number of highly capable general practitioners applying to work at it. This was in a large part due to Pinsent's enthusiasm, with Michael Drury (1926–2014) stating that his 'genius was for inspiring others'.

Throughout his career Pinsent received a number of accolades. In 1962, he delivered the ninth James Mackenzie Lecture, entitled 'James Mackenzie and research tomorrow', and was appointed OBE in 1970. He wrote his doctoral

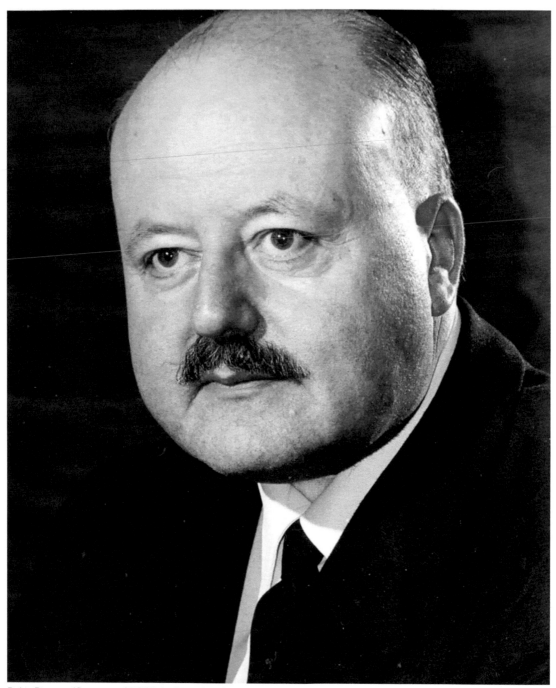

Robin Pinsent. (Courtesy of RCGP Archives, London.)

thesis from general practice in 1971 on the topic of morbidity recording. In recognition of his remarkable work in general practice, he received the inaugural Baron Dr Ver Heyden de Lancey Memorial Award in 1977 from the RCGP, named after the Dutch dentist, doctor and lawyer. Pinsent also has a biennial memorial lecture in his own name, started in 1992, by the Midland Faculty of the College.

Aside from the impact he made on research and general practice, Pinsent was also interested in homeopathy. He was the chairman of the British Homeopathy Research Group for six years, an organisation he founded in 1977. He examined the impact of the environment on health and his insistence on bringing attention to the possible interplay between the two was an example of his vision. He initiated the Tamar Valley Project that investigated the link between the unusual water supply of the town of Tavistock and the distribution of gastric cancer. This was of particular interest as his father had developed cancer whilst residing in the area. Whilst he was unable to gain any definitive evidence of cause and effect in this study, an awareness of the difficulty surrounding environmental research was gained. Further studies have suggested that regional abnormal mineralisation may be the causative factor.

Pinsent had a number of health issues throughout his life. Firstly he developed atrial fibrillation around 1954. In the late 1960s, he was diagnosed with laryngeal cancer and required a total laryngectomy. However, this did not deter him from continuing to speak publically and working until his retirement. His desire to help others with a similar affliction was shown by attempts to produce a teaching manual for those struggling with oesophageal speech.

Pinsent retired to his native Devon in 1978. He spent his retirement tending to his garden, fly-fishing and spending time with his wife Ruth. However, his enthusiasm for research and literature did not cease and he continued to stimulate others in conducting research and edited his local parish magazine. He was invited to become the provost of the new Tamar Valley Faculty of the RCGP in 1980, a position which he took. During his last year of life Pinsent stepped back from his activities and died in Tavistock on Christmas Day 1987.

Further Reading

Davies AE. R. J. F. H. Pinsent, OBE, MA, MD, FRCGP, FRACGP, MFHOM. *British Homeopathic Journal* 1988;77(2):143–44.

Diabetes Survey Working Party. A diabetes survey. *British Medical Journal* 1962;5291:1497–503.

Drury M. R.J.F.H Pinsent. *The Journal of the Royal College of General Practitioners* 1988;38(307):88.

Fry J, Hunt Lord of Fawley, Pinsent RJF (eds.). *A History of the Royal College of General Practitioners: The First 25 Years*. Lancaster: MTP Press; 1983.

Pinsent RJFH. Research Newsletter No.1. *Research Newsletter* 1953:1.

Pinsent RJFH. *An Approach to General Practice*. Edinburgh: E. & S. Livingstone; 1953.

Pinsent RJFH. James Mackenzie and general practice tomorrow. *The Journal of the College of General Practitioners* 1963;6(1):5–19.

48 DONALD LASCELLES CROMBIE (1922–2000)

Philippa Banks and Stuart Pinder

Donald Lascelles Crombie was born in Greenock, Scotland, on 23 November 1922 to Donald and Margret Crombie. Crombie did not initially set out studying medicine, having enrolled in the foundation mathematics course at the University of Glasgow when 15 years old. In 1940, his family relocated from Scotland to Birmingham, and along with moving home, Crombie moved his field of study to medicine, qualifying with BChir in 1945 from the University of Birmingham.

Crombie began work as a general practitioner in 1946 in Harborne, Birmingham, and continued to work there until his retirement in 1989. In addition to his work as a general practitioner, Crombie was the medical officer at the Blue Coat School in Birmingham (1952–1959). He also completed his doctorate in medicine at the University of Birmingham in 1955, writing his thesis on the assessment of medical care in general practice.

Crombie was inspired by Professor Lancelot Thomas Hogben (1895–1975), who was involved with medical statistics at the University of Birmingham, and, in 1957, with Robin Pinsent (1916–1987), the then chair of the College of General Practitioners Research Committee, Crombie set up a research unit in Birmingham. This was initially called the Statistics and Records Unit and is now known as the RCGP Research and Surveillance Centre. The aim of this unit was to establish and develop a recording system for epidemiologic research in general practice and this still remains the case today. The studies and research produced by the research centre are world acclaimed. Crombie remained a director of the facility until his retirement in 1992 and continued to act as a consultant advisor until his death.

Medical literature was aided greatly by Crombie. He was involved in large studies on diabetes, mental health, outcomes of pregnancies and many more. Between 1971 and 1972 and then between 1981 and 1982 his RCGP Birmingham Research Unit organised the second and third National Morbidity Surveys, following the first survey in 1956. These surveys provided a valuable insight into disease prevalence in the United Kingdom, allowed the analysis of trends in co-morbidities, provided information for service planning and enabled the examination of social and regional inequalities. His research was internationally renowned and did much to help give the Birmingham research centre its stellar reputation.

In 1971, Crombie delivered the 18th James Mackenzie Lecture entitled 'Cum sciencia caritas' which is the motto of the RCGP, meaning 'Science with compassion'. The topic of his lecture was about the short fallings of the profession and the importance of medicine as a vocation, not a 'science'. He went on to speak of his belief that 'the major function of this college should be the reinstatement of the holistic view of medical care'. Holistic care is still the aim of many general practitioners, and he was a strong advocate for the reduction of paternalistic medicine in favour of patient-centred care and improvement of a rounded medical education. Perhaps most interestingly, he spoke of the emotional components of illness, the links between health and mental wellbeing and the importance of recognising the context of a patient's life and emotions in their presentation to general practitioners.

Internationally, Crombie contributed to the International Association of General Practice and the World Organization of National Colleges, Academies, and Academic Associations of General Practitioners/Family Physicians (WONCA), where as part of the classification committee he helped develop the International Classification of Heath Problems in Primary Practice (ICHPPC-II). In 1978, under Clifford Kay, he also formed part of a team who reported on the possibilities of computers within general practice. This work was the start of the technological phase of medicine, with the development of software for safe prescribing, patient records and tasks.

During such a long and distinguished career Crombie was decorated with several awards, acknowledgments and key roles. With the College he was awarded fellowship, and was chair of the research committee (1953–1966). In 1963, he became president of the General Practice Section of the Royal Society of Medicine, and, in 1967, was appointed OBE for his contributions to medicine. He was awarded the Baron Dr Ver Heyden De Lancey Memorial Award in 1982 and the Kuenssberg Prize in 1998. He also worked as an honorary senior lecturer at the University of Birmingham and became a visiting associate professor of family medicine to the University of Western Ontario between 1983 and 1985.

At 77 years old, Crombie died on 26 January 2000. He was survived by his wife Gwenyth (1922–2010), to whom he had been married since 1947, and his three children.

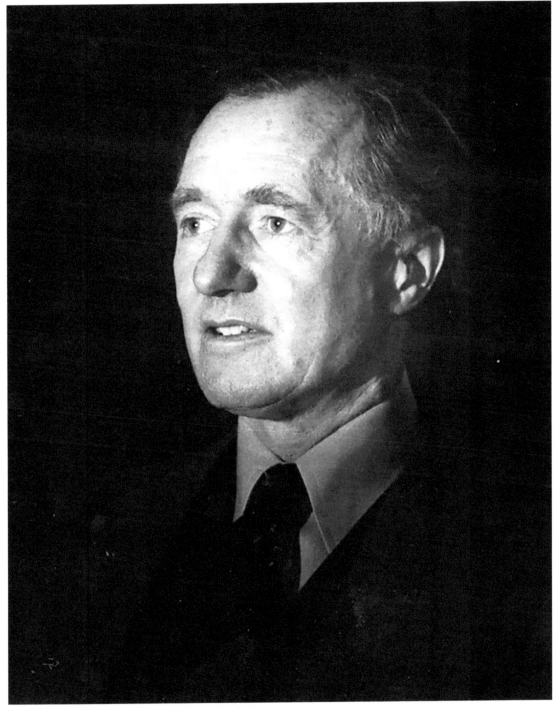

Donald Crombie. (Courtesy of RCGP Archives, London.)

Further Reading

Crombie DL. Diabetes mellitus: Incidence, causation and management. *Proceedings of the Royal Society of Medicine* 1962;55(3): 205–11.

Crombie DL. James Mackenzie Lecture 1971: Cum scientia caritas. *The Journal of the Royal College of General Practitioners* 1972;22(114):7–17.

Fleming DM. Donald Lascelles Crombie Obituary. *British Medical Journal* 2000;320:876.

49 GEORGE IAN WATSON (1909–1979)

Mohammedabbas Khaki, Sayyada Mawji, Armaan Iqbal and Neil Metcalfe

The son of epidemiologist Sir Malcom Watson (1873–1955) and Lady Watson, George Ian Watson was born on 9 March 1909. He studied medicine at the University of Cambridge as an undergraduate, and subsequently studied at St Thomas' Hospital in London, qualifying with MBBChir in 1933. He was then appointed to houseman jobs in Plymouth and Glasgow. Additionally, he completed a diploma in Tropical Medicine and Hygiene in 1937 and was awarded MD in 1940.

From 1939 to 1945, Watson served in the Second World War (1939–1945) with the RAMC in Burma, rising to the rank of lieutenant colonel. During the war he worked with an entomologist to study malaria. This work involved investigating its local prevalence as well as the biting times and flying heights of various types of mosquitos. After his involvement in the war, he decided to return to England and enter general practice. Based in Peaslake in Guildford, Surrey, he was characterised as 'a family doctor… above all' with his first concern being 'always the welfare of his patients'.

Having achieved further postgraduate qualifications in tropical medicine and hygiene following the war, this, together with his medical experiences in the war, led him to develop a keen interest in clinical virology. Through shrewd observation, he identified and defined symptom patterns of epidemic diseases in his practice to ensure others could also study their distribution and spread. One of the first symptom patterns he identified, presenting with pyrexia and diarrhoea, he named 'Shere fever' based on the village near Guildford where he had encountered it whilst in practice. Following a report from his colleague working at the Virus Reference Laboratory in Colindale, James Macrae (1911–1987), Watson postulated that there may be a link to Coxsachie virus, which presented in a similar way, though there was no evidence published to denote that the viruses were of a similar strain. Some of his findings were published in *Research Newsletter* in 1953.

An inquisitive person, Watson used to carry red pocket books to write notes about anything that he came across which sparked his interest. His dedication to research can be highlighted through his creation of the Epidemic Observation Unit at the University of Surrey in 1953. This was used as a way to gather and analyse information reported by other general practitioners, which mainly concerned, but was not exclusive to, infectious diseases. He also managed to receive funding for his work for a number of years whilst being part of the Medical Research Council (MRC). At the time, his appointment to the MRC committee in itself was significant as not many general practitioners were being appointed to the committee. The work that he did was recognised through the Sir Charles Hastings Clinical Prize, which he first received in 1954 for an essay he had written on measles and again five years later in 1959 for an essay on the clinical epidemiology of Asian influenza.

In 1961, Watson was part of the board that took over the running of the bacteriological service administration of the Public Health Laboratory which was associated with the MRC. The main aim of the Public Health laboratory was to study infectious diseases using laboratory investigations. In the same year, he was awarded the James Mackenzie Prize by the College. A few years later, in 1966, he gave the 13th James Mackenzie Lecture entitled 'Learning and teaching by family doctors'.

From 1952, Watson was a member of the Foundation Council of the College before becoming the president of the RCGP in 1970, one of the roles which he is most memorable for. At a Council dinner in front of Sir Keith Joseph, the Secretary of State, Watson was remembered for having delivered an effortless speech, having memorised it entirely. His contributions to both College and then when it became RCGP included forging links with the other Royal Colleges, as well arranging for a gavel to be made for the College. It was unclear if Watson intended to use the gavel, a small mallet commonly struck against a sound block to call to attention, for functional or ceremonial purposes. By liaising with the Greek Ambassador, His Excellency Monsieur Basile Mostras, Watson was able to source a gavel from the wood of an ancient plane tree from the island of Cos, where Hippocrates, the 'father' of medicine, had taught and practised. The gavel was subsequently stolen but Watson managed to arrange a replacement from the same source in 1971. Watson continued to serve his role as President of the RCGP 1970 to 1972, but his presidency was restricted by one year to permit HRH Prince Philip, the Duke of Edinburgh, a one-year presidency from 1972 to 1973. During this period Watson acted as Prince Philip's deputy, and it was during this year that the Royal Charter was presented to the College. Watson's other roles involved working overseas and attending international conferences. Even after his retirement from the Council he continued to work on behalf of the College, acting as a College ambassador to the Gulf States.

Away from medicine Watson assumed various roles in Guildford, one of which was leading a fundraising project for the doctor's stained-glass window that was erected at Guildford Cathedral. In addition, Watson was knowledgeable about subjects outside of medicine and was always keen to discuss Mesolithic artefacts near where he lived. Watson died on 3 June 1979, aged 70, in Surrey, survived by his wife Caroline to whom he married in November 1939. According to an obituary published in *The Lancet* at the time, he was described as 'friendly and kind' with it being by the 'help he gave to others… that he will be remembered'.

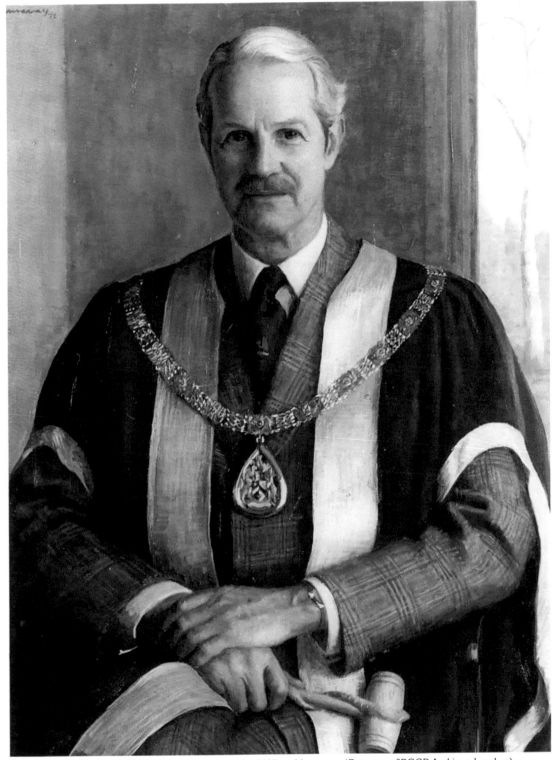

RCGP presidential portrait of George Ian Watson. Artist: William Narraway. (Courtesy of RCGP Archives, London.)

Further Reading

Anon. GI Watson, OBE, MA, MD, FRCGP, DTM&H. *British Medical Journal* 1979;2(6182):137.

Fry J, Hunt Lord of Fawley, Pinsent RJF (eds.). *A History of the Royal College of General Practitioners: The First 25 Years.* Lancaster: MTP Press; 1983.

Pinsent RJFH. G.I. Watson, OBE, MA, MD, FRCGP, FRACGP, DTM&H. *The Journal of the Royal College of General Practitioners* 1979;29:506.

Pinsent RJFH. George Ian Watson, O.B.E., M.A., M.D. Cantab., F.R.C.G.P. *The Lancet* 1979;1(8130):1358.

Watson GI. Progress Report: (2) Epidemic observation scheme. *Research Newsletter* 1953;os-1(2):5–6.

Watson GI. Learning and teaching by family doctors. *The Journal of the College of General Practitioners* 1967;13(1):3–21.

JOHN FRY (1922–1994)

Hannah Louise Regan

John Fry was born as Jack Freitag on 16 June 1922 in Lublin, Poland, into a Jewish family. His parents Anczel and Basia Freitag (née Mintzman) moved to England in December 1929, following his father's completion of medical examinations at King's College Hospital and purchase of a practice in South Norwood, Croydon. He undertook his secondary school education at Whitgift Middle School in Croydon between 1932 and 1939, proceeding to medicine at Guy's Hospital, London from where he graduated and qualified as a doctor in 1944.

Fry entered general practice in March 1947, a year prior to the creation of the NHS, working briefly alongside his father, whilst searching for a practice. In July 1947, Fry purchased and moved to his own practice, St James's practice, at 36 Croydon Road in Beckenham, Kent. Despite showing an initial interest in surgery and having been awarded FRCS in November 1947, he remained in general practice. He balanced his work as the sole general practitioner alongside working part-time at the Croydon General three days a week for numerous years. His first assistant general practitioner, Colin Coole (1919–), joined him in practice in 1956. Throughout his professional life, Fry remained at the St James's practice, leaving only to retire in Colin Coole (b.1919).

Fry joined the forum of general practitioners created by the Royal Society of Medicine in 1951. Through this he became integrated with those determined to found a college of general practitioners, namely John Hunt (1905–1987) and Fraser Rose (1897–1972), who co-founded the College at the end of 1952. He wrote various letters supporting its establishment. However, he had not attended the BMA General Practice Review Committee in October 1951 from which seven doctors subsequently joined the steering committee for the College.

Fry's MD thesis was entitled 'Clinical patterns of respiratory tract diseases in a general practice: 1950–1954'. His interest in respiratory illnesses, he wrote, was due to the fact 'they account for over 25% of all work in general practice'. He wrote the first textbook of clinical general practice, collaborating with eight general practitioners in 1953, entitled *Clinical Medicine in General Practice*. This was regarded at the time as 'a training manual to assist a new speciality to emerge' by the 1951 BMA president, Lord Henry Cohen (1900–1977). One of Fry's major articles, 'Are all 'T's and A's' really necessary?', was published in the *BMJ* in 1957 and it queried how many tonsillectomies and adenoidectomies in children were actually required. It was one of the first papers to question standard practice, a seed of evidence-based medicine. Subsequently he published a further book, *The Catarrhal Child* (1961) which indicated that tonsillitis was a self-resolving disease and that the anxiety levels of parents regarding the condition was not an indication for surgery. Having earned respect for his publications, he was appointed as an editor for *Medical Care*, which was founded in 1963.

An avid writer, Fry co-introduced the popular general practice magazine *Update* which aimed to provide recent information on the latest management of common ailments. He was later appointed as editor of *Update*, *Update Review* and the international version in 1974, contributing until 1983. He also edited *Primary Care* (1980) and *Scientific Foundations of Family Medicine* (1978). He wrote *Profiles of Disease in Childhood* (1966) and *Common Diseases: Their Nature, Incidence and Care*, the latter originally published in 1974 and currently extending to five editions. Furthermore he co-authored an exam-style question book aimed at those sitting the membership examination for membership of the College called *A Comprehensive Guide to Preparation and Passing the MRCGP Examination* (1978).

One of Fry's notable influences on general practice was the initiative of extensive work on data collection and analysis. He was famed for clinical research based upon his consultations: utilising this information and his observations he began to reach conclusions about the epidemiology of diseases in his patient population. The first paper that he published used this method and was in the *BMJ* in 1951. It was based on erythema nodosum. He had approximately 9000 patients on his register enabling him to build up a large dataset of findings which he proceeded to publish in several papers including 'Infection mononucleosis: some new observations from a 15-year study' (1980), and an update entitled 'Infectious mononucleosis: 25 years observation' (1989). Fry maintained meticulous note taking throughout the entirety of his career, culminating in the practice's first annual report for the period of 1990 to 1991. This annual report delineated all details of the practice including its history, aims, staff members, demographics of the population served and the problems Fry and his team had faced.

Continuing his research Fry presented a paper, in 1985, at a medical statistics seminar at Guy's Hospital in London entitled 'Morbidity statistics' based on his experiences as a general practitioner, he identified that the data available on morbidity was poor and that this was mainly due to the 'gross inaccuracy of mortality data', exemplified by studies over-relying on death certificate information. He noted in 'Morbidity statistics' that data were incomparable where different sources had used differing coding systems to record diseases, despite the establishment of the International Classification of Diseases. He stated that 'the frequency and the cost of morbidity is more important than mortality', which may indicate why he pursued recording morbidity statistics. He believed that if the NHS gathered morbidity

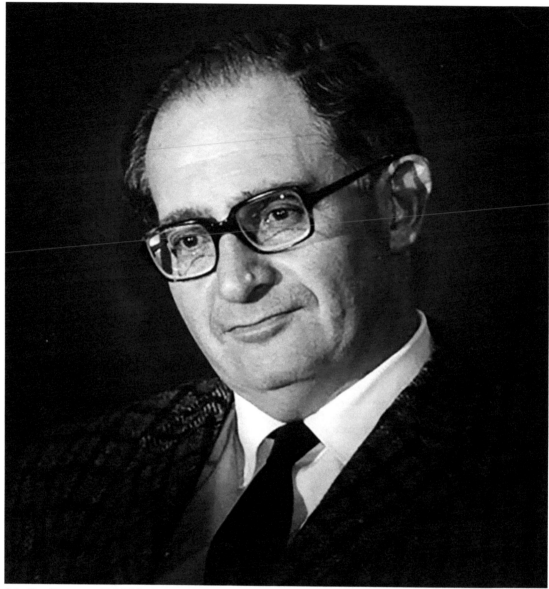

John Fry. (Courtesy of RCGP Archives, London.)

data from all available sources, this could be used to create and enforce guidelines for treatment of such diseases, showing his forward thinking.

Fry held several posts at the College during his career. He was a member of College Council from 1956 to 1990 and represented the South East Thames Faculty. He also sat on the *College's* Research Committee (1956–1967 and 1971–1972), who during his time there, helped develop the *Journal of the College of General Practitioners* from the initial research committee's newsletter *Between Ourselves*. Moreover, he joined the Postgraduate Education Committee (1956–1959), which inaugurated postgraduate teaching to newly qualified doctors. This interest in postgraduate teaching was seen in his assisting the provision of monthly lectures and seminars at Canterbury to over 100 colleagues. He continued practising his commitment to education in joining the Examinations Committee (1961–1963) and organising a five-day course at the RCGP in 1969 to educate general practitioners in basic statistical and research methods. He also sat on the Undergraduate Education Committee in 1963. He joined the Practice Organisation Committee (1962–1971) of which he became vice-chairman on three occasions: 1964, 1967 and 1969 to 1971. The main focus of this committee was to raise standards of accommodation and facilities provided by practices on a national scale. Furthermore, he was chairman of the Board of Censors from 1975 to 1978, and delivered the 22nd James Mackenzie Lecture in 1976 on 'Common sense and uncommon sensibility'.

Fry was concerned with reviewing the stability and future needs of the NHS as a part of the Medical Services Review Committee (1958) and served as one of six members on the Porritt Committee led by surgeon Sir Arthur Porritt (1900–1994). *The Porritt Report* (1962) aimed to review the provision and organisation of medical services 10 years after the NHS had started. The principal finding of the report was that the NHS did need reorganisation of services including local lead administrative units for each area to plan and develop services in these areas. These suggestions later formed the basis of the Green Paper on NHS reorganisation in 1968 proposed by the then Minister of Health, Kenneth Robinson.

Fry and John Dillane (1928–2013), a partner at St James's from 1961 to 1988, proceeded to research 30 practices in 1962, analysing the efficiency of each. Dillane was intent on researching practices with a good reputation and investigating the underpinning organisational methods, which made them successful, including management and the utilisation of resources. This pilot study led to Fry persuading the College to research this on a nationwide scale. The research was led by Ann Cartwright (1925–), who was sponsored by the Nuffield Provincials Hospitals Trust, with Fry serving as adviser. The compilation of this data resulted in the report, *General Practice in 1963, its conditions, contents and satisfactions* (1963), which suggested doctors wanted 'better premises' as well as improvements in both the organisation of services as well as access for their patients to treatments in hospital.

Following Fry's recommendation of a group of doctors to audit general practice and assess how it could develop nationwide, a Present State and Future Needs Committee was formed in July 1964. The committee was appointed by the College Council and was chaired by him. The *Present State and Future Needs Report* was published in 1965. It reported how workload and operational efficiency needed review, as the morale of general practitioners was low and many were emigrating due to this. Of note, observations made included that general practice needed to move away from being provided by single-handed doctors and towards a team approach to make the most of available resources. Fry also commented how resistance to teamwork, education and prevention strategies was delaying general practice development. With regard to preventative measures, children's immunisations were reported to not be done routinely in 27 per cent of surgeries, and educating patients on health and providing birth control were low on the priority list of general practitioners.

Fry undertook futher roles. He was consultant to the army between 1968 and 1987. At the Royal Society of Medicine he was vice-president (1956–1959,1964–1967), as well as serving as president (1962–1963 and 1988–1989) of their General Practice Section. In 1963, he addressed the need for better patient records to be held by general practitioners at the BMA conference. Working alongside general practitioners Michael Drury (1926–2014), and Jock Anderson (1926–2000), he aided the creation of the syllabus for a medical secretary preparatory course, which was piloted at Bromsgrove College of Further Education between 1962 and 1963 and other colleges followed suit nationwide. He was a committee member of the MRC (1965–1988) and was elected annually to the GMC between 1970 and 1992. Furthermore, he served as an advisor on the Disciplinary Committee of the GMC in 1974, and was appointed as senior treasurer in 1976. Between 1981 and 1982 he was chairman of the Preliminary Proceedings Committee for the GMC.

Internationally, Fry was keen on participating and working with the WHO. A travelling fellowship was awarded to him by the WHO in 1960, which led to him travelling to Denmark, Holland and Sweden comparing methods of general practice. He completed a report on this in 1960. His findings included the benefits of direct access to investigations as part of routine care given to general practitioners, particularly in Copenhagen, as well as how nurses enabled general practitioners to manage large volumes of patients in areas where general practitioners were few. He noted their massive contribution to care compared with in the United Kingdom. In latter years, he visited North America and the USSR. In 1964, he was invited to Geneva in order to help contribute to the *WHO Technical Report 267* formed by the Expert Committee on General Practice. Fry was given the position of consultant of general practice to the WHO in 1965. He was an advisor to the WHO (1965–1983) and received a WHO fellowship in 1969.

Fry was appointed OBE in 1975 for his contributions to general practice. His other accolades include being awarded the Sir Charles Hastings Clinical Prize of the BMA twice, in 1960 and 1964, the first occasion being in recognition of his observations aiding the diagnosis of asthma. The James Mackenzie Medal from the RCP of Edinburgh was awarded to him in 1965 for his work in the science of general practice. He also received Guthrie and Hunterian Gold Medals, the Abercrombie Award from the RCGP (1977) and the Baron Dr Ver Heyden De Lancey Memorial Award (1984). For his time spent as a trustee to the Nuffield Provincial Hospitals Trust he was awarded Her Majesty Queen Elizabeth the Queen Mother Fellowship. He also received the Foundation Council Award in 1993, after serving 34 years on the College Council.

Fry was an inspirational figure, reflected in the research awards given in his name today. King's College London currently offers the John Fry at Guys scholarship to help undergraduate medical students who have an interest in general practice who are experiencing financial hardship. The RCGP presents the John Fry Award annually to a general practitioner undertaking research in the field of general practice and the Nuffield Trust offer a John Fry Fellowship to a senior academic or practitioner to write and lecture on a subject in the field of general practice.

Descriptions of Fry portray him as a warm and gracious character. He was described in his obituary in the *BMJ* to be 'always full of humour, with a twinkle in his eye, he had time for everybody'. Despite many achievements, he was renowned for his humility, and enjoyed morning jogs, gardening and supporting his local football club Crystal Palace. Altruistically, he donated his entire personal collection of books to the RCGP.

Fry married Joan Sabel (1921–1989) on 2 April 1944, and they remained together until 1989 when she pre-deceased him. Together, they had two children. Shortly after his wife's death, he remarried in September 1989 to a family friend, Trudy Amiel (née Scher). In his later years, he struggled with fibrosing alveolitis, as his father had. He died on 28 April 1994, aged 71 years old in Farnborough, Kent.

Further Reading

Anon. Porritt Report on N.H.S. *British Medical Journal* 1962;2:1171–73.

Blythe M. *Almost a Legend: Leading Reformer of General Practice*. London: Royal Society of Medicine Press; 2007.

Fry J. Are all 'T's and A's' really necessary? *British Medical Journal* 1957;1:124–28.

Fry J. *The Catarrhal Child*. London: Butterworth; 1961.

Fry J. Common sense and uncommon sensibility. *The Journal of the Royal College of General Practitioners* 1977;27(166):9–17.

Fry J. Infectious mononucleosis: Some new observations from a 15-year study. *The Journal of Family Practice* 1980;10:1087–89.

Fry J. Morbidity statistics. In: Aslib Biological & Agricultural Group Seminar. *Medical Statistics* 29 November 1985; Guy's Hospital Medical School, London, Great Britain Aslib Proceedings, June/July 1986;38:187–92.

Fry J. *The Fry Papers Collection: Box B/FRY.* RCGP Archives, London.

Fry J, Dunachie PD, Wagstyl JW. Infectious mononucleosis: 25 years' observation. *Update* 15 September 1989;520–23.

Fry J, Hunt Lord of Fawley, Pinsent RJF (eds.). *A History of the Royal College of General Practitioners: The First 25 Years*. Lancaster: MTP Press; 1983.

Pereira Gray DJ. Obituary: J Fry. *British Medical Journal* 1991;308:1367.

RCGP Archive. *The Fry Papers Collection: Box B/FRY*. London: RCGP.

Tait I. John Fry (1922–1994). In: Matthew HCG, Harrison B (eds.). *Oxford Dictionary of National Biography*. Volume 21. Oxford: Oxford University Press; 2004.

51 ROBERT EDGAR HOPE-SIMPSON (1908–2003)

Mehreen Mahfooz

Robert Edgar Hope-Simpson was born on 31 January 1908 to Sir John Hope-Simpson (1868–1961) and Lady Quita Hope-Simpson (1870–1939) and was the fourth of their five children. He attended preparatory school at Heddon Court in Hertfordshire from 1913 to 1919, and then Gresham's School in Norfolk from 1919 to 1925, where he won a prize for natural history, a field in which he would go on to excel in during the rest of his life.

Hope-Simpson spent a year studying Natural Sciences at the Faculté des Sciences, Grenoble, France (1925–1926), before choosing to study medicine at St Thomas' Hospital, London in 1926. He chose to intercalate in Physiology during his medical studies and it was during his time in the laboratory that he met his first wife, Eleanor Mary Dale (1906–2000), daughter of Sir Henry Dale. In 1932, Hope-Simpson qualified with MRCS and LRCP from St Thomas' Hospital and also married Eleanor. His first training post was at Dorset County Hospital in Dorchester, where he was the RMO. This was followed by a post at a general practice in Beaminster and he remained there during the Second World War (1939–1945), refusing to fight as a conscientious objector, due to his Quaker beliefs. During this time, he also developed an interest in epidemiology and how the health of the community around him was affected in different ways.

After the war, in 1945, Hope-Simpson moved to Cirencester, Gloucestershire, where he ran his own successful practice and where he was to remain for most of his life. Following his newfound interest in epidemiology, he set up the Cirencester Research Unit, an epidemiological research team based around his practice, using his patient list of around 3500 as a basis for most of his work. In addition to this, he also chaired a committee for the MRC, which was based at Cirencester. During the 1940s and 1950s he was able to use these two roles to help him write various papers on epidemiology, many of which were published in prestigious journals, such as *The Lancet* and the *BMJ*. He was particularly interested in the epidemiology of infectious diseases, two of his main focuses being shingles and influenza.

It was widely accepted contemporaneously that chickenpox and shingles were related in some manner. Yet it was Hope-Simpson's research that eventually proved that both diseases were a result of the same virus and not two different organisms as previously suggested. Together with his Research Unit he travelled in 1953 to a small, closed community on the Island of Yell, one of the north isles of Shetland, Scotland. There they carried out an 11-year longitudinal study which involved following up every single recognised case of chickenpox or shingles within that group. He was hugely aided by the members of that community and their excellent memories regarding these conditions. As well as this, coinciding scientific research elsewhere in the United Kingdom provided him with new microbiological research techniques. This helped him reach his eventual conclusion, which was that shingles was caused by the reactivation of the varicella virus, the organism that is responsible for chickenpox primarily.

Hope-Simpson reported his conclusion in June 1964 at the first Albert Wander Lecture, organised by the Royal Society of Medicine. This report was published the following year in *Proceedings of the Royal Society of Medicine* as 'The nature of herpes zoster: A long-term study and a new hypothesis'. The later-termed 'Hope-Simpson hypothesis' was also a result of his research. This stated that being exposed to chickenpox helped 'boost' the immune system to delay the onset of shingles.

Hope-Simpson also became interested in the epidemiology of influenza following an epidemic in 1932 and 1933, which was shortly after he had started in general practice. By using research from his own practice as well as data from previous studies, he hypothesised that there must be seasonal influence on the transmission of influenza. With subsequent research, he demonstrated the involvement of vitamin D in this disease process. In 1992, he published a textbook on the topic entitled *The Transmission of Epidemic Influenza* (1992).

For his contributions to epidemiology and general medicine, Hope-Simpson was awarded various honours. He was appointed OBE in 1963 for his contributions to public health and was also given the Stewart Prize from the BMA for his work in epidemic disease. He received two separate honours from the RCGP: the Kuenssberg Prize (1983), for the herpes zoster research project that directly resulted in a demonstrable change to clinical practice; and the George Abercrombie Award (1999), for significant literary contributions to the field of general practice. As well as this, in 1999, the Varicella-Zoster Virus (VZV) Foundation awarded him with their gold medal, for outstanding research in the field.

Hope-Simpson cared for his first wife, Eleanor, during her ongoing illness, until she died in 1997. He remarried when 93 years old to Julia Hardy. He continued to live his life based on his Christian beliefs to the very end, and was a popular, welcoming figure at the Society of Friends. In his spare time, he enjoyed painting and writing poetry.

Hope-Simpson died of old age when 95 years old on 5 July 2003, leaving behind his widow, a daughter and four grandchildren. His written work and his contributions to clinical practice continue to be of use in medicine today. He is fondly remembered by many as one of the best doctors of all time, with Sir Denis Pereira Gray (1935–) declaring

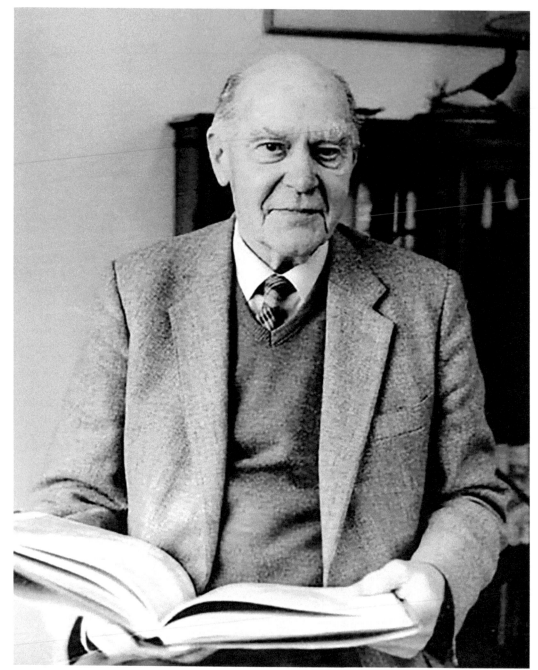

Robert Hope-Simpson. (Courtesy of RCGP Archives, London.)

in Hope-Simpson's obituary that 'Hope-Simpson was one of the outstanding General Practitioner researchers of the twentieth century'.

Further Reading

Hope-Simpson RE. The nature of herpes zoster: A long-term study and a new hypothesis. *Proceedings of the Royal Society of Medicine* 1965;58(1):9–20.

Hope-Simpson RE. *The Transmission of Epidemic Influenza.* New York: Plenum Press; 1992.

Pereira Gray D. Robert Edgar Hope-Simpson. *British Medical Journal* 2003;327(7423):1111.

RCGP Archive. Letters of Hope-Simpson donated to RCGP 1962–66. Box B/HOP. London: RCGP; 2003.

52 RICHARD SCOTT (1914–1984)

Abigail Gittens and Neil Metcalfe

Richard Scott was born on 11 May 1914 in Newtongrange, in the Parish of Newbattle, Midlothian. His parents were Richard Scott, a colliery manager, and Beatrice Scott (née Aitken), who married in 1912. Both parents were upright folk and very active in their local church. He was educated at Beath High School, in the coalfields of Fife, which has a proud record of producing a number of distinguished former pupils, such as the Nobel prizewinner Sir James Black and the United Kingdom's first Minister for the Arts, Jennie Lee, who was married to Aneurin Bevan, Minster of Health at the start of the NHS. Scott went on to study medicine at the University of Edinburgh, graduating MBChB in 1936. In 1938, he was awarded MD with commendation for his thesis 'Anaemia in women of the childbearing period'. In the same year, he received the Lewis Cameron postgraduate prize.

Prior to the outbreak of the Second World War (1939–1945), Scott, in 1939, had spells of work as an assistant in general practice, in Fife, and in hospital medicine, in Edinburgh and Greenock. As a pre-war member of the Territorial Army, he was called up in 1939. He served in the United Kingdom until 1942 and thereafter in North Africa, Sicily, Italy and India, almost entirely in hospital work, latterly as a venereologist. He attained the rank of Lieutenant Colonel.

On demobilisation Scott studied in Edinburgh for a diploma in Public Health and was awarded the medal for the best student. He was then invited, in 1946, by Professor Frank Crew (1886–1973) to become a lecturer in the Department of Public Health and Social Medicine at the University of Edinburgh. Crew recognised that with the imminent arrival of the NHS, in 1948, public dispensaries, which were charitable care services for the sick and poor and used for medical student teaching, would no longer be necessary, as everyone would be entitled to free access to a general practitioner. He realised that this would result in major losses to the education of medical students. Crew encouraged Scott to undertake a project to explore the medical and social needs of families in sickness and health. The objectives of the project were to be the provision of medical services to patients, teaching for medical students and facilities for long-term studies of illness in families. The project was referred to as the 'laboratory in the community'.

The NHS came into being on 5 July 1948. During this year Scott, along with a medical assistant, a dentist, a nurse and an almoner (medical social worker) took over the Royal Public Dispensary of Edinburgh in West Richmond Street and created a teaching practice. Scott was the director of the project and the first students were accepted in October 1948. Each year 30 students attended a course lasting three months with clinical instruction about the social impact of sickness and health.

In March 1950, *The Collings Report* was published in *The Lancet*. It revealed poor standards and training of general practitioners. On 2 December 1950, also in *The Lancet*, Scott published 'A teaching general practice'. In it, he explained how the teaching of general practice had been set up, and how its phased teaching programme gave students some responsibility for patients' care and an understanding of the differences between hospital and general practice. The paper described the change in patient numbers throughout the initial years of the practice, increasing from 195 patients at the end of July 1948 to 1200 in July 1950. Scott decided that the maximum number of registered patients would be around 2000. The practice bordered an overcrowded slum area of the city. Therefore, the majority of the patients were still the very poor who had originally attended the dispensary. However, registration of patients from other areas and university staff created a more diverse list. The inclusion of 400 complete families created an easy resource for teaching and research. The paper stated that the primary concern in teaching was to illustrate the social aspects of health and sickness. He explained that by adopting a team approach the practice was able to look at and manage the social determinants of health as well as disease. The practice even set up a social club for patients and families, an initiative which reflected an interest of Crew's in the Peckham Experiment.

In 1951, Scott obtained a travel bursary from the Rockefeller Foundation that made it possible for him to spend three months in the United States and Canada studying various teaching and community research projects. Later, in 1952, the Rockefeller Foundation gave financial support for the development of general practice as an academic discipline. With this funding, a second University of Edinburgh teaching practice was set up in Edinburgh's Cowgate, based in what had been the Livingstone Memorial Dispensary. This development led to the establishment of the university's General Practice Teaching Unit, with Scott as its director and an enlarged team of doctors and other workers.

In 1956, the General Practice Teaching Unit became the Department of General Practice, an independent department within the University of Edinburgh Medical School. It was the first such department in the world. Then, in 1963, Scott became the first professor of general practice for anywhere in the world, when he accepted the James Mackenzie Chair of Medicine in relation to general practice at the University of Edinburgh. This was a post he held until he retired in 1979, when the university conferred on him the title of professor emeritus. In 1969, the trustees of the Royal Dispensary donated the premises and their remaining funds to the University of Edinburgh. The premises were refurbished as a modern general practice teaching centre and renamed Mackenzie House.

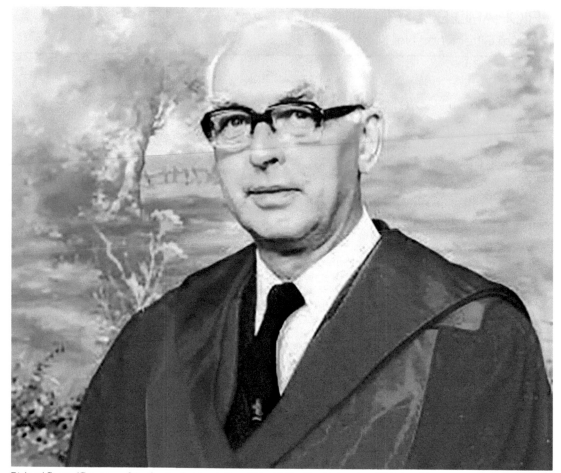

Richard Scott. (Courtesy of the Centre for Population of Health Studies, University of Edinburgh.)

Closest to Scott's satisfaction in creating a first-class University department was his pleasure in helping found the College. He was a member of the steering committee, whose work resulted in the creation of the College, and was a member of its Foundation Council in 1952 to 1953 and remained a Council member until his retirement. He was the first Honorary Secretary of the College's Scottish Council (1953–1968), chairman of the Undergraduate Education Committee (1957–1962, 1968–1972), the 11th Mackenzie Lecturer in 1964 when he gave his lecture entitled 'Medicine in society', awarded fellowship of the College in 1967 and was chair of the RCGP Scottish Council between 1971 and 1974. The RCGP Tartan, presented in 2002, is based on the set of the Scots Tartan in recognition of its contribution to general practice and the RCGP.

Scott was appointed advisor and subsequently consultant to the WHO in 1961 and was elected a member of the College of the Family Physicians of Canada in 1972. In 1979, he was awarded FRCP of Edinburgh. As well as pioneering trainee programmes in the South East of Scotland, he helped transfer the College's Undergraduate Education Committee to the autonomous Association of University Teachers of General Practice of which he was chairman of in the year prior to his retirement. He was awarded the Baron Dr Ver Heyden De Lancey Memorial Award in 1979 for the promotion of efficiency and dignity in general practice.

Scott married Mary Ellen Maclachlan (1918–1987) in 1939. They had three sons and two daughters. Once described as 'never much of a one for top tables', he was witty and engaging in private. At home, when not entertaining visitors to his department from all over the world, he presided over mealtime discussions on every possible subject; he told his family stories and encouraged them to do the same. He liked aphorisms, which he deployed sometimes for comic effect, at other times in all seriousness, such as 'Time spent in reconnaissance is seldom wasted', 'Proficiency at billiards is the sign of misspent youth' and 'Man's chief end is to glorify God and enjoy Him forever'. He loved to cook on the weekends, almost always a pasta dish, inspired by his time in Sicily with the army. Summer holidays and weekends were in a house, cottage or caravan in one of the many beautiful parts of Scotland. He enjoyed watching football with members of his family. He attached great importance to his involvement with the Samaritans, the Cyrenians and, in his retirement, with the Edinburgh University Settlement.

People who knew him well have highlighted Scott's quiet modesty and unselfishness, often resulting in credit for his ideas and actions going elsewhere. They also mention the tenacity of purpose and strength of will, which lay behind the deceptively quiet exterior. His career is still admired, being acknowledged posthumously when on 15 June 2017 the RCP in conjunction with the University of Edinburgh unveiled a blue plaque for Scott at Mackenzie House.

Scott was no showman, but he tirelessly pled the case for general practice to be given the attention it required. He wanted general practitioners to be given the 'time, tools and training' to do their job. He died at 69 years of age on 28 November 1983. His minister, at the funeral, spoke of the three attributes that made up the greater part of him: physician, teacher and family man. When Scott retired, his successor Professor John Howie (1937–) quite simply said of him that he had taken academic general practice from nowhere to somewhere. The profession owes him much.

Further Reading

Anon. Richard Scott MD Edin, FRCP, FRCGP. *The Lancet* 1984;323(8367):58–59.

Howie J, Whitfield M (eds.). *Academic General Practice in the UK Medical Schools, 1948–2000: A Short History*. Edinburgh: Edinburgh University Press; 2011.

Milnes-Smith P. Professor Richard Scott: Celebrating the first professor of general practice in the world. *British Journal of General Practice* 2017;67(662):410.

Scott R. A teaching general practice. *The Lancet* 1950;2(6640):695–98.

Scott R. Medicine in society. *The Journal of the College of General Practitioners* 1965;9(1):3–16.

Thomson DM. General practice and the Edinburgh Medical School: 200 years of teaching, care and research. *The Journal of the Royal College of General Practitioners* 1984;34:9–12.

53 RICHARD MAURICE SOTHERON MCCONAGHEY (1906–1975)

Chanu Gunasekara and Neil Metcalfe

Richard Maurice Sotheron McConaghey (well known as Mac) was born in India in 1906 to a military family. Following his family's legacy, McConaghey served the RAMC during the Second World War (1939–1945). During this time he rose to the rank of lieutenant colonel, which was a reflection of the discipline and perseverance he possessed as an individual. He was known to be a family man and was very much supported by his wife who was a woman with formidable resilience who accommodated the demands that the College made of him. He was also an intellectual with a great passion for reading and acquiring knowledge. This enabled him to foresee the need for the establishment of a separate college and a journal for general practice.

Following his contribution to the Army during the war, McConaghey completed his MD at the University of Edinburgh in 1947 and began his interest in medical writing. His thesis was titled 'Headache – A study of pain' and was based on notes on 100 cases he observed in his own practice throughout 1946. Following this he moved to Dartmouth in Devon where he worked as a general practitioner. He was also part of the standing committee of the Devon local medical committee and on the standing committee of the Devon and Exeter executive committee, the predecessor to the family practitioner committee. By being part of these governing bodies he was able to gain much experience of the various complaints against doctors, which he identified as an after-effect of the lack of an academic basis and the urgency of its formation.

In 1952, McConaghey was approached by John Hunt (1905–1987) and was given the opportunity to be part of the Foundation Council of the College. Accepting this invitation was the highlight of his career, giving him the opportunity to become one of the 23 who sat on the first council that year. By serving and chairing committees such as the awards committee, the library committee, the publications committees and the editorial board, he played a pivotal role in the early days of the College. In 1953, he was elected vice-chairman of the first faculty board of the South West England Faculty and subsequently became provost in 1958.

McConaghey is best known for his editorship of the *Journal of the College of General Practitioners*. At a time when the work of general practitioners was not recorded or passed down the generations, the formation of the College facilitated the existence of a research committee. This committee quickly identified the need for communication between general practitioners and a newsletter entitled *Between Ourselves* was introduced under the guidance of Robin Pinsent (1916–1987). McConaghey worked alongside Pinsent for the third edition of the newsletter. In 1954, McConaghey was asked to take up the post of editor when Pinsent fell ill.

Looking back on when the College was founded McConaghey expressed in the *BMJ* that 'Everything that is worthwhile is worth the struggle and hard work necessary for its attainment. It is up to general practitioners themselves to start work at once'. When he took over from Pinsent he stated that he did so with much apprehension and 'with no previous experience of editing, little of writing, a complete ignorance of the niceties of punctuation and an inherent inability to spell, I felt singularly ill-equipped for the job'.

McConaghey worked as the second honorary editor of *Between Ourselves* from 1954 to 1957. Members of his first editorial board all had the striking resemblance of having obtained MD, and with their support he worked diligently to make the newsletter to be more than just a vehicle for communication. Although he had the liberty of creating a journal which would act as a vehicle either for news, review or original articles of scientific record, he purposefully chose the most difficult and challenging choice: he chose a journal of scientific record. One of the first revolutionary changes he made was to campaign for the removal of the 'not for publication' mark and expand the limited circulation of the newsletter between members of the research group to include all members of the College. By 1958, the newsletter was renamed as the *Journal of the College of General Practitioners Research Newsletter* (*Journal*) and the pages were first sewn together and a spine was created on which the title appeared.

McConaghey also fiercely insisted that all articles published in the *Journal* were peer-reviewed. Peer-reviewing was a relatively new concept at this time and most college members did not comprehend the need for peer-review of articles by general practitioners. Articles submitted were also of poor quality and many were hand written and lacked references. As committed as he was to his role as the editor, at numerous occasions he took it upon himself to rewrite papers and add references from his own extensive library. He also published supplements when he felt it was needed. He was always greatly helped and loyally supported by the *Journal's* first business manager, Miss Irene Scawn. He strove for quality rather than quantity and the *Journal* became the academic voice of general practice.

In 1961, McConaghey's diligence and commitment to the *Journal* led it to be accepted by the *Index Medicus*. At the time this was the hallmark of acceptance of a scientific journal and gave the *Journal* the honour of being the first internationally recognised scientific journal of general practice.

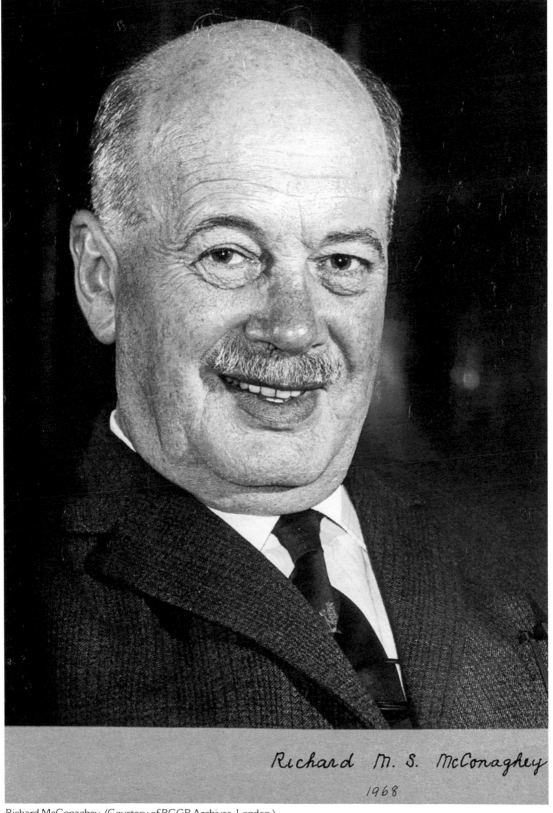

Richard M. S. McConaghey

1968

Richard McConaghey. (Courtesy of RCGP Archives, London.)

With every little effort adding up McConaghey was able to bring the *Journal* to become a working example of steadily rising academic standards. The *Journal* gave British general practitioners a head start in publishing, encouraging them to write for it. In 1964, he noticed a rise in the quality and quantitiy of the material he was receiving and justified an increase of the publication of the *Journal* from quarterly to bimonthly without a significant increase in his editorial board or staff. In 1967, the prefix 'Royal' was incorporated renaming it the *Journal of the Royal College of General Practitioners* and the publication frequency was increased to monthly volumes.

Further roles were undertaken and awards earned. McConaghey was Chairman of the Board of Censors (1955–1959) which later became the College's Assessment Committee. In 1964, he had the honour of delivering the Gale Memorial Lecture entitled 'Medical ethics in a changing world' and the 12th James Mackenzie Lecture thereafter, in 1965, entitled 'Medical practice in the days of Mackenzie'. In the same year he was appointed OBE. He was on the first list of Fellows of the College in 1967, and, in 1970, was the first ever recipient of the George Abercrombie Award, given for exceptional contribution to the literature of general practice.

In 1971, McConaghey retired from his post as editor of the *Journal*. In his 17 years in this honorary role, a length of service in this particular role that has not since been equalled, he was able to achieve his ambition of creating a scientific journal for general practitioners, written and edited by general practitioners. Away from medicine he played a big part in the life of Dartmouth, where he worked with the St John's Ambulance Brigade and founded the Dartmouth League of Friends and the Dartmouth Rotary Club. He also helped to create the Northcott Medical Foundation. His presidency of the Dartmouth Swimming Club was illustrated to his many visitors who were often pressed to join him in a cold early morning bathe in the Dart.

On 21 August 1975, McConaghey died, aged 67 years old in his home in Dartmouth, leaving behind his wife and two daughters. Prior to his death the Editorial Board arranged for the *Journal* to carry the words 'Founding Editor: RMS McConaghey' and his successor took a proof to him so that he saw it before he died. In June 2008 the RCGP unveiled their first ever blue plaque in his honour.

Further Reading

McConaghey RM. Medical practice in the days of Mackenzie. *The Journal of the College of General Practitioners* 1966;11(1):3–20.

McConaghey RM. Proposals to found a Royal College of General Practitioners in the nineteenth century. *The Journal of the Royal College of General Practitioners* 1972;22(124):775–88.

McConaghey RMS. Si monumentum requiris, circumspice [Editorial]. *The Journal of the Royal College of General Practitioners* 1972;22(114):1–4.

Pereira Gray D. Mac. Editorial. *The Journal of the Royal College of General Practitioners* 1975;25:627–29.

Pereira Gray D. The emergence of the discipline of general practice; its literature and the contribution of the College Journal. McConaghey Memorial Lecture 1988. *The Journal of the Royal College of General Practitioners* 1989;39:228–33.

54 JOHN FRENCH BURDON (1915–2000)

Odon Nsungu and Neil Metcalfe

John French Burdon was born on 15 March 1915 in the town of Hartlepool, County Durham. His father was a house and church decorator and his mother a housewife. He attended Durham University College of Medicine, from where he qualified MBBS, in 1938.

After qualifying, Burdon joined the RNVR in 1940, where he served as acting surgeon-lieutenant for six years. Whilst serving in the RNVR, he developed an interest in psychiatry, documenting his observations and events that occurred whilst he was deployed. Two of his publications discussing the psychological changes he experienced and the psychiatric conditions experienced by naval personnel were published in *The British Journal of Psychiatry* and *Journal of the Royal Naval Medical Service*. After leaving the RNVR, he opened a general practice in Paignton, Devon, where he practised until his retirement. In 1956, he received a diploma in Anaesthetics and began administering anaesthetics at the hospital in Paignton.

The College was founded on 19 November 1952. The *Annual Report* was published annually from the College's creation and had the aim to outline the activities of the College, the Council, committees and faculties. The report was sent to fellows, members and associates of the College. John Hunt (1905–1987), the Honorary Secretary of the council, was the editor of the *Annual Report* (1952–1958) and Burdon became the assistant editor in 1957. In 1959, Burdon became the honorary editor of the *Annual Report* and remained in the position until 1981, making him at the end of his service the then longest serving honorary editor for the College before Denis Pereira Gray (1935–) elapsed this when contributing 25 years of such service. He became a member of College Council in 1967, which he served until 1979.

In order to help general practitioners publish and share their research on subjects relevant to general practice, the College started producing *Research Newsletter* in 1953. *Research Newsletter* was produced four times a year and Richard McConaghey (1906–1975) was elected as editor. In the years that followed, the *Research Newsletter* developed from containing solely research to general material on general practice. This change was marked when, under McConaghey, the title changed in 1958, in the 18th issue, to *Journal and Research Newsletter*. In 1960, the name changed again, this time to *Journal of the Royal College of Practitioners* (*Journal*) and Burdon was named the assistant editor of it. In 1967, he joined the Editorial Board which was the same year that the journal's name changed to the *Journal of the Royal College of General Practitioners*.

Burdon felt strongly about vocational training and the continued education of general practitioners. He made several suggestions on how postgraduates could be trained for a career in general practice. Through journal articles, he emphasised the importance of starting general practitioner training at an early stage. He proposed that this be done by exposing medical undergraduates to general practice and teaching them the key skills they would require on a daily basis. He highlighted several key skills that doctors needed to acquire. He, first of all, saw the first skill being excellent communication skills. He saw communication skills as vital for dealing with the variety of situations that general practitioners faced. Secondly, training in prescribing medication was another key skill that needed to be covered. Thirdly, he focused on educating medical students on the challenges they might face, such as pressure from the patient to prescribe a medication that might not be necessary or pressures from pharmaceutical representatives. Furthermore, he believed medical students, potential future general practitioners, needed a strong understanding of the NHS and the services available for patients. In 1959, he proposed the use of an examination for membership in the College by writing an article in the *Journal of the College of General Practitioners Research Newsletter*. The purpose of the examination would be to:

Test knowledge of family doctoring, and thus serve to indicate technical competence.
Provide a syllabus which would influence future standards of skill and scope for the family doctor.
Give additional prestige and academic status to the College.
Make entry more difficult, even for those the College would welcome as members.
Make membership more valuable, thus offsetting the effect of making it more difficult to obtain.

Burdon went on to remark 'the vital question now facing the College would seem to be: When do we start examining?' He became chairman of the Board of Censors (1963–1967), later the Assessment Committee, whose work did a lot in the preparation and creation of the MRCGP. The policy of creating the MRCGP had multiple supporters as well as opponents but his work and that of the Board of Censors is credited with the aid of hindsight as having been far-sighted. The MRCGP came into use in 1965 and was then adopted as the sole entry to membership of the College in 1967, which was the same year that was awarded College Fellowship.

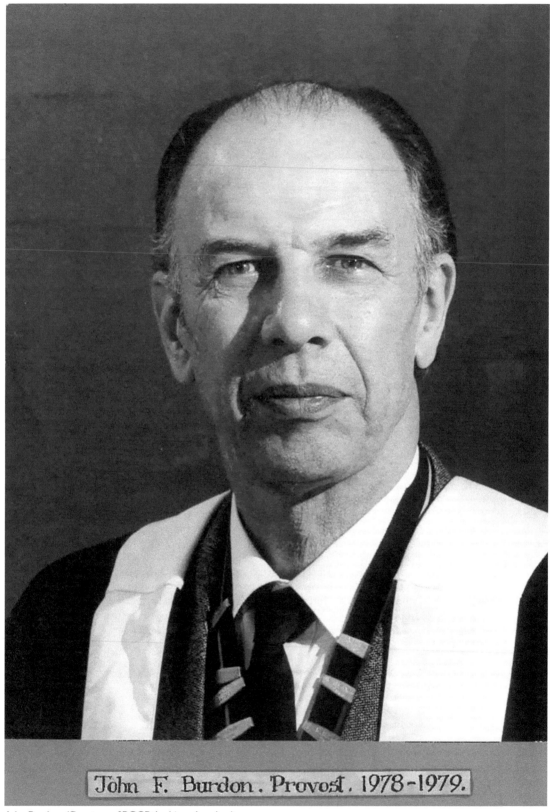

John F. Burdon. Provost. 1978-1979.

John Burdon. (Courtesy of RCGP Archives, London.)

Burdon had further roles within the College. He was an active member of the College's South West England Faculty and served as the chairman of that faculty from 1974 to 1976 and was also provost from 1978 to 1979, the highest honorary post in one of the biggest Faculties in the College. He was involved with arranging undergraduate education such as lectures, discussions and student attachments to practices. He was awarded the George Abercrombie Award in 1982 for his contribution to the literature of general practice.

Away from his activities with the College, Burdon was also one of the 44 doctors and managers who had an input into the Medical Services Review Committee. This committee produced the *Porritt Report* in 1962. It was one of the first reports to scrutinise the NHS and was part of the Hospital Plan of the Minister of Health, Enoch Powell. The Report criticised the separation of NHS services into hospital, general practices and local authorities and called for them to be reorganised. The Hospital Plan approved the development of large district general hospitals for population areas of about 125,000 people. This was a massive project never seen before. Cost and time implications were severely underestimated though the introduction of postgraduate centres improved the training and career prospects for both doctors and nurses.

When he retired to Denbury near Newton Abbot, Burdon edited the parish magazine with his usual care and became a general handyman to the parish. He died on 5 January 2000 leaving behind his wife, Elizabeth. He was an influential figure in the early years of the College. He was a far-sighted college activist who worked hard for the College nationally and locally in developing criteria for entry for MRCGP and who edited the Colleges *Annual Reports* for many years with rare attention to detail.

Further Reading

Anon. Porritt Report on N.H.S. *British Medical Journal* 1962;2:1171–73.

Burdon JF. Foreign service neurosis. *The British Journal of Psychiatry* 1944;90(380):746–52.

Burdon JF. A psychiatric survey of naval personnel. *Journal of the Royal Naval Medical Service* 1945;31:248–52.

Burdon JF. Entry by examination. *The Journal of the College of General Practitioners Research Newsletter* 1959;2(3):299–300.

Fry J, Hunt Lord of Fawley, Pinsent RJF (eds.). *A History of the Royal College of General Practitioners: The First 25 Years*. Lancaster: MTP Press; 1983.

55 CUTHBERT ARTHUR HARRY WATTS (1910–1998)

Joanna Legg

Cuthbert Arthur Harry Watts (well known as Arthur) was born in Shildon, County Durham, on 6 January 1910. He was the only son and youngest of six children born to Harry and Mary Watts. His father was a clergyman and they lived on Swinburne Road in Darlington with their servant. His grandfather was also a clergyman and the vice-principal of Durham Training College of Clergymen. Although Watts did not follow in the family tradition and become a clergyman himself, his Christian faith was important to him throughout his life.

Watts completed his medical training at the Durham University Medical School, where he graduated in July 1934 with MBBS. In June 1937, he married Beatrice Mary Axton (1911–1988), the two of them having met when both at medical school.

Immediately after qualifying, Watts undertook two house appointments at the Royal Victoria Infirmary (RVI), Newcastle. These were in both surgery and medicine and he was paid £50 a year for these appointments. He was especially keen to experience working in the maternity unit as his ambition was to become a general practitioner with a specialist interest in obstetrics. However, during his house appointments, he began to develop an interest in psychiatry. During his time there he worked under Horsley Drummond (1881–1959), a physician who influenced psychiatry at the RVI. He witnessed Drummond using Corrigan's Button, which was cautery used for a shock treatment in psychiatric patients, and Watts was largely unimpressed by this technique.

Watt's Christian faith influenced his next decision to move to South Africa in 1938 where he began working at St. Mary's Hospital. This was a missionary hospital in Zululand. He continued to work there alongside his wife until the outbreak of the Second World War (1939–1945). At this time, he joined the South African Medical Corps (SAMC). It was whilst serving in the army that Watts furthered his interest in mental health; he was invited to go on a psychiatric course at the Neuropsychiatric Centre of the SAMC at Potchefstroom. He spent a year working at the centre where he was able to observe a large range of psychiatric illnesses and was able to practise psychotherapy. At heart, he was a family doctor and he never wanted to become a full-time psychiatrist but instead wanted to use his experiences in the field and apply it to general practice once the war was over.

Upon demobilisation in 1946, Watts settled into a country practice at Ibstock in Leicestershire. Here he realised that psychoneurosis was not rare. Many of these patients looked to him for the help that they were unable to receive at the hospital, where they were treated with an attitude of rejection and seen as a nuisance.

Over time Watts developed a strong interest in depression. He was one of the first doctors to recognise it as a medical condition and identify its symptoms. He noted that the books available on psychiatry were largely unreadable by the ordinary doctor, and succeeded in changing this, publishing several books during the course of his career. His first book, *Psychiatry in General Practice*, was published in 1952 and in it he mentions that for each case of depression there are several more undiagnosed. This is something he realised, on reflection many years later, and due to his interest in the condition, that he had missed a case of severe depression in his earlier career when investigations on a male patient with constipation were negative, he had granted the patient a clean bill of health only for the patient to go straight home and commit suicide by placing his head in a gas oven. His book, however, also described how he hoped for greater consideration of psychiatric patients and removal of the associated stigma that they had. Within the same book he also challenged the idea that psychiatric patients were solely the responsibility of psychiatrists. He emphasised the importance of managing such patients in general practice, stating that only a tenth of these patients would require the input of a consultant.

Watts not only helped spread mental health knowledge into general practice but in 1952, he became one of the founder members of the College. He was very active in his membership and was one of the first members to be made a fellow. He was appointed OBE in 1969. He was awarded the James Mackenzie Award in 1971 and, in 1993, the George Abercrombie Award for his contribution to the literature of general practice. He was also commended by the Royal College of Psychiatrists and was made an Honorary Fellow of that college on his retirement. He is still recognised today by the Leicester Faculty of the RCGP who award the Arthur Watts Prize to an outstanding fourth year medical student for best overall performance in all aspects of the clinical methods course.

Watts retired in 1975 and enjoyed his retirement filling it with travel and walking holidays especially in the Lake District. He also enjoyed playing bridge and entertaining his many friends. Although he had spent his life as a practising Christian, in his later years he became dissatisfied with the ritual of conventional worship and turned to the Quakers, whose companionship and simple style of worship he found great comfort in. He was predeceased by his wife and died on 1 January 1998. He was survived by his four children, including his daughter Margaret Frances Williams (1940–) who became a general practitioner, 10 grandchildren, including Jane Povey (1968–), a general practitioner and two great grandchildren.

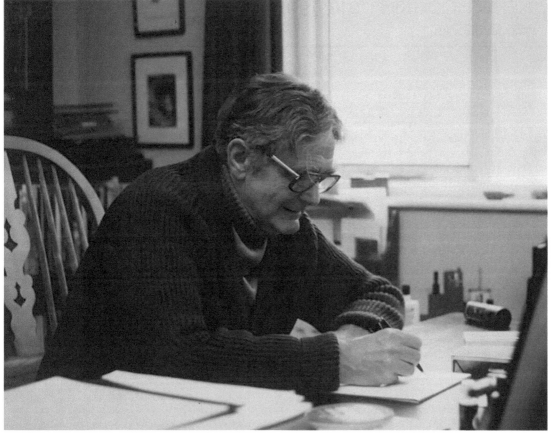

Arthur Watts working in his study. (Courtesy of Margaret Frances Williams; née Watts.)

Further Reading

Cooter R, Pickstone J. *Companion to Medicine in the Twentieth Century*. London: Routledge; 2003.

Watts CAH, Watts BM. *Psychiatry in General Practice*. London: J & A Churchill; 1952.

Watts CAH. *Depressive Disorders in the Community*. Bristol: John Wright & Sons; 1966.

Watts CAH. General practice. *British Medical Journal* 1979;2:1055–56.

Williams MF. Obituary Arthur Watts. *British Medical Journal* 1998;316(7135):941.

56 KEITH HODGKIN (1918–1999)
Imogen Monks

George Keith Howard Hodgkin was born on 30 May 1918 to parents George and Mary. Just over three weeks later his father died of typhoid. His early life was spent in Banbury, Oxfordshire, where he lived until 1933 and he attended the Dragon School, a large co-educational prep school. In 1931, he attended Gresham School, until his mother remarried and the family moved to Edinburgh. After finishing school, in 1936, he began his university studies at Magdelan College, University of Oxford, where he remained between 1936 and 1939. He gained a second-class degree in physiology and then went on to study medicine, graduating BM in 1942 and then doing his house jobs at Hammersmith Hospital. When the Second World War (1939–1945) broke out, Hodgkin declared himself to be a conscientious objector, but as he was a medical student who had been born before 1 June 1918 he was in a group exempted from conscription. However, in 1943, he changed this decision and became a surgeon lieutenant in the navy, serving from 1943 to 1946. After this, in 1947, he worked in Oxford as a pathologist for a year. In 1946, he married Ro (née Candler) and this partnership lay at the centre of all his subsequent happiness and success.

Hodgkin became a general practitioner in 1949 and began this part of his career in Stockton, Durham. In 1952, he moved to Redcar and founded a practice. The practice at Redcar was where he began to develop his most notable book, *Towards Earlier Diagnosis* (1963) with the help of his partners there. The inspiration for the book came from his difficulties and mistakes he made whilst starting his career, and indeed later on, as a general practitioner. He mainly blamed this on his hospital-based medical training, which he felt ill-prepared graduates for work as a general practitioner. As quoted from this book:

> Firstly many of the common problems of general practice are never encountered in hospital so that the new entrant is forced to learn his job by time-consuming trial and error methods. Even the basic principles are of limited use until the doctor is aware of the different emphasis of his new environment, e.g. the simple guide *that common diseases occur most often* cannot be applied until he *knows* the common disorders.

He recognised that the types of illness seen in general practice were broadly dissimilar to those seen in hospital, and the need to diagnose conditions in their earliest forms in general practice was a challenge for those who had only experienced hospital medicine. The book went on to have five editions and is credited with influencing the distinction between the work of hospital medicine and general practice.

Hodgkin's contribution to record-keeping in general practice has significantly influenced the way general practitioners document in the medical records of patients today. He attributed his early habit of record-keeping to one of his professors at medical school, Sir Arthur Hirst (1879–1944). Hirst suggested to Hodgkin that the best way to learn medicine was to keep your own records on every 'case' seen. This sparked his extensive and thorough record-keeping throughout his career for which he is widely known and led to his aforementioned book *Towards Earlier Diagnosis*. In 1953, he realised that record-keeping in general practice was unsatisfactory and that there was a need to document the diagnostic reasons for all the actions they were advising. He saw the lack of simple summaries of diagnosis and treatments as inextricably linked to poor record-keeping:

> These failures will only be corrected when the profession ceases to pay lip service to the importance of the record and accepts the simple truth that good medicine cannot be practised without logical, well-kept practical records, in which diagnostic predictions and problems are clearly stated and related to clinical findings and managerial decisions.

Later on in his career Hodgkin had a variety of roles. He moved to Newfoundland, Canada, where he became professor and chair of family medicine at the Memorial University from 1973 to 1978. There he was able to set up a department of general practice and revelled in the opportunity this gave him to watch ospreys fishing outside of committee meeting windows.

On his return to England he took an active role at the RCGP. This was not a new association for he had been the 16th James Mackenzie Lecture in 1969 when he presented 'Behaviour: The community and the general practitioner'. However, his contribution on his return was mainly with the Examination Committee and he helped develop oral and written parts of the exams from 1978 to 1985. By then he had co-authored *Problem-Centred Learning: the Modified Essay Question in Medical Education* (1975). He also became a visiting professor for Glasgow Medical School (1973), Dundee Medical School (1978) and also lectured at the University of Western Australia (1982). Towards the end of his career he took up the position of medical advisor for *Reader's Digest*. For his contribution to medical literature he was awarded the George Abercrombie Award in 1986. This did not mean the end of his writing for he enthusiastically pursued 'The uncertainties, mistakes, dilemmas and other contributions to a happy and shared family life', which he wrote in the years 1992 to 1994. He even joked with family and friends about writing a book on 'electronics for the elderly' just before he died. He died of coronary heart disease on 2 June 1999, leaving his wife and three children with his son Paul (1951–) ultimately following him into general practice.

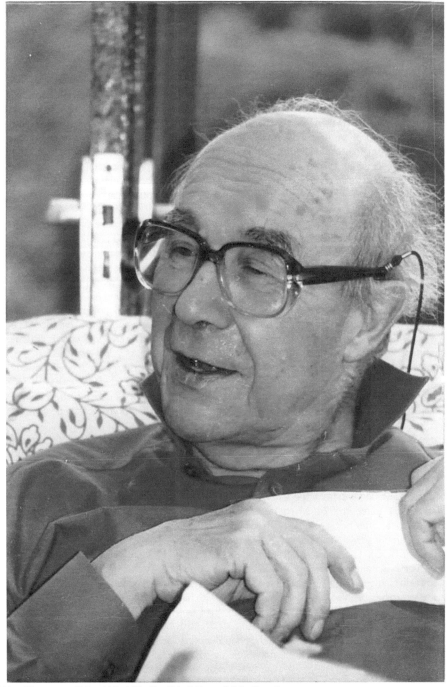

Keith Hodgkin. (Courtesy of Hazel Hodgkin, Paul Hodgkin and Julie Steer.)

Further Reading

Hodgkin GKH. Behaviour: The community and the general practitioner. *The Journal of the Royal College of General Practitioners* 1970;90:5–11.

Hodgkin K. *Towards Earlier Diagnosis: A Family Doctors Approach*. London: E&S Livingstone; 1963.

Hodgkin K, Knox JDE. *Problem-Centred Learning: The Modified Essay Question in Medical Education: A Handbook for Students, Teachers and Trainers*. London: E&S Livingstone; 1975.

Wellcome Library Archive. Reference box GP/25/1. *Keith's family record 1918–1994. The uncertainties, mistakes, dilemmas and other contributions to a happy and shared family life.*

57 DAVID MORRELL (1929–2012)
Adam Davies and Mason McGlynn

David Cameron Morrell was born on 6 November 1929 in Wimbledon, London, to parents William and Violet Morrell. His background was that of a strictly adherent Roman Catholic, both at home and his schools which were Presentation College (now Elvian School, Reading) and then Wimbledon College, London. He began his medical training at St Mary's Medical School, London, in 1947, one year before the start of the NHS. He graduated in 1952, shortly before marrying Joyce (née Eaton-Taylor), with whom he raised five children.

Following his graduation, Morrell performed a short service at the Royal Air Force Hospital, Ely, Cambridgeshire, between 1954 and 1957. During his service he was promoted to Flight Lieutenant, and was awarded MRCGP in 1955. In 1957, following his time at Ely. He began his first job as a general practitioner at a practice in Hoddesden, Hertfordshire, where he worked for five years.

In 1963, Morrell moved to Edinburgh. Here he undertook a role in the general practice department at the university, a department amongst the first of its kind in the development of medical education and practice-based research. It was here, in 1963, that he was first introduced to Richard Scott (1914–1983), the world's first professor of general practice. These two, amongst others, worked in a practice on West Richmond Street. This was a unique establishment combining clinical practice with teaching and research. Morrell would later transport this model of practice, and work to refine it at Guy's and St Thomas' Hospital in London, when he relocated to Lambeth in 1967.

In 1966, Morrell published *The Art of General Practice*, a seminal work in the development of teaching general practice, and arguably one of his most important contributions to academic medicine and general practice. The book would go on to have many further editions and was to be translated into Arabic, Dutch and Swedish. It comprised chapters on the characteristics of general practice: problem solving, history taking, physical examination, prognosis and treatment, the prevention of disease and the primary care team. The book was an early representation of the academic and clinician that he wanted himself to be, standing very much alongside his previous work with Scott, on research, teaching and clinical practice. Whilst itself didactic, this book, a compendium of case histories, yielded what he had learnt in the early portion of his career. It was intended in this sense as a tool for medical students and young doctors.

When Morrell moved to Guy's and St Thomas' Hospital in 1967, he developed the first department of general practice to exist there, bringing with him the aforementioned model of academic clinical practice. Here he was appointed as senior lecturer. The department was expanded following the publication of four papers describing the critical differences between care in the hospital and care in the community. The papers led to Sir George Godber (1908–2009), amongst others, requesting further development from the Wolfson Foundation in conjunction with the British Academy for growth of the department. Later, in 1974, Morrell was appointed as a Wolfson professor of general practice at Guy's and St Thomas' Hospital, after being awarded FRCGP in 1972. Here he worked with Martin Roland (1951–), a general practitioner in Cambridge who had recently worked with a team to develop the Cambridge Community Based Clinical Course (CCBCC). The course involved students following individual patients from the community through the course of their hospital stays. The CCBCC contributed to an increased cognisance and prominence of academic general practice in Cambridge. Following this, a national shift in attitudes around teaching methods employed within general practice was to be observed. This, very much in line with his work and aspiration, enabled him to work with Roland, and the two continued their work as academics and clinicians for those around the Lambeth Walk and Kennington Road area.

Over his career, Morrell made many further noteworthy contributions to academic general practice. One of these involved a collaboration with Professor Walter Holland (1929–) in the field of epidemiological research. Holland, himself head of the department of clinical epidemiology at St Thomas', and his team provided much of the academic support for Morrell's research in 1979, which later led Morrell to co-edit the book *Teaching General Practice* (1981), as well as editing *Epidemiology in General Practice* (1988), a book based on his own research. The book went on to be deemed a 'landmark' publication in the field and was met with favour by readers and publishers alike.

Morrell received numerous accreditations in recognition for his advancement of academic general practice later in his career. In 1979, he was invited to deliver the William Pickles Lecture, which he did, entitled 'Now and then'. In 1982, he was appointed OBE in commemoration of his service to general practice, and in the same year received a papal knighthood, for contributions to the care of the sick and disabled on the Lourdes Pilgrimage. He was awarded the Baron Dr Ver Heyden De Lancey Memorial Award in 1985 and was appointed the first chairman of the academic advisory board in general practice at the University of London. He was later appointed sub-dean at St Thomas' Hospital Medical School from 1984 to 1989, and chairman of the Education Committee of the United Medical and Dental Schools of Guy's and St Thomas'. He was also made a Fellow of the Faculty of Public Health in 1986,

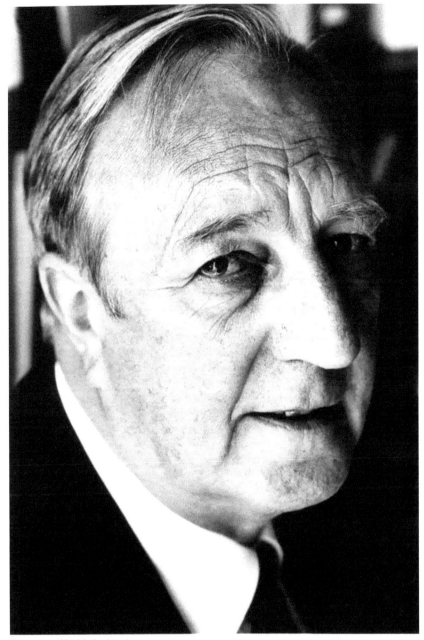

David Morrell. (Courtesy of BMA Archive.)

and was appointed chairman deputy of general practice for the United Medical and Dental Schools, London, from 1988 until his retirement.

In 1993, Morrell published *Diagnosis in General Practice: Art or Science* shortly before retiring. The publication was centred on the development of diagnostic techniques in general practice over the 40 years that Morrell had worked within the field. In 1994, following his retirement, he was elected president of the BMA, a post he occupied between 1994 and 1995. In his presidential address, on 6 July 1994, he concluded: 'Can the BMA – and that means not just the Officers, but all its Members, as in 1965, lead us out of the mire of market place medicine to the high ground of professional medical care? That is the end to which I will address myself during my period of office as your President'.

Morrell died on 19 March 2012. His obituary published in the *BMJ* reflected on his presidential address by describing it as 'a prescient, almost prophetic comment, perhaps containing the key to the enormous impact David made on all aspects of academic primary care'. The obituary described him maybe not the last, 'but he was certainly the embodiment of the now almost extinct three stranded clinical academic-clinician, researcher and teacher. He changed the course of general practice in all three areas'.

Further Reading

Holland W. *Improving Health Services Background, Method and Applications*. London: Edward Elgar Publishing; 2013.

Howie J, Whitfield M (eds.). *Academic General Practice in the UK Medical Schools, 1948–2000: A Short History*. Edinburgh: Edinburgh University Press; 2011.

Jones R. David Morrell. *British Medical Journal* 2012;344:36.

Morrell D. *The Art of General Practice*. London: Faber; 1966.

Morrell D. William Pickles Lecture 1979. Now and then. *The Journal of the Royal College of General Practitioners* 1979;29(205):457–65.

Morrell D. *Diagnosis in General Practice: Art or Science?* London: Nuffield Provincial Hospitals Trusts; 1993.

Petchey R. General practice under the National Health Service, 1948–1997. *British Medical Journal* 1998;317:357.

Thomson DM. General practice and the Edinburgh Medical School: 200 years of teaching, care and research. *The Journal of the Royal College of General Practitioners* 1984;34:9–12.

58 SOLOMON WAND (1899–1984)

Alaina Halim

Solomon Wand was born in Manchester on 14 January 1899, the son of a merchant. He attended Manchester Grammar School before reading medicine at the University of Manchester. He was awarded an overall distinction for his medical degree, which he received in 1921. Upon qualifying as a doctor, he worked in Balsall Heath in Birmingham in a practice which has since been renamed The Wand Medical Centre to commemorate him. Over the next 50 years, he undertook a fulfilling career with various roles that helped to influence the future of health care for generations to come.

Wand joined the BMA Council in 1935, a move that essentially shaped the rest of his career. He was an active member of the council and played a part in many committees throughout his 37 years with the BMA. In the same year as the formation of the NHS in 1948, he became chairman of the GMSC. The fundamental feature of the NHS was the '100% principle', which meant that it would be a free health service available to everyone in the country. Wand was known to regret the acceptance of this principle as he, and many other doctors, felt that changes were being made too quickly. Regarding the introduction of the NHS, he later recalled in 1978, 'I had the feeling that he [Bevan] wanted to be the architect of the finished structure. That is why he went for the lot. That was the biggest mistake and we urged him to go slowly. He should have done it step by step'.

Before the establishment of the NHS, Wand was happy with the structure of general practice in Birmingham, particularly the Birmingham Public Medical Service. This service allowed the collection of regular prescriptions and offered lower fees to those with special circumstances. Moreover, free hospital care was available to a certain extent, which led to the establishment of the Birmingham Accident Hospital. Although general practitioner earnings were relatively low, the service seemed to work well for the community, and so his reluctance for the '100% principle' NHS to take over has been contemplated to have been possibly justified.

In 1948, general practitioners in the United Kingdom agreed to work in the NHS, but there were disagreements surrounding their remunerations. Wand, due to his role with the GMSC, argued that this should be 100 per cent, but the Ministry of Health disagreed. After much disagreement, this resulted in the Danckwerts Award of 1952, when Wand and Derek Stevenson (1911–2001), then Secretary of the BMA, between them trounced the government of the day and achieved a victory for general practice. This was that the 'betterment' to be applied to the 1939 remuneration of general practitioners should be 100 per cent, unequalled before or since. This increased the pay of general practitioners and it was mentioned in Wand's obituary in the *BMJ* that the Ministry of Health had likely never forgiven him for his victory.

As remuneration negotiations were taking place, Wand's wife, Claire, became terminally ill and passed away in 1951. The couple had two children together: their daughter, Jill, and their son Laurence (1924–2012), who became a general practitioner. This was a difficult time for Wand as he was understandably devastated by his loss. He and Stevenson received monetary awards for their services to the medical profession in 1953 and they decided to set up a trust fund, which would help to further the education of general practitioners and provide scholarships. The pair agreed to name it the Claire Wand Fund.

In 1954, the BMA awarded Wand their gold medal, the highest award they offer. This medal was in celebration of his achievements for both the BMA and for general practice as an entity. Additionally, the BMA wanted it to be a means of thanking him for his dedication to it and his participation in an unparalleled number of positions in various committees throughout the years. Although not known at the time of this award, Wand was later to become the only person to have held all three of the senior positions in the BMA: chairman of the Representative Body (1951–1954), chairman of Council (1956–1961) and treasurer (1963–1972).

Although he was best known for his work within medical politics and general practice, Wand was also concerned with other aspects of the community. In addition to his membership of the Education Act Committee and the Financial Hardship Committee of the BMA, he was a prominent member of the Occupational Health Committee, which produced a report on the industrial health in factories, considering the health care needs of labourers. Wand also participated in work with Family Doctor Publications for many years; he later became chairman and oversaw the production of *You and Your Baby* in 1968, an informative book for new parents. Furthermore, he was on the Committee of Medical Schools and became Honorary Vice-President of the British Medical Students Association in 1959, a role which he took great pleasure in, as he was eager to help young people to achieve their ambitions of becoming the doctors of tomorrow through mentoring and support.

Throughout his career, Wand received multiple forms of recognition for his achievements. This included honorary degrees, such as a doctorate of civil law from Durham University in 1957, and an LLD from Queen's University in Belfast in 1962. However, he was said to be most proud of his honorary LLD from University of Birmingham in 1984, as this was the city in which he spent the majority of his career. Additionally, Wand received fellowship of the College in 1964, and, in 1980, he became a Fellow of the BMA. He was appointed OBE in 1983.

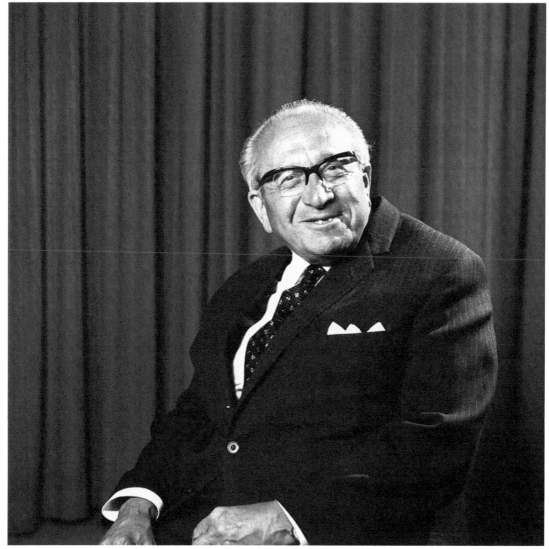

Solomon Wand. (Courtesy of BMA Archive.)

He was widely known as a strong negotiator with a good-willed character. Through his passion for general practice, he was highly motivated in his work and helped to mould the NHS into what it is today. His loyalty to his colleagues and his profession was admired by those who knew him and he received some of the most prestigious forms of recognition for his medical work. He married his second wife, Shaunagh, in 1960 and they spent 24 years happily married, enjoying shared hobbies such as travelling. He died on 16 September 1984. He is notably remembered for his dedication to the BMA and contributions to the medical profession.

Further Reading

Anon. Forty million pounds. *British Medical Journal* 1952;1(4760):697–98.

Anon. Thirty years ago: Six doctors recall the birth of the NHS. *British Medical Journal* 1978;2(6129):28–33.

Marks J. *The NHS: Beginning, Middle and End? The Autobiography of Dr John Marks*. Oxford: Radcliffe Press; 2008.

RG. Obituary of Dr Solomon Wand. *British Medical Journal* 1984;289(6448):841–42.

Rubinstein W, Jolles M, Rubinstein H. *The Palgrave Dictionary of Anglo-Jewish History*. Basingstoke: Palgrave Macmillan; 2011.

Wand S. Claire Wand Fund. *British Medical Journal* 1981;282(6275):1552.

59 DAME ANNIS GILLIE (1900–1985)

Jessica Dunphy

Katharine Annis Calder Gillie was born 8 August 1900 in Eastbourne, Sussex. She was the eldest of four children born to the Reverend Dr Robert Gillie, a minister in the Presbyterian Church, and his wife Emily Japp. She was educated at Wycombe Abbey School and University College Hospital, London, graduating MBBS in 1925. She was awarded MRCP in 1925 and joined a general practice in London as an assistant to a partnership of three women.

When one partner died and the others retired, Dame Annis single-handedly ran the practice from her home in Connaught Square, London. During the Second World War (1939–1945). Dame Annis moved out of her London home to Pangbourne, Berkshire, but continued to visit her patients in London and the surrounding countryside. She has been described by Dame Albertine Winner (1907–1988), a contemporary of Gillie and the first female deputy chief medical officer of the Department of Health, as 'quite the best general practitioner in London during the late 1930s and early 1940s'. Dame Annis had many distinguished clients on her list including Sir Hugh Casson, president of the Royal Academy, and Lord Clark, author and broadcaster. She resumed partnership in 1954, which continued until her retirement in 1963.

Gillie was heavily involved in the renaissance of general practice following the war. With the College Dame Annis was a member of the Foundation College and was Council Chair from 1959 to 1962. During this time she delivered the eighth James Mackenzie Lecture in 1961 entitled 'James Mackenzie and general practice today'. She was president of the College from 1964 until 1967, when the College received its Royal Charter, and was the only woman to hold the post until Lotte Newman (1929–) commenced the post in 1994. During the time that Gillie held office, many important decisions about the College were taken. These include the decision to include an examination as a prerequisite for membership and the decision to purchase 14 Prince's Gate, home of College headquarters until 2010. She was awarded Honorary Fellowship of the College in 1966.

In parallel with her work at the College, Gillie was involved in another enterprise, which would profoundly influence the course of British medical practice. Following the war, there was a negativity within the general practice community. Morale was low with recruitment falling and many general practitioners emigrating, in part due to a feeling that the specialty was neglected and underfunded. In response to these difficulties and exacerbated by a strained relationship between the College and the BMA, the Standing Medical Advisory Committee set up a subcommittee to study the future scope of general practice.

Gillie was appointed chairman of the subcommittee, the aim of which was to predict the course along which general practice should develop and grow over the next decade, following similar, recently published 10 year plans for hospital and local authority health services. The committee published *The Field of Work of the Family Doctor*, also known as *The Gillie Report*, in 1963. The report broke precedent as the chapters were written, at Gillie's insistence, by members of the committee, rather than the usual government departmental officials. The report noted the discontent within the general practice community and emphasised the importance of general practice within the wider health service. The report stressed the value of training and education at all stages and the need for a formal and structured postgraduate training pathway for general practice trainees. Furthermore, it highlighted the importance of integrated health care, both between general practice and hospital care and between medical and auxiliary health professions. The report, however, determined that an administrative unification of the NHS was not essential to achieving these aims. This conclusion was the opposite of *The Porritt Report* (1962), a review of medical services in the United Kingdom published the previous year, which had deemed the unification of general practice, hospital and local authority services necessary for the future of the NHS. Ministry of Health officials were relieved at the outcome of *The Gillie Report*, as there was little support for unification of services within the department. *The Gillie Report* profoundly influenced the Family Doctor's Charter agreed between the BMA and the Minister of Health in 1964, which helped to restore the fortunes of general practice by improving working conditions and increasing pay. Furthermore, recommendations in *The Gillie Report* impacted greatly upon the Report of the Royal Commission on Medical Education 1968, which recognised general practice as a separate medical specialty with dedicated postgraduate training.

In addition to her work with the College and the Standing Medical Advisory Committee, Gillie was also a member of several other statutory bodies concerned with medicine. She was a member of the GMC (1946–1948), the Medical Practices Committee, the Executive Council of London and the Central Health Services Advisory Council. She was a member of the BMA Central Ethical Committee (1952–1963) and of the BMA Council (1950–1964). She was elected a Fellow of the BMA in 1960 and Vice-President of the association in 1968, becoming the first woman to hold the post. She championed women in medicine and was president of the Medical Women's Council from 1954 to 1955. She also served on the North West Metropolitan Regional Hospital Board, and later on the Oxford Regional Hospital Board. Many other honours came her way. She was awarded FRCP in 1964 and received an honorary MD by the University of Edinburgh in 1968. She was appointed OBE in 1961 and Dame Commander of the Order of the British Empire (DBE) in 1968.

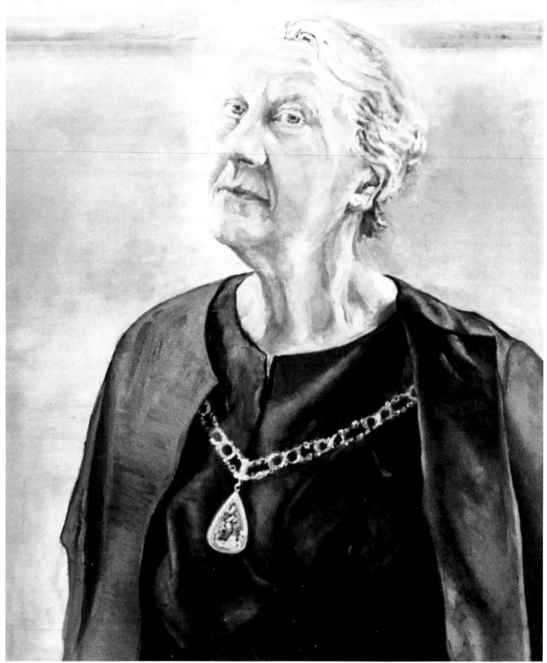

RCGP presidential portrait of Dame Annis Gillie. Artist: Mimi Winter. (Courtesy of RCGP Archives, London.)

Gillie has been described by Winner and Ekkehard von Kuenssberg (1913–2000) as a 'model' chairman of conferences and organisations. They went on to report that she had a gentle but firm manner and was skilled at facilitating and encouraging others. She controlled hostilities at meetings and was able to silence unconstructive contributions, but always did so with courtesy. Her concise and knowledgeable summaries at the end of debates helped progress and understanding, generally persuading committees to produce sensible and well-balanced conclusions.

In 1930, Gillie married architect Percy (Peter) Chandler Smith (1902–1983). His practice was destroyed during the war and he was rejected for military service, so for many years Gillie was the main breadwinner in the household. In later years, as her husband became increasingly incapacitated with multiple sclerosis, she gradually withdrew from medical organisations and devoted herself to looking after him. They moved to Bledington, a Cotswold village, and took great pleasure in converting an old bakehouse into a country home with an extensive library and garden. Together they had two children, a son and a daughter, the latter Julia Dawkins (1932–1973). She died on 10 April 1985 at her home in Oxfordshire.

Further Reading

Blake R, Nicholls CS (eds.). *Dictionary of National Biography 1981–1985*. Oxford: Oxford University Press; 1990.

Central Health Services Council, Standing Medical Advisory Committee. *The Field of Work of the Family Doctor: Report of the Sub-committee*. London: HMSO; 1963.

Drury VWM. Gillie [*married name* Smith], Dame Annis Calder (1900–1985). In: Matthew HCG, Harrison B (eds.). *Oxford Dictionary of National Biography*. Volume 22. Oxford: Oxford University Press; 2004.

EVK. Dame Annis Gillie FRCP FRCGP. *British Medical Journal* 1985;290(6478):1360.

Gillie A. James Mackenzie and general practice today. *The Journal of the College of General Practitioners* 1962;5(1):5–21.

Loudon I, Horder J, Webster C (eds.). *General Practice under the National Health Service 1948–1997: The First Fifty Years*. Oxford: Oxford University Press; 1998.

RJFHP. Annis Calder Gillie DBE, MB Lond, FRCP, FRCGP. *The Lancet* 1985;325(8435):996.

60 SIR JAMES CAMERON (1905–1991)
Matthew Betts and Rohin Reddy

In 1964, Alfred Bentley Davies (1902–1971), chairman of the GMSC between 1958 and 1964, resigned leaving a population of general practitioners tired, disillusioned and in need of new leadership. Solomon Wand's (1899–1984) work as the head of the GMSC from 1948 to 1952 had seen the Danckwerts Award go some way to alleviating concerns by increasing pay for general practitioners, but many still believed there were improvements to be made. Reductions in undergraduate admissions, alongside only a 20 per cent increase in qualified graduates, compared to a doubling in hospital consultant numbers, exacerbated the already considerable stress caused by unsystematic pay from a global resource pool levied against general practitioners. Alongside this, many general practitioners were on the brink of retirement, which compounded the recruitment crisis at a time when patient numbers were increasing, particularly amongst the young and old. Furthermore, premises and equipment were inadequate and greater numbers of ancillary staff were required. These salient issues were highlighted in a landmark juncture by Annis Gillie (1900–1985), chair of the sub-committee set up by the Standing Medical Advisory Committee. *The Gillie Report* (1963) quantified 'the barely tolerable pressure on the family doctor', a quandary evidenced by much correspondence in contemporaneous issues of the *BMJ*.

The 1966 General Practice Contract was a landmark juncture that changed general practice in the United Kingdom. Before, it had been argued that there were no safeguards to practice and, despite the Danckwerts Award, pay was severely lacking in comparison with hospital consultants whose career earnings were 48 per cent higher contemporaneously. There were talks of strikes and mass resignation and newly appointed Minister of Health, Kenneth Robinson, who in 1977 was awarded Honorary Fellowship of the RCGP, remarked that general practice was in a state of 'absolute turmoil'. The contract included prioritising adequate time for patients as well as better pay and working hours. It also attempted to forward the notion that general practitioners were specialists in a field of his or her choosing. It was James Cameron, then working as a general practitioner in Wallington, London, who embodied much of the driving force behind the implementation of the contract. Consequently, he is widely regarded as one of the architects of modern general practice.

Born on 8 April 1905 at Bridge of Earn, Perthshire, Sir James was educated at Perth Academy before qualifying as a doctor at St Andrews University in 1929. He was lauded for distinguished service as a captain in the RAMC for service in the Second World War (1939–1945) attached to the 1st Battalion, Rifle Brigade, during which time he was a prisoner of war for five years following the fall of Calais in 1940. It was following the war, however, that his influence came to bear, as he translated his gregarious activity as a member of the BMA, which he joined in 1947, to general membership of the GMSC in 1956, and latterly to BMA Council in 1961.

It was during the early years of Sir James' tenure on the GMSC that general practice underwent much modification. He was one of the many general practitioners making home visits on a daily basis that numbered into the dozens, alongside just as many consultations in surgery. The foundation of the College in 1952 gave hope to those feeling that the rewards were not justifying efforts, alongside much needed support for the nation's general practitioners in the drive towards the contract, overstretched and underappreciated, as they were.

Cameron rose to oversee the GMSC with election to chairman in 1964. He led from the front as a key negotiator between general practitioners and government; from his position at the head of the GSMC talks were heralded to usher in a brand new contract. His appointment could not have come at a more volatile time for general practice in the United Kingdom; shortly after assuming his role, a group of two dozen Birmingham-based general practitioners resigned from the NHS to set up an alternative community service that ultimately did not survive. Sir James recognised the risk of a dearth of faith in general practitioners across the country should reactionary politics continue. The petition for a new future for general practice was mounted, alongside which undated resignations were furnished and sent to BMA House totalling 14,000 within a fortnight of the call. As a result, over a weekend in Hove with the help of colleagues, he penned the landmark *Charter for the Family Doctor Service* for immediate submission to the BMA, who adopted the programme as its own at the eleventh hour. The programme called for much-needed modernisation of equipment and premises, auxiliary help in the form of practice nurses to aid with home visits, a top-down reassessment and reorganisation of time-heavy self-certification methodologies and a wholesale reduction in the number of patients to be looked after. Alongside these requests, the programme made the case for an independent financial body established in the understanding that pay should coincide 'realistically' to a general practitioner's 'workload and responsibility' hand-in-hand with a limitation to a reasonable working day, week and year.

On account of the 10-point programme, Sir James successfully oversaw the termination of the 'pool' system of payment which had been so enormously contentious. Having been denigrated by the Socialist Charter for Health as a 'cottage industry' as a result of their desperate plea for change, general practice in the United Kingdom seemed to have found its guardian. State subsidies and the contract guidelines would soon ensure that the BMA's newly

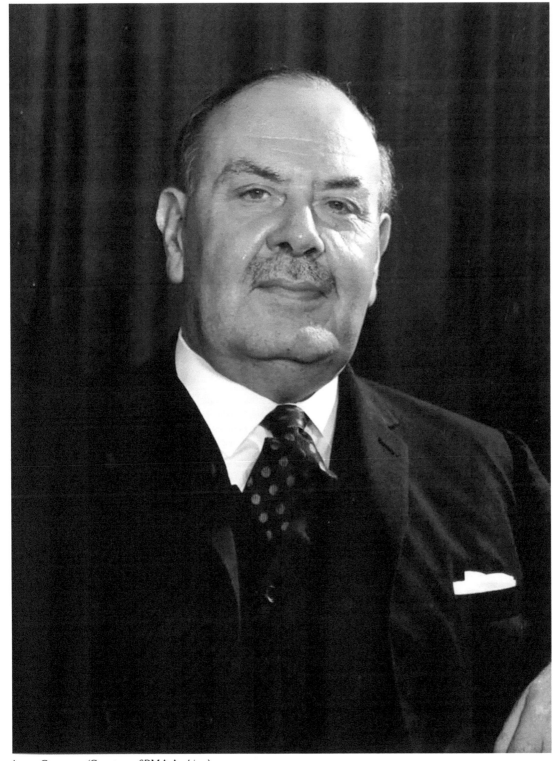

James Cameron. (Courtesy of BMA Archive.)

adopted Charter for the Family Doctor Service successfully underpinned the ability of a general practitioner 'to give the best service to his patients'. This was a result of better equipped and better staffed premises, greater autonomy, basic practice allowances for general practitioners with patient lists exceeding 1000 patients and pension provisions. Additionally, the new 'red book' payment system allowed general practitioners to claim back 70 per cent of staff costs and 100 per cent of the cost of their premises from the NHS. Cameron stood stalwart at the helm of the committee that mapped out the core ideology of the contract that would go on to stand as foundations underpinning fruitful negotiations with the aforementioned Robinson.

Cameron resigned from his position in 1974, and was duly granted a gold medal citation from the BMA in recognition of his valuable influence and achievement. Earlier, in 1966, he had been awarded Fellowship of the College. A knighthood was appointed to him in 1979. However, his career was far from over, and he was successfully elected to the post of BMA Council Chairman in 1976, having turned 71 years old. He held the position for three years, continuing to spread his talents across a number of related fields, nationally and internationally.

Cameron's legacy is celebrated by the Cameron Fund, which was set up in 1970 with the sum of £800,000 remaining from the days of the pool payment system. Despite the Treasury's eagerness to retain the money, Sir James was instrumental in securing the wherewithal to do so, thereby making the idea of a charitable fund in aid of general practitioners in financial difficulty a reality. The Cameron Fund's continued work serves as testament to his fight for the cause of the general practitioner, and recalls the Orwellian retort he is famed for employing: 'all doctors are equal, but some are more equal than others', when division within the fraternity was rife, and the threat of removal of general practice from the national system all too real. He was regarded as a zealous defender of the profession who was keen to ensure that the interests of patients remained at the forefront of the minds of general practitioners.

Sir James was husband to Irene, who passed away in 1986, and father to a son and two daughters. He died on 20 October 1991, following a distinguished career as a trailblazer in his field.

Further Reading

Anon. Charter for general practice. *British Medical Journal* 1965;1(5436):669–70.

Anon. Step by step. *British Medical Journal* 1965;2(5452):1.

Anon. *Royal Commission on the National Health Service*, Chapter 7. London: Stationery Office; 1979.

Anon. Towards a better family doctor service. *British Medical Journal* 1965;1(5439):875.

Culver G. *The 1966 GP Contract and Sir James Cameron*. London: The Cameron Fund; 2016.

Fraser B. Sir Bruce Fraser on 'The Doctor and the Administrator'. *British Medical Journal* 1968;2(5604):553–54.

Gullick D. Obituary: Sir James Cameron. *British Medical Journal* 1991;303:1130.

Lewis J. *Independent Contractors: GPs and the GP Contract in the Post-War Period*. Manchester: National Primary Care Research and Development Centre; 1997.

Macpherson G. Reviving the fortunes of general practice: James Cameron and Kenneth Robinson. *British Medical Journal* 1982;345:26–29.

Socialist Medical Association. *Charter for the Family Doctor Service* [pamphlet]. London: Today and Tomorrow Publications; 1965.

61 IAN DINGWALL GRANT (1891–1962)
Mariam Altheyab, Stuart Pinder, James Parry-Reece and Neil Metcalfe

Ian Dingwall Grant was a former Chairman of BMA Council (1961–1962) and former president of the College between 1956 and 1959. In these positions his main objective was to improve general practice, using the wealth of knowledge he accumulated during his over 40 years of being a general practitioner in Glasgow.

Grant was born on 6 June 1891, and raised in Nigg, a town in the Scottish Highlands where his father, Reverend Evan Grant, worked as a church minister. He was educated at Bellahouston Academy in Glasgow, and later attended the University of Glasgow where he graduated with MBBCh in 1913.

Grant's working career started in Glasgow hospitals. He worked as a house surgeon at the Victoria Infirmary and assistant gynaecologist in the dispensary. In 1914, he travelled to India, where he joined the Indian Medical Service in which he served throughout the First World War (1914–1918) and was mentioned in despatches. He stayed with the Indian Medical Service until 1920. After the war he returned to Glasgow, where he worked until 1960 as a general practitioner.

Much of Grant's efforts were with the BMA. He became president of the Glasgow and West of Scotland branch from 1939 to 1943. In 1942, he was elected to the BMA Council, and served in a significant number of central and local committees of the BMA. These included being chairman of the Scottish Committee (1949–1952, now known as BMA Scottish Council), the Representative Body (1954–1957), the International Relations Committee (1957–1961) and the Private Practice Committee (1948–1953). In his role as chairman of the International Relations Committee, he assisted with the development of general practice in South Africa, Kenya, Nigeria and Australia. In 1955, he was appointed as Honorary Secretary for general practice when the BMA held its annual meeting in conjunction with the Canadian Medical Association in Toronto. Three years later, his distinguished service to the BMA was further recognised when he was elected as Vice-President. He was Chairman of BMA Council from 1961 to 1962.

In addition to his work for the BMA, Grant also did much work with the College. He was a member of Foundation Council, First Provost of the West of Scotland Faculty (1954–1956) and, in 1956, was elected as the second ever president of the College, succeeding William Pickles (1885–1969), when nominated for the position at the fourth annual general meeting. He was described contemporaneously by his colleagues on College Council as the ideal general practitioner who served the highest ideals and who's altruism and devotion to professional activities made him worthy of the honour. Whilst president in 1956, he delivered the third James Mackenzie Lecture. His lecture, entitled 'Our heritage and our future', emphasised the importance of professional unity, and the necessity of maintaining some private practice in the welfare state due to his concerns over the NHS. On a separate occasion on this topic he suggested 'we should never have agreed that so intimate and personal a matter as health should be placed under the control of the politicians. Health, like religion, should be outside party politics'. In 1958, he travelled to South Africa where he gave lectures on the activities of the College. That same year, the College created faculties in South Africa, which increased both membership and international recognition of the College and its work. He then served as president until 1959. In the same year he was awarded an honorary fellowship of the College and a fellowship of the Australian College of General Practitioners.

Grant wrote a number of articles on general practice and his involvement with the Colleges of General Practice in both the United Kingdom and abroad; these included 'The college of general practitioners', 'In other lands: The College of General Practice of Canada' and 'General medical practice in Australasia and Britain'. Much of his writings came from his concerns with the evolution of the role of the general practitioner. In an article published in the *BMJ* entitled 'Status of the practitioner, past, present, and future', he communicated his dismay that general practice was losing its place in hospital medicine and noted that many general practitioners were losing much of their clinical work to hospital outpatient departments. He felt that medicine was becoming commercialised and mechanised in its specialisation and regulation by the state, commenting that many general practitioners felt they 'lost our freedom in medicine and became cogs in the administrative machinery'. It was presented at the annual general meeting of the Fellowship for Freedom in Medicine in 1961. Furthermore, whilst he was the President of the College and Vice-President of the BMA, he wrote an article entitled 'The British College of General Practitioners' in which he laid out the aims of the new college in advocating for general practitioners, promoting education and promoting research in general practice.

Grant received multiple awards throughout his career, and, in 1958, was presented with a portrait of himself by members of the College. That same year he received an honorary MD by the University of Birmingham; the public orator that presented him with his MD described him as a person who used all of his time in the service of his profession, and who's humility probably did not allow him to realise how much he deserved all the honours that were granted to him. Thereafter, he was appointed CBE in 1960.

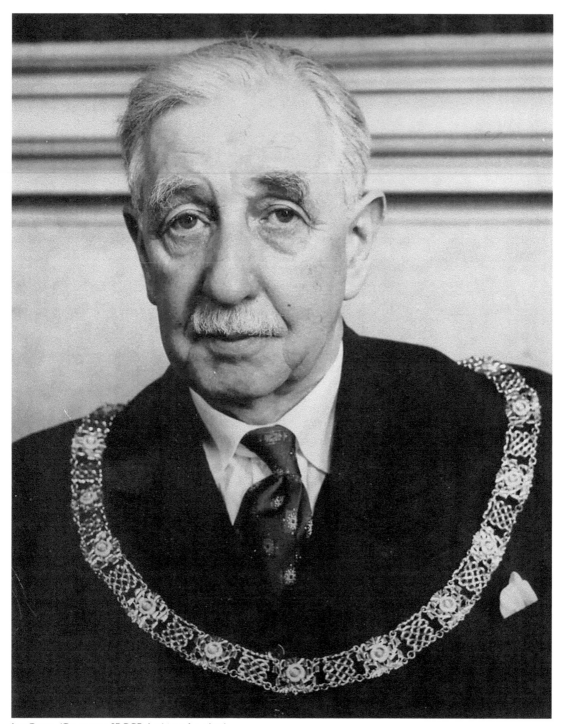

Ian Grant. (Courtesy of RCGP Archives, London.)

Friends and colleagues described Grant as a kind, wise and dignified man, who dedicated his life to improving medical care not only locally or nationally, but on a global scale. He died on 17 April 1962, aged 71 years old, whilst in post as chairman of the BMA. He was taken ill in his flat at the BMA House, Tavistock Square, London. He was survived by his wife and son, Charles Grant (d. 2015), who followed his father into medicine. In memory of Grant and in recognition of his work, the Ian Dingwall Grant Award was established in 1967 by The Scottish Council of the RCGP and was made possible by a donation from the Caledonian Medical Society upon the winding up of its affairs. It is awarded to encourage young postgraduates preparing for a career in general practice to add to their experience.

Further Reading

Anon. Obituary: Ian D. Grant, C.B.E., M.D. *British Medical Journal* 1962;1:1210.

Fry J, Hunt Lord of Fawley, Pinsent RJF (eds.). *A History of the Royal College of General Practitioners: The First 25 Years*. Lancaster: MTP Press; 1983.

Grant ID. In other lands the College of General Practice of Canada. The College of General Practice in Canada. *College of General Practitioners Research Newsletter* 1957;16:235–38.

Grant ID. The Third James Mackenzie Lecture. Our heritage and our future. *Research Newsletter* 1957;4:7–23.

Grant ID. The British College of General Practitioners. *South African Medical Journal* 1958;32(43):1044–47.

Grant ID. General medical practice in Australasia and Britain. *Journal of the Royal Society of Health* 1960;80:305–09.

Grant ID. The College of General Practitioners. *Postgraduate Medical Journal* 1960;36:302–5.

Grant ID. Status of the practitioner, past, present, and future. *British Medical Journal* 1961;2(5262):1279–82.

62 SIR RONALD GEORGE GIBSON (1909–1989)

Sophie Moriarty

Ronald George Gibson was born in Southampton on 28 November 1909. He was the only child of George Edward Gibson, a pharmacist, and Gladys Muriel, née Prince. He was educated at Osbourne House School in Romsey and then Mill Hill School in London before attending St. John's College, University of Cambridge. He finished his medical studies at St Bartholomew's Hospital from where he qualified in 1937. At the same hospital he undertook his first medical posts of casualty officer and physician for the paediatric department. For the majority of his life and career he resided in Winchester. A lover of all things British, he loved nowhere more than his home city of Winchester, and was an active pillar of its community.

Gibson's initial entry into general practice was interrupted by the Second World War (1939–1945). He served as the principle medical officer at the rank of Lieutenant Colonel in the RAMC from 1940 to 1945 in Kenya and later in Somaliland. His experience working with young soldiers sparked his interest in adolescent health and led him to work as medical officer to Winchester College and to St. Swithum's Girls School on his return to general practice in 1945.

The main result of Sir Ronald's service during the war, however, was his new passion for medical politics. His main concern was with reforming the constitution of BMA Council and its working methods within the new post-war United Kingdom. Involving himself initially at a local level, he quickly rose to Honorary Secretary (1946–1950), then chairman (1952–1953) of the Winchester division before then being secretary (1959–1960) and later president of the Wessex Branch (1962–1963). He also became a member of BMA Council in 1950 and was chairman of the Organisation Committee (1956–1962). In this role he recognised that the BMA was void of opportunities for junior members to voice their concerns and aspirations.

This led him to quickly establish the first junior member's forum in 1958. Eliciting and addressing the sentiments of all in the profession, not only of the senior members, was something he was noted for throughout his BMA career. On becoming Chairman of BMA's representative body (1963–1966), before being elected Chairman of BMA Council which he undertook between 1966 and 1971, he regularly toured the country to allow doctors' voices to be heard. During his five years in this role he avoided large presentations and speeches to mass audiences, though the delivery of the 14th James Mackenzie Lecture in 1967 was an exception, preferring instead to confer with smaller groups in order to gain a greater understanding of their situation and the contexts in which their concerns arose. This display of respect, in addition to his efforts in safeguarding junior doctors, earned him the trust and respect of the profession according to those who knew him. This proved to be key in future negotiation with the government and in establishing the public image of the BMA as a trustworthy and caring organisation.

Sir Ronald was Chairman of BMA Council during difficult times and he was constantly conducting difficult negotiations with numerous health secretaries. He was known for his firm but fair approach. In his view, the most important key to success in these situations was the professional unity of doctors, which he secured by touring the country and by working in close collaboration with the royal colleges and other bodies. Wanting to enhance the BMA's reputation not only amongst the public but also the scientific community, he established the Board of Science in 1968, which promoted the BMA to be regarded as having a notable view on medical, social and ethical issues. He himself contributed numerous papers to the scientific literature on various subjects: from venereal disease in African women to the ethics and management on terminal conditions. From his roles within the BMA, he worked closely with the *BMJ*. He began sitting on the *BMJ* Committee in 1971, elected Deputy Chairman of the Committee in 1973 and continued in such a role until 1985.

Known by his colleagues for his organisational skills, Sir Ronald was still very engaged with his local community and other organisations. Despite his roles on a national level, general practice remained his primary interest. His meticulous eye for originality enabled him to apply novel ideas from visits to other centres of excellence to his own work. He built a successful practice in Winchester, which at the time was one of the first to integrate nursing care and community health workers, something which has contributed to a change in British General Practice.

Sir Ronald was awarded various prizes, honours and degrees. In 1956, he was awarded the College's Butterworth Medal for his essay on the care of the elderly. In 1961, he was appointed OBE and then CBE in 1970 for his dedication and service to his work and community. He was awarded FRCGP in 1968 as well as FRCS by election in the same year. He was Chairman of the Standing Medical Advisory Committee of the Department of Health. It was following this appointment, and his membership of an important enquiry into prison brutality against IRA members in Northern Ireland in 1971, that he was appointed Knight Bachelor in 1975.

On retirement, Sir Ronald became involved in a new project called Brendoncare. Sir Ronald himself referred to the state of elderly care at the time as 'a 'scandal', and he believed that the elderly should have access to the dignified and respectful care they required. Along with a generous benefactor, Mrs Phoebe Bacon, he created Brendoncare, which

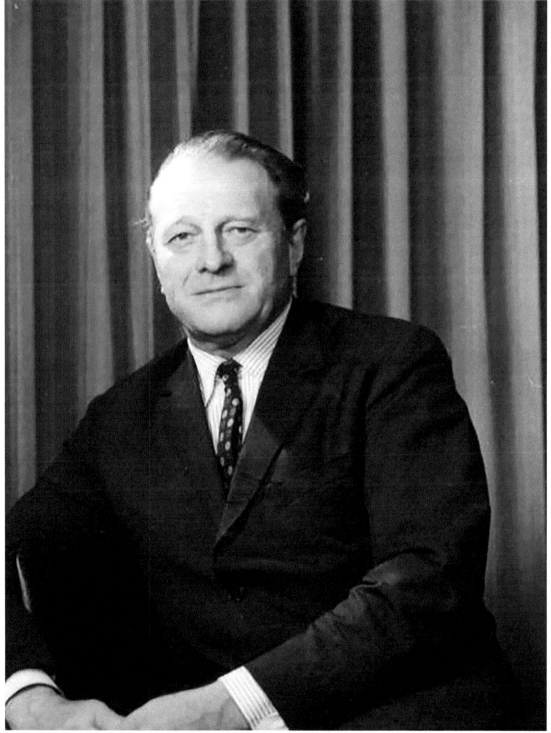

Ronald Gibson. (Courtesy of BMA Archive.)

was one of the first dually registered nursing homes in the United Kingdom. Contrary to other retirement homes of the time which had strict regimes, Brendoncare took a more flexible and autonomous approach to care: there were no shared rooms and residents were encouraged to bring their own furniture. Up until her death in 2002, Queen Elizabeth the Queen Mother was Patron.

Sir Ronald was regarded by all who knew him as a 'gentleman'. An active part of the community and a deeply religious man, he was president of the Winchester Amateur Operatic Society and was appointed High Steward of Winchester Cathedral. He became the Deputy Lieutenant for Hampshire towards the later years of his life for his commitment to local affairs. His other interests included cricket, gardening and music; he was said to have been at his happiest whilst playing piano. He married Elizabeth Alberta Rainey in 1934 with whom they had two daughters. Following his death in 1989, aged 79 years old, a memorial service was held in Winchester Cathedral.

Further Reading

Gibson R. Lucerna pedibus meis. *The Journal of the Royal College of General Practitioners* 1968;15(1):3–22.

Gibson R. *Family Doctor: His Life and History*. London: Allen & Unwin; 1981.

DS, Sir Ronald George (1909–1989). *British Medical Journal* 1989;298:1574–5.

PART 4: FEATURED GENERAL PRACTITIONERS FROM THE LAST 50 YEARS (1967–2017)

This final section looks at the 50 years of general practice from 1967 to 2017. By 1967, the quantity and quality of research in general practice had increased dramatically from the mid-twentieth century and there were several chairs of general practice. A new general practitioner contract had come into force from 1966 and the College had been given a Royal Charter in 1967, thus becoming RCGP. Teaching at postgraduate and undergraduate levels was still in the developing stages and general practice was still different from how it is today. Some of the contributions of general practitioners to medical education, research, medical literature, medical politics and society will again be presented.

Postgraduate General Practitioner Training

The concept of vocational training had been prioritised in the 1960s and led to a significant *Report of the Royal Commission* in 1968.[1] The education committee of the College was small but included various leaders in this field, such as Annis Gillie and Ekke Kuenssberg amongst others, and was chaired on different occasions by Bill Hylton, Pat Byrne and John Horder.[2] Later further support came from Paul Freeling, Conrad Harris, Donald Irvine, Marshall Marinker, John Stevens (d. 1982) and Ian Tait (1926–2013).[2] Together, the committee produced the first report from general practice called *Special Vocational Training for General Practice* (1965),[3] and the following year published *Evidence of the College to the Royal Commission on Medical Education*.[4] Invited to answer questions to the Commissioners and representing the educational committee and the College was Horder, who did much to impress upon them of a general practice being a discipline in its own right and hence the need of specific training for it.[2] This led to the Commission virtually accepting all of the College's Report in the *Report of the Royal Commission* in 1968, with it recommending a formal postgraduate training programme of five years.[2]

The first half of the 1970s then saw further reports and a notable book that helped vocational training progress. Irvine produced the first report on the characteristics of trainers and their practices in his RCGP report *Teaching Practices* (1972),[5] though the most notable publication came from one he co-authored. *The Future General Practitioner: Learning and Teaching* (1972)[6] included the following contributors: it was chaired by Horder, who wrote the first chapter on health and disease; Byrne, who wrote on the consultation; Freeling, who wrote on human development; Harris who wrote about human behaviour; Marinker who wrote on medicine and society and Irvine, who wrote on practice organisation. It was the first book to put learning before teaching as well as to comprehensively define the content of general practice. RCGP pressure to keep aiming for legislation was continued and summarised in Irvine's William Pickles Lecture in 1974 when he reported 'general practice is no longer prepared to be the dustbin of medicine!'[7] Considering that training in Ireland fell under the GMC until 1978 and the RCGP had an influence there until the Irish College of General Practitioners was formed in 1984, the influence of James McCormick was also paramount at this time. He was chairman of the Consultative Council on General Medical Practice which produced the report *The General Practitioner in Ireland* (1974),[8] also referred to as the *McCormick Report*. Amongst its 107 recommendations was one regarding a three-year training of general practitioners in a combination of community and hospital settings.

Several ideas initially conceived by Kuenssberg also helped move training forwards. In terms of training the actual trainers and thus permitting general practitioners to have a part in their own continuing education, he conceived a course funded by the Nuffield Provincial Hospitals Trust which was led by Freeling together with Suzie Barry.[2,9] It stimulated interest in educational theory and the optimum conditions for adult learning as well as the theory and practice of learning in interactive small groups.[2,9] Furthermore, it was Kuenssberg who identified the need for an organisation to oversee the training that was being proposed. This was achieved when his proposal to join the RCGP Vocational Training committee with the BMA's GMSC, now known as the General Practitioners Committee (GPC), was accepted, creating a new body, recognised by government, called the Joint Committee on Postgraduate Training for General Practice (JCPTGP) in 1975.[2] The JCPTGP provided regional inspectors rather than those inspecting at an individual practice level. This was something which was held as an exemple by many, including successive chief medical officers of England, and helped higher standards of training.[10] This training became mandatory following the NHS Vocational Training Act 1976, which required doctors wishing to enter general practice in the NHS to produce evidence that they had acquired suitable medical experience. This was consolidated in the NHS Act of 1977 and amendments led to stipulations that from 15 February 1981, doctors pursuing a career in general practice must have undertaken a year as a trainee in general practice. In addition, from 16 August 1982, it was compulsory to have completed three years full-time employment in specified posts.[11] This was just 11 years from the publication of RCGP's *Special Vocational Training for General Practice* and was perhaps RCGP's most striking example of policy role. Various courses had been created by this time to permit such training, one of which, for example, included the first postgraduate university department of general practice in Europe at the University of Exeter which had been established by Denis Pereira Gray.[12,13] This meant that a general practitioner principal from 1982 needed to have been through such a scheme before being issued with a certificate from the JCPTGP.

The quality of entry into general practice was the next step required in the development of postgraduate general practitioner training. There was no objective standard of entry into general practice when obtaining the certificate of the JCPTGP. The MRCGP examination was non-compulsory and only around 0.2 per cent from over 7000 applications to the JCPTGP were noted in the report *Quality in General Practice* (1985) to have been refused.[14] This report had been overseen by Alastair Donald, who was chairman of the JCPTGP between 1982 and 1985. Ultimately this situation led to the 'three chairman letter' when the then Chairmen of the GMSC, JCPTGP and RCGP, Ian Bogle, Irvine and Pereira Gray, respectively stated that completion of vocational training should mean the achievement of a satisfactory level of competence rather than a completion of time served.[2,15] A working party under Irvine at the JCPTGP then prioritised setting up an objective assessment and by November 1995 the then JCPTGP chairman, Pereira Gray, announced the acceptance of summative assessment of vocational training and hence an expected minimum standard of a general practitioner trainee when finishing their training.[2] This started in September 1996, when the JCPTGP was able to say with confidence that general practitioners practising in the United Kingdom were at an assured standard of clinical skill and that they were being presided over by ever-increasing standards for both practice and hospital-based trainers.[10] The JCPTGP's role eventually was taken over by the Postgraduate Medical Education and Training Board (PMETB) in September 2005 and then the GMC in 2010. Summative assessment has now been phased out when from 2007 a new version of the MRCGP became the sole method to obtain a certificate of completion of training.

Undergraduate General Practice Training

University departments of general practice were developed in this time frame. In 1968, the *Todd Report*[1] had taken into account the GMC's recommendation[16] for the GMC and the RCGP undergraduate Education Committee that medical schools should have general practice teaching as well as the RCGP's own undergraduate education committees recommendations. It concluded that general practitioners involved in teaching undergraduates should be offered senior academic appointments.[1] In that year, a paper revealed that there were 27 undergraduate medical schools in the United Kingdom from which there were a total of five departments of general practice.[17] It also showed that 12 of the medical schools had all students being taught in general practice.[17] Originally, these were NHS practice-based departments as exemplified by Byrne at the University of Manchester, where he was to become the first professor of general practice in England, and David Morrell at Guy's and St Thomas' medical school. The first attempt at a non-undergraduate general practice-based department was at the University of Aberdeen where Ian Richardson, originally appointed as a reader in 1968 before being appointed professor in 1970, laid the foundations of a research-based department using his background in public health.[18] Within four years there had been roughly a doubling of the development of undergraduate general practice: in 1972, of 29 undergraduate medical schools, there were 11 departments of general practice and 22 medical schools had all students being taught in general practice.[19]

There are other people that helped with the development of general practice within medical education. For a full account of the topic readers are advised to look particularly at *Academic General Practice in the UK Medical Schools, 1948–2000* (2011)[20] but for this section two names are included. The first is Michael Drury, who, prior to being the first professor of general practice at the University of Birmingham, provided innovative teaching and assessing of communication skills, including the use of video, which influenced the curricula of all medical schools in the United Kingdom. He co-authored *Introduction to General Practice* (1979)[21] which was written at an appropriate level for the medical student and expertly showcased the specialty to all. The other name is John Howie, who led the University of Edinburgh's department from 1981 to 2000. Some aspects of his contributions to research are described later but what is also relevant for undergraduate general practice was how a 10-year campaign of persistence from 1981 led to the boosting of finances for teaching and research to university departments in the United Kingdom. For a long time such roles were occasionally provided on an ad hoc basis necessitating much good will for low remuneration. Howie instead helped secure for academic general practice a percentage of the Service Increment for Teaching monies, with which the NHS was supplementing teaching hospital budgets in England and Wales, and similarly the Additional Cost of Teaching (ACT) budgets in Scotland. These monies helped provide high quality teaching in general practice within medical schools, and by 1996 resulted in all of the 29 undergraduate medical schools having departments of general practice and all medical students being taught in general practice.[19]

Research

As an individual researcher Julian Tudor Hart was an inspiration to many. He had developed epidemiological expertise through his association with the MRC and then spent 30 years as a general practitioner in a declining Welsh mining community. He wrote numerous papers and books though he is best known for describing of the 'inverse care law' in

1971.[22] This law, he explained, was that the patients with the greatest need receive the poorest health care, particularly where health economies are subject to market forces. He was also interested in cardiovascular disease and is credited with being the first general practice to routinely measure blood pressure. He was able to demonstrate it was possible to reduce premature mortality in high-risk patients by almost 30 per cent.

Staying in Wales but looking at research from a general practice department perspective, the work of Robert Harvard Davis and Nigel Stott was influential. They both worked at the University of Wales College of Medicine. Davis had been particularly involved when chairing the Standing Medical Advisory Committee which, in 1971, produced a report known as the *Harvard Davis Report*.[23] This made several conclusions about the organisational aspect of general practice, including limiting patient list sizes to 2500 per general practitioner. Stott co-authored important research on antibiotic use in general practice. He showed that antibiotics did not help recovery times from uncomplicated lower respiratory tract infections and published on the over prescribing of antibiotics for upper respiratory tract infections in winter.[24] Both Stott and Davis collaborated to produce the Stott and Davis consultation model (1979),[25] or 'the exceptional potential in each primary care consultation model'. They suggested there are four areas that can be systematically explored each time a patient consults, including the management of presenting problems, modification of help-seeking behaviours, management of continuing problems and opportunistic health promotion.[25] It is a model still of relevance and taught today.

With the increasing number of general practice departments, as well as funding, research also increased from these areas. From the names featured in this section the work of Pereira Gray and Howie are included. Pereira Gray researched and has been publishing on continuity of care,[26,27] generalism and the doctor–patient relationship. Howie led research on epidemiology and public health and has worked on the links between personal continuity and the quality of general practitioner consultations. He was able to prove that longer consultations are better consultations.[28] This work, like that from Pereira Gray, was seen as being highly influential in demonstrating the importance of the nature and quality of the doctor-patient relationship.

Research groups provided further help. Various research funding charities and the pharmaceutical industry assisted with research about general practice as well as 'in' general practice in this time.[18] One of the most influential has been the MRC. It helped support the RCGP's 'Oral contraceptive study', proposed by Kuenssberg and then masterminded by Clifford Kay (1927–) from the RCGP's Manchester Research Unit that had been founded in 1968. This study started in the same year and used 1400 general practitioners to enroll 46,000 women, half of whom were using oral contraceptives at the time, into a follow-up study. Meticulous observations over many years have produced important information about the morbidity and mortality rates of such a class of medication.[29,30] The MRC later appointed Martin Roland to Chair its Health Services Research Committee in 1994. This appointment of a professor of general practice confirmed that such a large research organisation recognised the ability of the top researchers from the discipline of general practice and the value of the generalist's vision.[18]

From the RCGP perspective, the '*What Sort of Doctor*' initiative was an important document from the 1980s.[31] Instigated by the Board of Censors in September 1980, it aimed to develop assessment at general practices themselves. John Lawson was chairman of the first working group between 1980 and 1981 and when the report was published, in 1985, he was president of the RCGP.[31] The *Report of General Practice No. 23 What Sort of Doctor? Assessing Quality of Care in General Practice*[31] developed a framework for assessing quality in general practice through four areas: values, accessibility, competence and communication skills. It was felt to have a lot of impact on looking at overall outcomes of training, performance review, reviewing general practices at the practices themselves and had an effect on later establishing Fellowship by Assessment.

Further research to include is that in information technology (IT). Although more in relation to social welfare, one of the IT programmes to mention is that called the Lisson Grove Benefits Program, named after the practice where its creator, Brian Jarman, worked. This is a programme that calculates the distribution of social security benefits and eventually became adopted by local authorities, housing associations, citizen's advice bureaux and charities amongst others. Mike Pringle was shown the potential capabilities and use of IT in general practice in the 1970s. This led to a career-long interest in general practice information systems amongst others, and led to helping set up one of the world's largest databases of its type by accumulating over 24 million patient records from over 1300 general practices in the United Kingdom. This database, called QRESEARCH, has been used to develop new risk prediction algorithms to aid clinicians and act as a data provider for public health interventions. A separate system, PRIMIS, whose development was also helped by Pringle, is a system that assists general practitioners audit clinical data regarding patients with atrial fibrillation, chronic obstructive pulmonary disease and heart failure, as well as helping date information and the quality of patient records.

Other Contributors to Medical Literature

Many of the names already mentioned also produced praiseworthy research and publications for which more detailed information is available in their respective chapters. Two names not mentioned already include David Haslam and Roger Neighbour, particularly in terms of writing and that of books. Haslam has been a general practitioner since 1976 and has written over 1000 articles and 13 books, one of which was *Sleepless Children: A Handbook for Parents* (1984).[32] Three years later Neighbour published his seminal textbook on the doctor–patient consultation entitled *The Inner Consultation* (1987).[33] This is a book that Haslam, when chairman of the RCGP, reported as being 'one of the very few contemporary medical classics'.[34] It suggested five main parts to the consultation: connecting with the patient and developing rapport and empathy with them, summarising what the general practitioner has understood the problem to be, handing over or sharing with the patient an agreed management plan, safety netting with the patient by making contingency plans if something uncertain occurs and housekeeping, when the general practitioner stays in a clear mental focus for the next patient. Neighbour went on to publish *The Inner Apprentice* (1992)[35] and *Inner Physician* (2010).[36]

Palliative care has also been a topic written about effectively by general practitioners. Iona Heath has been a powerful writer with a regular column in the *BMJ* in which the Quality, deficiencies of the Quality and Outcomes Framework (QOF) scheme and the industrialisation of general practice have featured. Her essay 'The mystery of general practice' was published alongside 'Ways of dying' in her book, *Matters of Life and Death* (2007).[37] It discusses important issues on the role of the health care professional in the care of the dying and the idea of dealing with life and death being part of the art of general practice. Similarly Ann McPherson wrote much, with a lot of her success being related to her 30 books, including *The Diary of a Teenage Health Freak* (1987).[38] However, with regards to palliative care she chaired a project called health care professionals for assisted dying following an article she had written in the *BMJ*.[39] Attempts were made to change the law on assisted dying though no changes were made prior to her own death.

General Practitioner Involvement in Medical Politics and Allied Organisations

The BMA has seen various general practitioners be awarded the positions of chairman of the GMSC as well as chairman of BMA Council. During this section's time frame there was, as chairman of the GMSC, James Cameron (1964–1974), whose contribution has already been discussed in the previous section of this book, Bogle (1990–1997), John Chisholm (1997–2004) and Hamish Meldrum (2004–2007). Solomon Wand (1946–1951) and Ronald Gibson (1966–1971) are two general practitioners mentioned previously who have been chairman of council but two others have also undertaken this role and are mentioned in this section: Bogle (1998–2003) and Meldrum (2008–2012). Bogle and Chisholm did much that led to a new general practitioner contract in 2004 following a time when doctors had various grievances, the main ones being the on-going 100-hour working weeks for junior doctors and, with regards specifically to general practice, the government plans for headline-grabbing reforms such as NHS walk-in centres. The new contract was much lauded for items including an out-of-hours opt out. Meldrum later spearheaded two successive BMA campaigns against the privatisation of the NHS called *Support Your Surgery* and *Look after our NHS*. He reluctantly led a doctor strike in 2012 over pension changes which ultimately, the BMA was forced to back down.

Also linked to the BMA, but also particularly the Women's Medical Federation, was Rosemary Rue. At the start of her career she had been a general practitioner and towards the end of it she became President of both the BMA (1990–1991) and of the Women's Medical Federation (1982–1988). One of her greatest achievements was that she personally opened career opportunities for women doctors, by enabling them to work part-time whilst training to be specialists. In the mid-1960s she was assistant county medical officer in Oxford when she argued for funds to support four married women doctors in specialist training. This led to ten times that amount being successfully placed during that time and, by the end of the next year, 100 women were in post and 'the part-time training scheme for married women doctors' was born which evolved into the flexible training scheme now in use throughout the United Kingdom.[40]

Another female general practitioner featured is Mary 'Mollie' McBride. She held various regional health authority roles and was the first woman to hold the RCGP Honorary Secretary role (1989–1994). Following the death of her husband she honoured a mutual agreement and, in 1990, made the dramatic move from Chester to general practice in the east end of London. Many general practice leaders and politicians have spoken about social deprivation but only McBride moved purposefully to work where conditions were particularly difficult.[41] She took leading government officials and NHS leaders in person to her practice to see for themselves how difficult things were proving to be in socially-deprived areas.[41] Several of these visitors were profoundly influenced by seeing first hand the difficulties faced by general practitioners, often working in the shadow of multimillion-pound NHS institutions.[41]

Unsurprisingly, there have been contributions from general practitioners at the GMC. Irvine chaired the GMC's Committee on Standards and Medical Ethics that led to the publication of *Good Medical Practice*[42] that was first published in 1992. It is a document on core ethical guidance that the GMC provides to doctors, also intending to let the public know what they can expect from doctors. He was President of the GMC from 1995 to 2002. A separate committee, the GMC's Development Programme for Performance Procedures was chaired by Leslie Southgate. This scheme led to changes in fitness to practice policies as well as developments in workplace-based assessments, now part of the training of doctors both in hospital and general practice. Stott also served as deputy chair on the GMC committee on Professional Performance (2000–2004) and he chaired the GMC's Investigation Committee between 2004 and 2008.

It is important to note the involvement of general practitioners in international groups. Byrne was chairman (1973–1980) and Horder was Honorary Secretary (1974–1981) of the Leeuwenhorst Group, a group of university teachers of general practice that spanned 11 European countries. During this time the group defined the work of a general practitioner, as well as the broad education training goals which should be achieved by the time that a doctor enters independent general practice. This group had considerable success in the fact that its definition of general practice was accepted as a policy document, not only in the United Kingdom, but in most of the other countries represented in the group. Above all it was used in documents of the European Economic Community during the time when a Community Directive under the Treaty of Rome was being prepared.

Within WONCA, a number of general practitioners have had influential roles both past and present. However, with regards specifically to names in this part of the book, Stuart Carne was the WONCA president between 1976 and 1978 and Terry Kemple's work on recertification, when abroad, led to him receiving a RCGP International Travel scholarship to lead a workshop on the topic at a WONCA conference in 1995. Heath became an executive member of WONCA (2007–2013), as well as being both WONCA's WHO liaison officer and chair of Membership Committee (2010–2013). Finally, a leading name representing general practitioners from the United Kingdom abroad was Lotte Newman. She was the British representative of the Societas Internationalis Medicinae Generalis of which she became the first female president. She was also later vice-president of the European Society of General Practice (WONCA–Europe) during which she did much as part of a working party to create the European Society of General Practice and Family Medicine, established in 1995.

Several inquiries of note have either been aided by general practitioners or been about a particular general practitioner. Jarman became interested in mortality data research and he developed the Hospital Standardised Mortality Ratio, which compares the number of hospital observed deaths to the number of expected deaths over a period of time. He sat on the Bristol Inquiry panel that reported, in 2001, on paediatric surgical mortality for open heart operations.[43] Conclusions regarding numbers of surgeons and nurses, and a lack of leadership, accountability and teamwork were reached, leading to a reduction in mortality rates. The use of similar data, using a unit that Jarman helped develop, also led to an enquiry into the care at Mid-Staffordshire Hospitals Foundation Trust, between 2005 and 2009, after it had been noted that during that time between 400 and 1200 more patients died than would be expected for a comparable hospital. This led to a report in 2013 detailing 290 recommendations.[44] Due to the coroner noticing differences in the mortality rates at neighbouring general practitioner practices in Hyde, it was ultimately found that Harold Shipman had murdered an estimated 250 of his own patients. An enquiry into his case released six reports in total.[45] Over the series of reports a number of recommendations for the reform of various British systems occurred. It led to changes in death certification, the investigation of deaths and the regulation of controlled drugs in the community. Furthermore, it also split the GMC's role in both investigating and punishing doctors with fitness to practise hearings later being ran by an independent organisation.

General Practitioners Contributing to the Wider Society

The final general practitioners included in this section are those who have reached the highest levels in politics and sport. Liam Fox has been a MP since 1992 and at the time of writing is a cabinet member under Theresa May's leadership. He has had various political roles previously but currently is the Secretary of State for International Trade. From the sporting world there have been two Olympic gold medallists in Richard Budgett and Stephanie Cook. Budgett rowed to a gold medal as a member of the Men's Coxed Four at the Los Angeles 1984 Olympic Games and has gone on to have a successful career in Sport and Exercise Medicine, currently holding the post of Medical and Scientific Director of the International Olympic Committee. Cook won the women's modern pentathlon gold at the Sydney 2000 Olympic Games and when retiring, after becoming world champion a year later, returned to medicine. She undertook various sporting and Olympic Game roles when concurrently undertaking general practitioner training, and today works as a general practitioner.

References

1. Royal Commission on Medical Education 1965–68 (Chmn. Lord Todd). *Report of the Royal Commission on Medical Education (Cmnd 3569).* London: HMSO; 1968.

2. Pereira Gray D. Postgraduate training and continuing education. In: Loudon I, Horder J, Webster J (eds.). *Practice under the National Health Service 1948–1997.* Oxford: Clarendon Press; 1998.

3. College of General Practitioners. *Special Vocational Training for General Practice: Report from General Practice No. 1.* London: HMSO; 1965.

4. College of General Practitioners. *Evidence of the College to the Royal Commission on Medical Education: Report from General Practice No. 5.* London: HMSO; 1966.

5. Irvine D. *Teaching Practices: Report from General Practice No. 15.* London: HMSO; 1972.

6. RCGP. *The Future General Practitioner: Learning and Teaching.* London: RCGP; 1972.

7. Irvine DH. 1984: The Quiet Revolution? William Pickles Lecture. *The Journal of the Royal College of General Practitioners* 1975;25:399–407.

8. The Consultative Council of General Medical Practice. *The General Practitioner in Ireland.* Dublin: The Stationery Office; 1974.

9. Freeling P, Barry S. *In-service Training. A Study of the Nuffield Courses of the Royal College of General Practitioners*. Windsor: NFER-Nelson; 1982.

10. Keighley B. The JCPTGP: The passing of an era. *British Journal of General Practice* 2005;55(521):970–71.

11. Essex-Lopresti M. Vocational training for general practice. *British Journal of General Practice* 2012;62(605):646.

12. Pereira Gray DJ. The University of Exeter. In: Howie J, Whitfield M (eds.). *Academic General Practice in the UK Medical Schools 1948–2000: A Short History*. Edinburgh: Edinburgh University Press; 2011.

13. Pereira Gray DJ. *A System of Training for General Practice; Occasional Paper 4*. Exeter: RCGP; 1977.

14. RCGP. *Quality in General Practice: Policy Statement 2*. London: RCGP; 1985.

15. Irvine DH, Pereira Gray DJ, Bogle IG. Vocational training: The meaning of 'satisfactory completion'. *British Journal of General Practice* 1990;40:434.

16. GMC. *Recommendations as to Basic Medical Education*. London: GMC; 1967.

17. Harris CM. *General Practice Teaching of Undergraduates in British Medical Schools: Reports from General Practice*. No. XI. London: RCGP; 1969.

18. Howie J. Research in general practice: Perspectives and themes. In: Loudon I, Horder J, Webster J (eds.). *Practice under the National Health Service 1948–1997*. Oxford: Clarendon Press; 1998.

19. Hannay D. Undergraduate medical education and general practice. In: Loudon I, Horder J, Webster J (eds.). *Practice under the National Health Service 1948–1997*. Oxford: Clarendon Press; 1998.

20. Loudon I, Horder J, Webster J (eds.). *Practice under the National Health Service 1948–1997*. Oxford: Clarendon Press; 1998.

21. Drury M, Hull R. *Introduction to General Practice*. London: Baillière, Tindall and Cassell; 1979.

22. Hart JT. The inverse care law. *The Lancet* 1971;297(7696):405–12.

23. Davis RH (Chmn.). *The Organisation of Group Practice. A Report of a Sub-Committee of the Standing Medical Advisory Committee*. London: HMSO; 1971.

24. Stott NCH, West RR. Randomised controlled trial of antibiotics in patients with cough and purulent sputum. *British Medical Journal* 1976;2(6035):556–59.

25. Stott NCH, Davis RH. The exceptional potential of each primary care consultation. *The Journal of the Royal College of General Practitioners* 1979;29(201):201–5.

26. Pereira Gray D, Evans PH, Sweeney KG, Lings P, Seamark D, Seamark C et al. Towards a theory of continuity of care. *Journal of the Royal Society of Medicine* 2003;96:160–66.

27. Mainous AG III, Baker R, Love M, Pereira Gray D, and Gill JM. Continuity of care and trust in one's physician: Evidence from primary care in the United States and the United Kingdom. *Family Medicine* 2001;33:22–27.

28. Howie JG, Porter AM, Heaney DJ, Hopton JL. Long to short consultation ratio: A proxy measure of quality of care for general practice. *British Journal of General Practice* 1991;41(343):48–54.

29. RCGP. *Oral Contraceptives and Health*. London: Pitman; 1974.

30. Kay CR. The happiness pill? James Mackenzie Lecture 1979. *Journal of the Royal College of Practitioners* 1980;30:8–19.

31. RCGP. *What Sort of Doctor: Report of General Practice No. 23*. London: RCGP; 1985.

32. Haslam D. *Sleepless Children: A Handbook for Parents*. New York: Pocket Books; 1985.

33. Neighbour RH. *The Inner Consultation*. Lancaster: MTP; 1987.

34. Anon. 50 GPs who shaped (or will shape) General Practice. *Pulse* 2010;17 March:18–21.

35. Neighbour RH. *The Inner Apprentice*. Oxford: Radcliffe Publishing; 1992.

36. Neighbour R. *The Inner Physician*. London; 2016.

37. Heath I. *Matters of Life and Death: Key Writings*. Oxford: Radcliffe Publishing; 2007.

38. Macfarlane A, McPherson A. *The Diary of a Teenage Health Freak*. Oxford: Oxford University Press; 1987.

39. McPherson A. An extremely interesting time to die. *British Medical Journal* 2009;339:b2827.

40. Gray S. Dame Rosemary Rue. *The Guardian* 2005;12 January.

41. Pereira Gray D. Mollie McBride: An appreciation. *British Journal of General Practice* 2014;64(618):38.

42. GMC. *Good Medical Practice*. London: GMC; 1995.

43. Kennedy I (Chmn.). *The Report of the Public Inquiry into Children's Heart Surgery at the Bristol Royal Infirmary 1984–1995*. London: Stationery Office; 2001.

44. Jarman B. *Mid Staffordshire Public Inquiry Brian Jarman Witness Statements and Oral Hearing*. In: Francis R (Chmn.). The Mid Staffordshire NHS Foundation Trust Public Inquiry: Report of the Mid Staffordshire NHS Foundation Trust Public Inquiry. London: HMSO; 2013.

45. Smith J (Chmn.). *The Shipman Inquiry. (Reports 1 to 6)*. Norwich: Stationery Office; 2002–2005.

63 EKKEHARD VON KUENSSBERG (1913–2001)

Ivan Jobling

Ekkehard Von Kuenssberg was born in Heidelberg, Germany, on 17 December 1913. His parents, Professor Eberhard and Dr Katharina Von Kuenssberg, were respected academics in german law and biology respectively. The Kuenssberg family was aristocratic, claiming its family tree could be traced back to the time of Charlemagne. His mother's ancestry was Jewish, although she herself was brought up as a Protestant. She would survive the Second World War (1939–1945) hidden by friends and family.

Kuenssberg had four siblings and was educated at the boarding school Schule Schloss Salem, in southern Germany, where he became head boy. It was here, after listening to an organ recital by medical missionary Albert Schweitzer, that 16-year-old Kuenssberg first decided to undertake a career in medicine.

The Kuenssberg family was deeply opposed to the Nazi Party, and extremely concerned about the party's growing popularity in Germany. As a result of this, the then 16-year-old Kuenssberg moved to Austria and studied chemistry at the University of Innsbruck. During this time he developed his love of skiing, assisting refugees from the Nazi regime to escape over the Austrian mountains. However, when the Nazi Party came to power in 1933, he received an invitation from the Nazi Party's Schutzstaffe (SS) to join their ranks, probably due to his favourable aristocratic connections. Kuenssberg decided to leave Austria and live in England. Whilst travelling between the two countries he hid a considerable amount of money in a hollowed out tennis racket base and hockey stick.

For a time, Kuenssberg worked at the University of Cambridge as a lab assistant but wrote to every medical school in the country in order to secure a place to study. The University of Edinburgh replied, accepting Kuenssberg and waving his tuition fees as 'a present to Heidelberg University on its 400th birthday'. It was here that he met his future wife Constance Hardy (1911–2004) as well as taking time to set up the university's skiing and yacht societies. After university, he worked as a locum general practitioner in Granton, a deprived area of Edinburgh. During the war he was initially interned for five months but in 1944, he served in the RAMC in East Africa under the pseudonym 'Edgar Valentine Kingsley'. Here he eventually reached the rank of Lieutenant Colonel before returning to Granton as a full partner in 1946.

After the war Kuenssberg worked in the Granton area until 1981, ultimately helping to found nine new practices by the time of his retirement. He was famous for taking on a huge workload, travelling back regularly from meetings in London to do an evening surgery. His work in obstetrics and home deliveries was particularly respected. In 1958, he helped produce one of the first studies on cervical smears to be published by general practitioner practices. Furthermore, he helped start the RCGP Oral Contraception Study. This prospective cohort study started in 1968 and recruited 46,000 women. Follow-up finished in December 2006 and this study remains one of the biggest and most influential of its kind on the oral contraceptive pill. Importantly, the study showed oral contraception was not associated with an increased long-term increase in mortality. He was also notable for a letter, published in the *BMJ* in 1961 together with two neurologists working at the Northern General Hospital, which described the dangerous effects of Thalidomide before its effect on the foetus became clear. He was later invited to join the Dunlop committee, the only general practitioner on the first committee on the safety of drugs.

As well as having an impact clinically, Kuenssberg was a significant influence on medical policy in the United Kingdom. The 1950 *Collings Report* was particularly significant describing the state of general practice as 'bad and deteriorating'. In the years after the war general practitioners were extremely hard pressed, making up to 30 home visits a day and good practice suffered in many areas. It was partly as a result of this report that the College was founded and he did much in its early years. He was a founding member of the College in 1952, chairman of the Scottish Council Research Committee (1959–1962), chairman and Honorary Secretary of the Research Foundation Board (1960–1972), member of the research committee (1958–1965; 1967–1968; 1974–1982), chairman of Council (1970–1973) and president from 1976 to 1979. He was awarded the Foundation Council Award in 1967 and delivered the 17th James Mackenzie Lecture in 1970 entitled 'General practice through the looking-glass'.

Furthermore Kuenssberg, as the chairman of the Scottish General Medical Services Committee, was one of the four general practitioners who helped negotiate the 1966 General Practitioner Charter. This charter expanded the role of general practice, providing the funds needed for practices to improve premises and hire nursing and secretarial staff, amongst other changes. Due to the above described career, he was appointed CBE in 1969.

Kuenssberg strongly believed in increasing the involvement of nurse practitioners in general practice. He held a position on the Queen's Nursing Institute (QNI) committee until 1976. There, he was involved in developing an endowment, for a chair in community nursing and worked to obtain equal pay scales between ward and district nurses. He helped transform the role of the general practitioner in the United Kingdom from an isolated profession, often referred to as a 'cottage industry' to the constantly expanding one today.

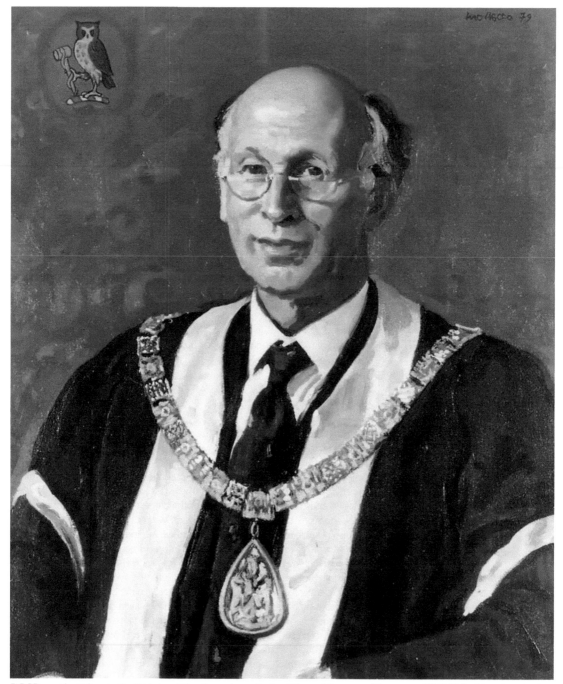

RCGP presidential portrait of Ekkehard Von Kuenssberg. Artist: Alberto Morrocco. (Courtesy of RCGP Archives, London.)

In 1981, the same year as his retirement, Kuenssberg was awarded FRCP and Fellowship of the Royal College of Obstetricians and Gynaecologists. The RCGP also named the Kuenssberg Award in his honour. This is awarded each year for an improvement in practice brought about due to an audit.

Kuenssberg died from Parkinson's disease and cancer on 27 December 2000 at Haddington, East Lothian aged 87 years old and was survived by his wife, two sons and a daughter. His attitude to his colleagues and work is captured well in his own words when resigning from the QNI board in 1976: 'I am only, too happy, at any time, to assist any projects the QNI might develop and many thanks for your gracious and forbearing welcoming of a troublesome member'.

Further Reading

Anon. Dr. Ekkehard Kuenssberg. *The Times* 2001; 4 January.

Anon. Obituaries. E. Kuennsberg. *Proceedings of the Royal College of Physicians of Edinburgh* 2001;31(4):369.

Kuenssberg EV, Simpson JA, Stanton JB. Is thalidomide to blame? *British Medical Journal* 1961;1(5221):291.

Kuennsberg EV. General practice through the looking-glass. *The Journal of the Royal College of General Practitioners* 1971;21(102):3–16.

Large A. Obituaries. Ekkehard Von Kuenssberg. *British Medical Journal* 2002;324(7337):617.

Wellcome Trust Library Archive. Dr. E V Kuenssberg. General Practitioner. Correspondence with QNI. 1976. Reference: SA/QNI/F.6/19:Box 58.

64 WILLIAM HAWKINS HYLTON (1903–1989)

Alan Gopal and James Parry-Reece

William Hawkins Hylton was born in Leeds on 6 March 1903. His initial foray into a profession began with engineering, not medicine. He read engineering at the University of Leeds and subsequently entered the family building firm. Some years later he decided engineering was not where he wanted to spend the rest of his working life and returned to the University of Leeds, this time reading medicine. He qualified in his early thirties.

Upon qualifying in 1939, he was called up to military service in the RAMC. He served in France, including Dunkirk, moving to India and Burma later, rising up the ranks to become a Lieutenant Colonel before he returned to England at the conclusion of the war. During his time in India he was introduced to, and subsequently married another doctor, Lorna Peterson (1914–2005). On their return, they set up a practice together in Clevedon, then part of Avon but now part of Somerset.

The lifetime contribution of Hylton to the College as a founding member and provost of the South West Faculty were substantial. Prior to 1965, general practice in the United Kingdom was regarded as in crisis. Eighteen thousand general practitioners were formally prepared to resign from the NHS, with the original agreement by general practitioners signed at the inception of the NHS about to be reneged. General practice was absent from the medical undergraduate curriculum in the majority of medical schools in the United Kingdom and the postgraduate alternative was unsatisfactory on both sides of the classroom. A third of newly qualified general practitioners were leaving the country to practise elsewhere as they struggled to fit into the national system. The efforts of the College to rectify this lacked backing from other medical specialities or the government and were nearly all met with failure. This had much to do with the fact that the College was occupied primarily with trying to establish itself; even the concept of general practice as an academic and vocational subject had yet to be widely acknowledged within the medical community at that point.

Hylton recognised this need for change. He became chairman of the Postgraduate Committee at the College to drive the College's efforts to rectify this situation personally. By 1964, it had acquired a large number of duties that it deemed best carried out by separate groups and was dismantled accordingly. Aside from the medical recording service and overseeing awards, vocational training and postgraduate education were the core two issues it served to advance. The Postgraduate Committee under Hylton recommended that College Council created a group to specifically oversee its development. The College approved its formation. When the Vocational Training Working Party (VTWP) was formed (the predecessor of the Vocational Training Subcommittee), Hylton was appointed its first chair.

The VTWP was established to help organise the development of a vocational training programme for general practice. It released a series of reports to help inform those who were developing local training schemes, and established a guide as to which hospital posts were most directly relevant to future general practitioners. Importantly it also influenced the Royal Commission on Medical Education. The broad principles of their vision were written in their preliminary report published in *The Lancet* in 1964 entitled 'Vocational training for general practice'. A second report was published which outlined a more detailed plan of this and included recommendations for how to use the failing remnants of previous schemes to shore up the newly proposed system of training. The conclusion of this report stated the need for an ambitious idealistic plan, rather than pragmatically trying to improve the ailing system of the time, as the flaws of that scheme would continue to haunt any overhaul.

The timing of the opportunity provided to the VTWP by the Royal Commission on Medical Education, popularly known as the *Todd Report*, was a tipping point to alter the state of the profession. Hylton and the VTWP took full advantage of it to radically alter general practitioner training in the United Kingdom. They presented a document on behalf of the College which was a culmination of their careful preparation to ensure that general practice became a core speciality in medical curricula. To do this, they looked to gain the backing of the government to enforce postgraduate training as a requirement of general practice. The evidence they provided aided the medical profession on the much needed reorganisation of medical education in the United Kingdom. The evidence was well received, and allowed the College to have a role within the postgraduate gateway into general practice.

By the time of the publication of the *Implementation of Vocational Training* report in 1967, Hylton had stepped down as chairman, but remained one of the core members, working with a notable array of general practitioners such as John Horder (1919–2012) and Patrick Bryne (1913–1980). In this report, a working model of vocational training was prepared, with recommendations for several concurrent regional experiments; no effort to formalise vocational training had ever been performed on this scale. These reports formed the basis of the general practice training scheme as it exists in the NHS today, legitimising the role of the College in their representation and regulation of the speciality through their guidance of undergraduate and particularly postgraduate education.

Aside from his commitments to the College, Hylton was involved with other organisations. He was President (1965–1967) and vice-president (1967–1968) of the Bath, Bristol and Somerset Branch of the BMA. His inaugural

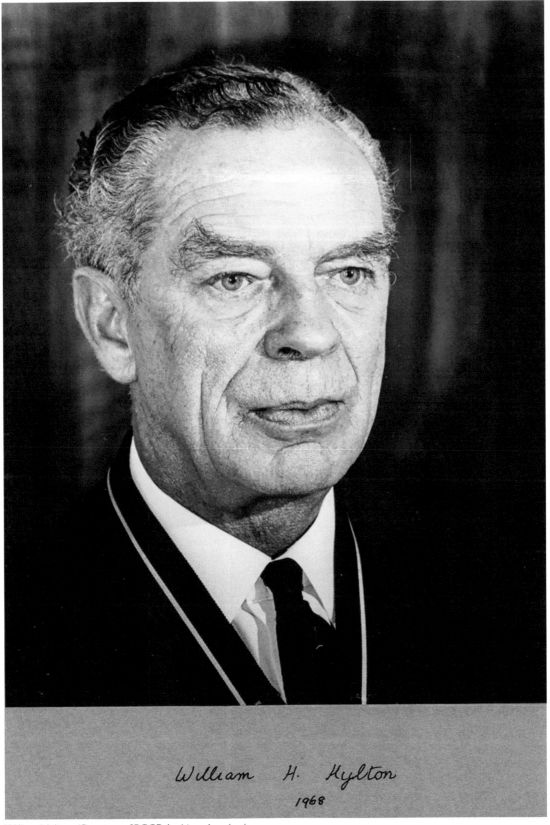

William H. Hylton

1968

William Hylton. (Courtesy of RCGP Archives, London.)

address was entitled 'General practice: Learning and teaching'. It looked at how to lay the foundations for a successful career in general practice, and how the profession could contribute to enhance hospital-based teaching. This was received with 'prolonged acclamation'. He was a Fellow of the Royal Society of Medicine, joining the general practice with Primary Health care section in 1964.

Hylton was known for his grounded decisiveness and compassion both inside and out of his practice. Outside of his working life, he enjoyed gardening and bird watching, making many trips abroad with Lorna. He continued to work at his practice until his early seventies, and spent his retirement in Clevedon until he died at 83 years of age on 20 March 1989. He was survived by his wife, five children and nine grandchildren.

Further Reading

Horder J, Swift G. The history of vocational training for general practice. *The Journal of the Royal College of General Practitioners* 1979;29:24–32.

JSM. Obituary. *British Medical Journal* 1989;298:1246.

Pereira Gray DJ. Postgraduate training and continuing education. In: Loudon I, Horder J, Webster C (eds.). *General Practice under the National Health Service 1948–1997*. London: Clarendon Press; 1998.

Swift G. Postgraduate education and training. In: Fry K, Horder J, Pinsent RJFH (eds.). *A History of the Royal College of General Practitioners: The First 25 Years*. Lancaster: MTP; 1982.

55 PATRICK BYRNE (1913–1980)

Imogen Monks and Neil Metcalfe

Patrick Sarsfield Byrne was born on 17 April 1913 in Birkenhead, near Liverpool, to parents John and Marie Byrne. His father was a butcher. He attended St. Edwards College, on the back of two scholarships won in Birkenhead, in Liverpool from 1923 to 1930. He then won a state scholarship to study medicine at the University of Liverpool. He graduated with MBChB in 1936. During this time, he had already shown himself to be a prolific prize winner and achiever, winning a gold medal in surgery and other clinical prizes. He was also the 'first holder of a cup for debating'; an early sign of his ability to hold his ground in the political sphere.

After medical school Byrne started work as a general practitioner in Milnthorpe, Westmorland. He worked there for 32 years. After this, other commitments took to the forefront of his working life, although he did remain active in general practice at the Darbishire House Teaching Health Centre until his retirement in 1978.

During his time as a general practitioner Byrne joined the College as a founding member. He was an active member of the College from 1952 to 1976. His roles there included being chairman (1966–1968) and provost (1968–1970) of the North-West England Faculty, chair of the amalgamated Education Committee (1964–1969), vice-chairman of the Council in 1966, chief examiner (1967–1973), chairman of the Board of Censors (1969–1975) and chairman of the Undergraduate Education Committee (1974–1975). Finally, he also became president of the College for three years from 1974 to 1976.

During his time at the College and its later incarnation the RCGP, Byrne made large changes to the way that general practice was taught and examined in the United Kingdom. Whilst chair of the Education Committee he recognised that educational changes were necessary in the speciality, specifically in the development of teachers of general practice. He delivered the twelfth Gale Memorial Lecture in 1968 entitled 'Preparation for teaching in general practice'. The main points of the lecture were to outline the practical aspects of undergraduate and postgraduate training in general practice and how these have been implemented at the University of Manchester, including an outline of the general practice curriculum and the successes and problems they encountered. He also contributed to a book published by the RCGP called *The Future General Practitioner: Learning and Teaching* (1972). This book aimed to give the general practice a framework, focusing on general principles and using examples to illustrate these.

Byrne was a pioneer in developing specific and vocational training for general practitioners. He helped change the way general practice was perceived, from being a specialty that was assumed could not be taught, to a subject where vocational experience as an undergraduate, postgraduate examinations and lifelong continuing education became essential. Only 20 years previously, the 'universities' denied that general practice was even an academic field. Byrne was instrumental in changing this opinion and he was the principal developer of the MRCGP in his role of chairman of the College's Board of Censors and chief examiner. During his time as president of the RCGP, he set up and chaired the first 'Postgraduate Committee of Council' which had the tasks of approving vocational training programmes, which led general practitioner trainees to be prepared for the aforementioned MRCGP examination.

At the persuasion of his friend, Professor Robert Platt (1900–1978), in 1965, Byrne began lecturing part-time at the University of Manchester, travelling the 70 miles each way between the university and his home. This led to him taking the post of director of general practice at the university and moving to Manchester in 1968. When he was appointed the first professor of general practice at the University of Manchester he was also the first ever professor of general practice in England. He was in charge of one of the largest educational departments of general practice in the United Kingdom.

Further to the Gale Lecture, Byrne gave several eponymous lectures both in the United Kingdom and internationally. He was the first speaker of some of these lectures, for example the William Pickles Lecture in 1968. This lecture was entitled 'The passing of the 'eight' train' where he presented the life of William Pickles (1885–1969) and went on further to discuss the advances in clinical training of general practitioners in Manchester. For the William Marsden Lecture at the Royal Free Hospital London in 1974, he presented 'Medical education and general practice' which began by paying homage to William Marsden (1796–1867) and moved on to discuss how general practice may be incorporated into medical education at undergraduate and postgraduate levels. In 1975, he was the David Lloyd Hughes Memorial Lecturer at Liverpool.

Byrne's commitment to the education of general practitioners extended worldwide. This was exemplified when working as chairman of the Leeuwenhost Group (1973–1980), a group of university teachers of general practice that spanned 11 European countries (see Appendix A for summary). The main aims of the group were to create definitions of general practice and of the general practitioner that were acceptable to all countries involved and to develop training programmes based on these definitions. The definition has continued to today. However, this was not the limit of his international acclaim. He took on the role of advisor to the British Council and many foreign governments,

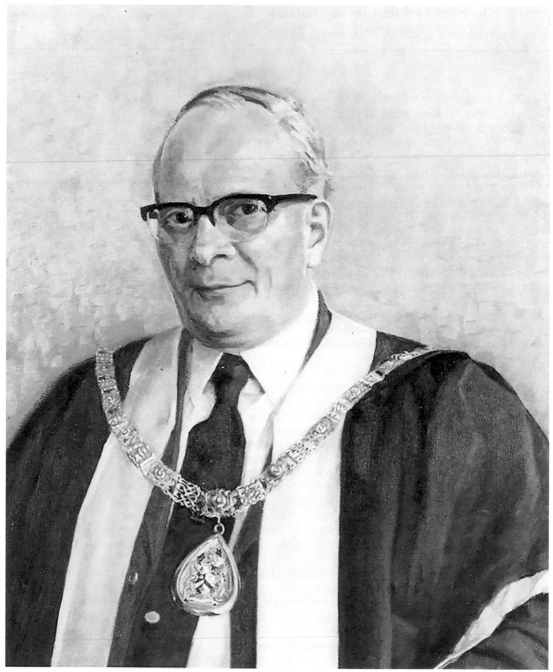

RCGP presidential portrait of Patrick Byrne. Artist: Ian Grant. (Courtesy of RCGP Archives, London.)

particularly on medical education and the establishing of departments or colleges of general practice. In 1971, he gave the W. Victor Johnston Memorial Oration to the College of Family Physicians of Canada. Notably, he was awarded the Hippocratic Medal of the International Society for General Practice in 1963, and the Sesquicentennial Medal of the Medical University of South Carolina in 1974. He was made an Honorary Fellow of the College of Medicine in South Africa and, in 1975, was given honorary membership of the College of Family Physicians of Canada in 1976.

Further roles were taken by Byrne in the United Kingdom. He advised the Department of Health and Social Security (now known as the Department of Health) on general practice in 1972. In 1978, he became a professor emeritus to recognise the service he provided to the development of the general practitioner. He was also appointed OBE in 1966 and CBE in 1975.

Byrne authored and co-authored a great number of publications. Perhaps the most influential piece was the book he co-authored with B.E. Long, *Doctors Talking to Patients* (1976). Together the authors studied over 2000 audio recordings and described six phases in the consultation which give it a logical structure. This included: the doctor establishes a relationship with the patient; the doctor discovers or attempts to discover the reason for the attendance; the doctor conducts a verbal and/or physical examination; the doctor, the doctor and patient or the patient (in that order of probability) consider the condition; the doctor and occasionally the patient detail further treatment or investigation; the consultation is terminated, usually by the doctor. They then divided the analysis of the 'consultation' into consultation and prescribing phases and also described a spectrum of consulting styles, one extreme being doctor-centred and the other, patient-centred. The model is useful for analysing 'dysfunctional' consultations where the patient may be misunderstood and dissatisfied whilst the doctor may be frustrated and today it is sometimes included in consultation training for general practitioner trainees. Other books he co-authored included *The Assessment of Postgraduate Training for General Practice* (1976); *The Assessment of Vocational Training for General Practice, Reports from General Practice No. 17* (1976) and *Learning to Care* (1976). In addition to this he co-edited *A Handbook for Medical Treatment* (1976) and *A Textbook of Medical Practice* (1977).

Away from work Byrne was an accomplished fisherman and also played cricket and golf. He very much enjoyed spending time with his family, which included his wife Kathleen (1913–2009), who was also a general practitioner, and his six children. Despite all his achievements he remained 'strangely sensitive to criticism' but nonetheless would stand out in the crowd with his keen political awareness and wit that would devastate his colleagues. He found time to enjoy himself with friends too, who described him fondly, as having the 'roar of a lion and heart of a lamb'. In 1980, he died suddenly aged 67 years old, only 20 months after his retirement. In his obituary in the *BMJ* it was written: 'He died just as he would have wished, suddenly, with friends, a glass in his hand, and an anecdote on his lips'.

Further Reading

Byrne PS. The passing of the 'eight' train. *The Journal of the Royal College of General Practitioners* 1968;15:409–27.

Byrne PS, Freeman J. *The Assessment of Postgraduate Training for General Practice*. London: Society for Research into Higher Education; 1976.

Byrne PS, Long BEL. *Doctors Talking to Patients*. London: HMSO; 1976.

Fry J, Byrne PS, Johnson S (eds.). *A Textbook of Medical Practice*. Lancaster: Medical and Technical Publishing; 1977.

Proctor HW, Byrne PS (eds.). *A Handbook of Medical Treatment*. Lancaster: Medical and Technical Publishing; 1976.

RCGP. *The Future General Practitioner: Learning and Teaching*. London: RCGP; 1972.

RCGP. RCGP Archive. Box Reference Number B/BYR.

Appendix A

'The General Practitioner in Europe: A statement by the working party appointed by the European Conference on the Teaching of General Practice, Leeuwenhorst, Netherlands 1974'.

'The general practitioner is a licensed medical graduate who gives personal, primary and continuing care to individuals, families, and a practice population, irrespective of age, sex and illness. It is the synthesis of these functions which is unique. He will attend his patients in his consulting room and in their homes and sometimes in a clinic or hospital. His aim is to make early diagnoses. He will include and integrate physical, psychological and social factors in his consideration about health and illness. This will be expressed in the care of his patients. He will make an initial decision about every problem which is presented to him as a doctor. He will undertake the continuing management of his patients with chronic, recurrent or terminal illnesses. Prolonged contact means that he can use repeated opportunities to gather information at a pace appropriate to each patient and build up a relationship of trust which he can use professionally. He will practice in co-operation with other colleagues medical, and non-medical. He will know how and when to intervene through treatment, prevention and education to promote the health of his patients and their families. He will recognise that he also has a professional responsibility to the community'.

66 JOHN HORDER (1919–2012)
Caroline Cartlidge

John Horder was born on 9 December 1919 and was raised by his family in Ealing, West London. His father, Gerald Morley Horder, was a quantity surveyor and his mother, Emma Ruth, née Plaistowe (1877–1973), was a professional violinist. He was educated in Sussex, after obtaining a classical scholarship to board at Lancing College, a high Anglo-Catholic school, which he attended from 12 years of age and attended church services twice a day. Although describing a love of churches, he considered himself agnostic, as detailed in his 1996 paper for the *Proceedings of the Royal College of Physicians of Edinburgh*, entitled 'I believe'. He was raised in a religious family, which he felt sparked an interest in philosophy, in amongst a passion for music and the arts.

Horder originally intended becoming a professional musician, which led him to train as a classical pianist and organist under Jean Roger-Ducasse, at the Paris Conservatoire de Musique. Horder remarked that he was taken to Roger-Ducasse's flat and played the Prelude, Chorale and Fugue of César Franck. It was also whilst in Paris that he met Elizabeth June Wilson (1920–2017) who, in 1940, became his wife and had a career as a general practitioner. He became accomplished on the piano but was encouraged to place his talents elsewhere. Therefore, he returned to read Classics at the University of Oxford in 1938.

Spurred on by his concern to study human nature, after a year Horder switched courses to read medicine. He assumed this would lead to a career in psychiatry, where he could focus on the psychological aspects of illness. His studies were, however, interrupted by the Second World War (1939–1945), where he became an officer in the King's Royal Rifle Corps. He described it as the 'worst moral problem' when he was called up to fight, especially when faced with the prospect of having to kill, as he was raised amongst pacifists. Consequently, he was discharged by the army, in 1942, after a period of illness where he was diagnosed with severe depression. He was treated throughout much of the rest of his life for this including being hospitalised for long durations on three occasions.

Despite initially describing this study of medicine as 'intellectually unsatisfying' compared to his previous studies, and wondering if he had made a mistake, Horder returned to Oxford, in the midst of the creation of the NHS, and qualified in 1948. In 1951, he worked as a locum general practitioner for a fortnight at the James Wigg Practice, where his wife was working. He ended up staying there for the next 30 years, ultimately becoming a senior partner at what became Kentish Town Health Centre, which he said provided him with fulfilment and opportunity. During the 1960s, American poet Sylvia Plath was one of his patients when she lived in Primrose Hill, North London. As detailed in his 2010 autobiographical articles, 'An account of my life', published in *London Journal of Primary Care*, most doctors of that era, he believed, gave little importance to psychological problems. Therefore, unlike many others, he felt that he took her depression very seriously, and acted diligently to support her care all the way until her suicide in 1963. Horder was a man of huge compassion which was exemplified with him continually asking himself 'was there anything more I could have done?' when interviewed retrospectively by *Camden New Journal*, in 2010.

Horder was involved in a couple of particularly influential books. He took a leading role in *The Future General Practitioner: Learning and Teaching* (1972), which was considered contemporaneously to be the most influential contribution to general practice education in both the United Kingdom and internationally at that time. It became the leading source document for postgraduate general practice training. Similarly, in 1994, he co-authored *Primary Care in an International Context* with his friend John Fry (1922–1994) and in 1998, co-edited *A History of the Royal College of General Practitioners: The First 25 Years*. He considered this latter book to have been his most comprehensive work.

Horder was highly influential and held a number of important roles and positions throughout his life, within many organisations. Most notably, he contributed in a major way to the RCGP. Initially, when he was with the College, he was an archivist in 1956 but ultimately became the president of the RCGP between the years 1979 and 1982. In addition, he fulfilled his duties as chairman of the RCGP Vocational Training Committee. On top of his already vast list of achievements, Horder became the first general practitioner from the United Kingdom to be appointed a WHO consultant, having links with other general practitioners and training schemes throughout Europe, and helped produce a report, published in 1960, which was circulated to every government in the world. During this post, he visited Portugal numerous times with a focus on redesigning general practice overseas to meet the needs of the population. He gave the William Pickles Lecture in 1969 and the RCGP has awarded the John Horder Award for exceptional contributions by RCGP staff since June 2008. Other roles included Honorary Secretary of the European Leeuwenhorst Group from 1974 to 1981, where they placed a lot of trust in his judgement when defining the job description of a general practitioner in European countries. Furthermore, he served as the president of the General Practice Section of the Royal Society of Medicine in the 1967 to 1968 session, and, in 1983, was appointed as visiting professor of the General Practice Teaching Group at the Royal Free Hospital School of Medicine for eight years.

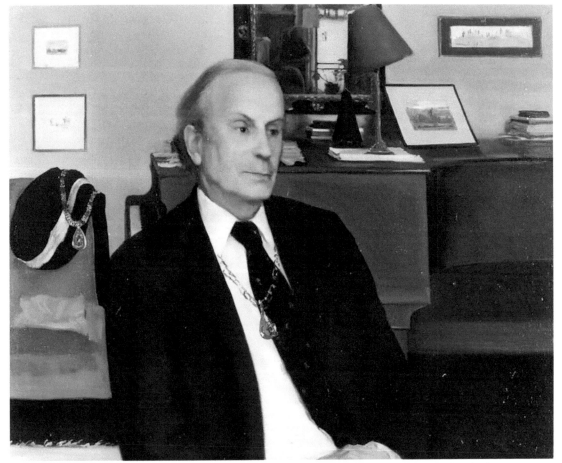

RCGP presidential portrait of John Horder. Artist: Robert Wraith. (Courtesy of RCGP Archives, London.)

Shortly after retiring from general practice in 1982, and completing his time as president of the RCGP, Horder committed to being the first chairman of the Centre for the Advancement of Interprofessional Education (CAIPE). Later, in 1994, he became President of CAIPE. Preceding a few unstable years, where CAIPE risked closure twice, their first national conference was held at Cumberland Lodge in the Windsor Great Park. Horder was seen as a very modest man that showed as he was the first to give credit to others for CAIPE's achievements. His desire for teamwork between professions was highlighted as a general practitioner when he recruited a 28-person strong multidisciplinary team in general practice. As a consequence, CAIPE, together with the General Practice and Healthcare Section of the Royal Society of Medicine, announced the John Horder Award for interprofessional teams working within primary health and social care that demonstrate outstanding principles of collaborative working. The annual award of £1500 was offered for the first time in September 2014 to honour Horder's lifetime work.

Horder received further honours. He was appointed OBE in 1971, CBE in 1981 and awarded the Foundation Council Award in 1998. As a result of his outstanding work in the realms of interprofessionalism, he was awarded honorary doctorates of science by Kingston University and the University of Westminster.

On 30 May 2012, Horder died of heart failure when 92 years old. He was survived by his wife, two daughters and two sons. He aimed to establish general practice as a respected speciality at a time when he believed it was seen as inferior to other medical professions. He taught the relevance of arts to the science of medicine and considered himself an 'artist from a family of artists', and his love of travel provided inspiration for his watercolour paintings, many of which were sold to raise funds for the RCGP. He also provided patient-centred care, looking at the patient as a whole and integrating all factors contributing to their ill health. For these reasons, and countless more contributions to medicine, he was given the title of 'Father of Modern General Practice' by Clare Gerada (1959–), former RCGP Chairman. His obituary in *The Times* stated that 'He was accessible and approachable, and inspired all those who knew him with the breadth of his knowledge, wisdom, and by his personal example'.

Further Reading

Fry J, Horder J. *Primary Health Care in an International Context*. Oxford: Nuffield Trust; 1994.

Horder J. The role of the general practitioner in psychological medicine. *Proceedings of the Royal Society of Medicine* 1967;60(3): 261–70.

Horder J. I believe. *Proceedings of the Royal College of Physicians of Edinburgh* 1996;26:466–71.

Horder J. Why I paint. *British Medical Journal* 1989;299:1577–78.

Horder J. An account of my life. *London Journal of Primary Care* 2008;1(1):51.

Horder J, Swift G. The history of vocational training for general practice. *The Journal of the Royal College of General Practitioners* 1979;29:24–32.

Howie J. Horder, John Plaistowe (1919–2012), General Practitioner. *Oxford Dictionary of National Biography*. Oxford: Oxford University Press. Available at http://www.oxforddnb.com/view/10.1093/ref:odnb/9780198614128.001.0001/odnb -9780198614128-e-106615 (accessed 25 January 2018).

Loudon I, Horder J, Webster C, (eds.). *General Practice under the National Health Service 1948–1997*. Oxford: Oxford University Press; 1998.

RCGP. *The Future General Practitioner: Learning and Teaching*. London: RCGP; 1972.

67 PAUL FREELING (1928–2002)

Fraser McMillan Brooks

Paul Freeling was born in London on 5 August 1928. In his early years, he attended Haberdashers' Aske's Boys' School in Elstree, Hertfordshire, excelling academically, and on the sporting field as captain of boxing and a notable competitor on the rugby pitch. This enthusiasm for competitive sport continued for many years and he became a keen bridge player. He won a scholarship to attend St. Mary's Hospital Medical School, now merged with Imperial College School of Medicine, and began training in 1947. He qualified as a doctor in 1952 and completed his national service with the RAF, spending time in Egypt and Kenya, where he captained the RAF rugby team.

Returning to the United Kingdom, Freeling worked as a general practitioner in Southall, before moving to work at St George's and Wandworth General Practitioner Surgery. From the start of his career, he was involved in general practice research and training. He worked with various general practice research groups, co-authoring several pioneering reports on general practice training. This work earned him a leading role within the RCGP's Nuffield Project, a residential training course beginning in 1974 which focused on preparing regional general practitioner trainers.

In September 1976, Freeling joined St George's, University of London as a senior lecturer in general practice in the Department for Clinical Epidemiology and Social Medicine. Here he continued to play and integral part in the transformation of general practice training through the subsequent decades. Two years later, a dedicated General Practice and Primary Care department was established. At the helm of this new department was Freeling who endeavoured to revolutionise the teaching of general practice within the medical school. Like other contemporary medical schools, general practice teaching was historically neglected at St George's, displaced by more specialised teaching. Freeling, alongside several like-minded general practitioners, fought to affirm the importance of general practice training and to carve out a place for its study within the medical curriculum. From humble beginnings as an offshoot of another department, whilst operating out of a semi-permanent portakabin on the St George's site, he employed four local general practitioners and secured greater incorporation of general practice placements into the medical timetable. The undeniable success of the new sub-department and its rapidly emerging research activity won it a promotion to permanent premises in the Jenner Wing at the heart of the hospital site. This led to Freeling being appointed professor of general practice at St George's Hospital Medical School in 1985. In recognition of his central role at St George's, he was named Vice-Dean in 1988, remaining in this role until his retirement in 1993. After playing an instrumental role in the establishment and successful development of the newly independent Department of General Practice and Primary Care, he retired from formal medical education, remaining an advisor to the school as Emeritus Professor.

Freeling found himself working during a pivotal time for the establishment of academic general practice training. As noted by John Howie (1937–), medical education programs in the decades following the founding of the NHS had failed to prepare trainees for a job role which a significant majority would take on. Medical trainees were denied formal general practice training and the principles of general practice were often disregarded. Many, rather derisively, considered general practice as mere summation of all specialities practised at a superficial level by amateur generalists. He played a pivotal role in altering this dynamic and demonstrating the worth of general practice as a valuable clinical discipline. In 1972, Freeling, alongside five RCGP Fellows, co-authored the landmark book *The Future General Practitioner: Learning and Teaching*, which sought to systematically define the academic and vocational content of general practice. *The Future General Practitioner: Learning and Teaching* was written the general practitioner educators but was considered by some as an important text for anyone with an interest in general practice. The book outlined five key themes central to general practice: health and disease, human development, human behaviour, medicine and society and the practice. The book particularly put emphasis on the importance of the psychosocial aspects of general practice and paved the way for the establishment of general practice as an academic discipline worthy of future research and refinement. Freeling's pioneering research into the dynamic role of the general practitioner and endless persistence as an advocate of general practitioner training has helped shape the United Kingdom's internationally regarded model of general practice education.

Aside from his work in the field of general practice training, Freeling made significant contributions to the research bodies of depression, asthma and AIDS within the community. His work improved the recognition, understanding and treatment of these conditions amongst general practitioners. Most significantly, in the field of depression, he played an integral role in the RCGP's ground breaking *Defeat Depression* campaign launched in 1992.

Freeling also authored several texts which challenged the contemporary culture of general practice. This included *The Doctor-Patient Relationship* (1967) and *The Special Function of the General Practitioner* (1964). Particularly in his work with Kevin Browne, a general practitioner from Hillingdon, he explored the dynamics of the doctor–patient relationship and encouraged general practitioners to consider their interactions with patients at a deeper more empathetic level.

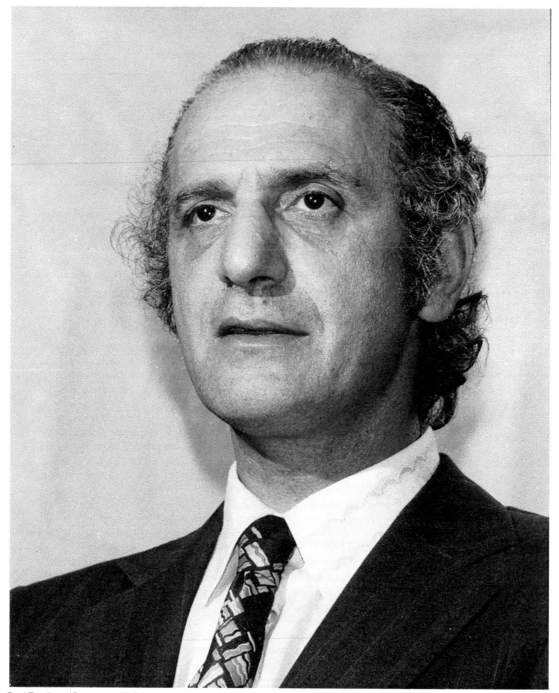

Paul Freeling. (Courtesy of RCGP Archives, London.)

Specifically, Freeling highlighted the holistic role of doctors and recognised their role in providing an opportunity for their patients to be listened to.

Freeling recognised and valued the importance of the role of the general practitioner. In a 1964 article, which he co-authored in *The Lancet*, the central role of general practice was highlighted to handle '90% of all episodes of illness'. He warned against the growing trend of hyper-specialisation, which, he believed, threatened the masterful, generalist approach to protecting the health of the population. The authors warned that 'when general competence is sacrificed to special ability, a skilled technician may be created but the doctor is lost'. Flying in the face of many contemporaries, he refused to devalue the gatekeeper role of the general practitioner or to underestimate the essential skills required to be a general practitioner. In another article he co-authored in *The Lancet* and published in 1965, the authors lamented the transformation of the general practitioner's role from that of the listener who offers sympathy, understanding and time, to the mechanical and impersonal process of symptom identification and removal. What is clear is that Freeling recognised the worth of the holistic and personable general practitioner, with whom each of their patients builds a unique relationship of trust and understanding.

In recognition of his services Freeling was honoured as the 1978 RCGP William Pickles Lecturer. Freeling titled his speech 'Those who can' and centred his talk on promoting better standards for vocational general practice training. Later, in 1981, recognising his many services to medicine, he was appointed OBE, whilst in 1992, he was presented the RCGP Foundation Council Award. He held visiting professorships in Australia, Finland, Israel and the United States. He died on 13 September 2002, after close to 50 years of shaping the philosophy of general practice. In the same year, he was posthumously awarded The President's Medal of the RCGP, which was accepted on his behalf by his wife. He was also survived by two children. He is remembered as an integral actor in the establishment of a holistic, patient-centred culture of general practice training, and recognised as a contributor to some of the principles and methods of modern general practice. Since 2004 the Paul Freeling Award has been awarded by the RCGP for innovative or meritorious work in the field of GP Specialty Training for general practice.

Further Reading

Browne K, Freeling P. The special function of the general practitioner. *The Lancet* 1964;283(7330):425–27.

Browne K, Freeling P. A basic misunderstanding. *The Lancet* 1965;285(7389):803–5.

Freeling P. William Pickles Lecture 1978: Those who can. *The Journal of the Royal College of General Practitioners* 1978;28(191): 329–40.

Freeling P, Browne K. *The Doctor-Patient Relationship*. London: Churchill Livingstone; 1976.

Howie J, Whitfield M (eds.). *Academic General Practice in the UK Medical Schools, 1948–2000: A Short History*. Edinburgh: Edinburgh University Press; 2011.

RCGP. *The Future General Practitioner: Learning and Teaching*. London: RCGP; 1972.

68 CONRAD MICHAEL HARRIS (1933–)

Ayesha Islam

Conrad Harris was born in 1933 in Liverpool. His father, Israel Harris (1900–1957), was a general practitioner and his mother, Bella Harris, was a housewife who was later appointed MBE for her voluntary work. He had one older sister, Mona Viviette Harris (1927–2003), who was also a general practitioner. He grew up in Bootle near Liverpool, one of the most deprived areas in the country. In 1939, his father went into the army and each time he was moved the family had to move to stay near him. Consequently, he attended many schools, so that Merchant Taylors' School, Great Crosby (Liverpool) where he started when nine years old was his thirteenth school.

Harris attended University of Liverpool Medical School in 1951, graduating in 1957. This is where he met his wife Malvina (née Max, 1934–1996), who was also a general practitioner. They married in 1957 and had three children. He also started his house jobs in 1957. During this time, he competed in the London–Seté car rally. En route, they passed through Andorra where they stayed for two days. They were greeted by the President of Andorra who made him a lifetime member of the National Car Club.

In 1959, Harris joined his late father's practice in partnership with his sister and brother-in-law Joseph Joel Rivlin (1921–2012). He enjoyed working in his hometown of Bootle and valued the level of trust put in him by his patients, many of whom had known him his entire life. The General Practice Charter in 1966 revolutionised the field of general practice. Amongst other changes, it made possible the creation of a larger team with a variety of roles within general practice. During this time he also served for six years as an elected Town Councillor for Bootle.

Harris showed an early interest in medical education, particularly in the teaching and training of general practice. He organised the general practice attachments of Liverpool medical students, and gained an Upjohn Traveling Fellowship to look at the extent of teaching in general practice for medical students nationally. He ultimately visited 14 medical schools in the United Kingdom and found that there were no formal departments in England, Wales nor Northern Ireland but that some general practitioners were organising small attachments of one to two weeks and running teaching method courses for the practices. This was published in his *General Practice Teaching of Undergraduates in British Medical Schools: Reports from General Practice* (1969). He also set up a teaching methods course for general practitioners in conjunction with the Department of Extramural Education of the University of Liverpool and ran teaching methods courses in the Department of General Practice at the University of Manchester. He also co-authored the influential *The Future General Practitioner* (1972). This book was designed specifically for the general practitioner teacher and added an entirely new dimension to the literature in this field. It offered the starting points from which any course organiser could have been happy to proceed. It was thought at the time to represent one of the most systematic attempts anywhere throughout the world to define the content of general practice itself.

In 1970, Harris decided to become a full-time academic, and spent four years at the University of Manchester as a senior lecturer in the first Department of General Practice in England. He was also a trainer and a Vocational Training Scheme organiser. His office was located nearby to a theatre through which he pioneered the use of professional actors, with video playback, in teaching consulting skills to undergraduates and trainees. This is now commonly used. Alongside his clinical work at Moss Side Medical Practice, he worked towards and obtained a masters degree in education in Education, in 1974, his dissertation *Measuring the Development of Professional Attitudes in Medical Students during the Undergraduate Period*. In this he described 'the anti-modelling effect', where it appeared that as medical students became more senior and reached their clinical years, their values differed compared to the values of their clinical teachers, although it was unclear whether this was a reaction medical students had to the threatening aspects of their teachers or simply generational. He also found that undergraduate years do socialise medical students into the profession. This was contrary to previous papers which had mainly focused on the American medical undergraduate system and theoretical in nature.

In 1974, Harris was asked to set up a department of general practice at St Mary's Hospital Medical School. Here, he continued the use of actors as simulated patients in the teaching of medical students. Alongside his clinical work in a practice in Fulham, he created a new style of re-registration rotation in the medical school, comprising four months each in medicine, surgery and general practice. The rotation proved to be very popular and its success persuaded the Department of Health to encourage similar schemes nationally.

In 1986, a separate department of general practice was created at the University of Leeds. Harris was awarded its foundation chair in general practice. His appointment signalled a major change in the education of medical students at Leeds Medical School as well as across the country. He and his team helped to establish a curriculum which emphasised the importance of teaching in general practice by expanding student placement allocation within the specialty. He also

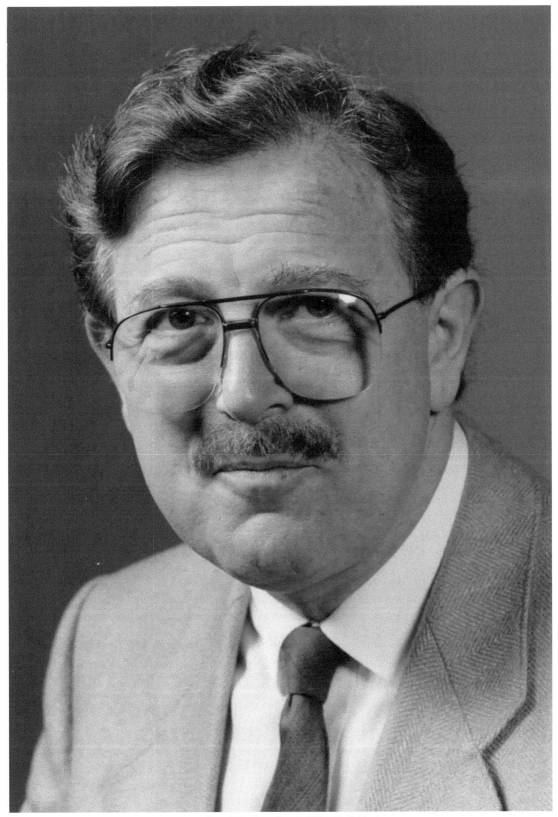

Conrad Harris. (Courtesy of the University of Leeds Archive, Leeds, West Yorkshire.)

organised a practical session entitled 'Use of the imagination as an investigative tool' greeted with enthusiasm by some students and with bemusement by others as this was not a commonly taught skill at the time.

As well as introducing new teaching methods, Harris also undertook research into the prescribing habits of general practitioners. In 1990, he was funded by the Department of Health to set up a National Prescribing Research Unit that made valued contributions to the understanding of a number of issues in general practice prescribing. These included the phenomenon of 'repeat prescribing' and the impact of general practice 'fund-holding' on prescribing patterns. The study aimed to see whether general practitioners would alter their prescribing habits if they were given feedback and the opportunity to discuss it with their colleagues. At the end of the two-year period, they found that the prescribing rate and expenditure had reduced in the groups who received feedback. With his colleagues Harris also explored the relationships of these prescribing patterns to unemployment and other socio-economic characteristics of the patients seen in general practice. They found that prescriptions were less expensive in the North of England but more frequently prescribed, in contrast to the more affluent southern parts of England.

Later, in 1996, Harris led a four year project funded by the European Union in Ulanbataar University, Mongolia, producing a new undergraduate medical curriculum to replace the existing 60-year-old Soviet model of medical teaching. Throughout his academic career he lectured in many countries and helped to shape medical education across the globe.

Away from medical curriculum work and teaching, Harris had other roles. He became a MRCGP examiner from 1968, Secretary of the RCGP Education Committee from 1969, a Member of RCGP Council also from 1969 and was awarded FRCGP in 1970. He was very active on four RCGP faculty boards and was President of the General Practice Section of the Royal Society of Medicine between 1984 and 1985. He wrote several books including *The Doctor-Patient Relationship* (1984) and *Lecture Notes on Medicine in General Practice* (1980) and published nearly 100 papers. In 1989, he gave the William Pickles Lecture on a topic relating to education entitled 'Seeing sunflowers' which highlighted the importance of research in general practice. He was the lead author of a paper published in *The Lancet* in 1986 which described a new discovery in one of his patients, who suffered from an imperfect sulphur metabolism. He found that because people with this disorder were unable to pass sulphur in their urine, they had to excrete sulphur in their sweat. These patients had a problem if they worked with clay rich in iron as the iron and the sulphur combined to make black marks on the ceramics they were making. At the time the cause of these black marks was unknown and the causes were outlined in his paper entitled 'The case of the black speckled dolls'. Furthermore he reports that he thoroughly enjoyed medico-legal work as an expert witness and always remained a practising general practitioner throughout his working career.

After retiring in 1998, Harris relocated back to London, gained a London University diploma in Asian Art and carried on collecting antique Chinese ceramics, Japanese woodblock prints and old Indian paintings until his flat could hold no more. He then took up cooking. Predeceased by his wife who died in 1996, he has three children and five grandchildren.

Further Reading

Freeling R, Harris CM. *The Doctor-Patient Relationship*. London: Churchill Livingstone; 1984.

Harris CM. *General Practice Teaching of Undergraduates in British Medical Schools: Reports from General Practice*. No. XI. London: RCGP; 1969.

Harris CM. Formation of professional attitudes in medical students. *Medical Education* 1974;8:241–45.

Harris CM. *Lecture Notes on Medicine in General Practice*. Oxford: Blackwell Scientific; 1980.

Harris CM. William Pickles Lecture 1989: Seeing sunflowers. *The Journal of the Royal College of General Practitioners* 1989;39(325): 313–19.

Harris CM. Patterns of prescribing. In: Griffin J (ed.). *Factors Influencing Clinical Decisions in General Practice. Papers of a Symposium Held in London on 23 April 1990*. London: Office of Health Economics; 1990.

Harris CM, Waring RH, Mitchell SC, Hendry GL. The case of the black-speckled dolls: An occupational hazard of unusual sulphur metabolism. *The Lancet* 1986;327(8479):492–93.

RCGP. *The Future General Practitioner: Learning and Teaching*. London: RCGP; 1972.

69 SIR DONALD HAMILTON IRVINE (1935–2018)

Sharon Messenger

Donald Hamilton Irvine was born in Newcastle upon Tyne in 1935. He practised in Ashington, a coal-mining community in Northumberland, for over 35 years. Sir Donald is widely known as one of the founders of vocational training for general practice and for his work on enhancing the quality of practice through clinical audit. He was the only general practitioner ever to be elected president of the GMC.

The key words that spring to mind when trying to summarise Sir Donald's professional contributions include 'patients', 'service', 'professional standards', 'quality', 'vocational training' and 'education'. These are all themes that have characterised his entire career, through his early professional life, his work with the RCGP, the GMC and, in retirement, the Picker Institute in Europe and the United States, and the Patients Association.

Sir Donald was born into a medical family. His father, Andrew Bell Hamilton Irvine (1901–1989), was a single-handed general practitioner in Ashington and was a founder member of the College. The father and son practised happily together for nine years, after which the father retired through ill health. At this point the young Irvine and three young colleagues in neighbouring practices decided to form a new, modern group practice. They established the Lintonville Medical Group from the outset as a modern multidisciplinary teaching general practice, one of the foundation teaching practices in the Northern Region.

Sir Donald's decision to study medicine was in part a result of being brought up in a medical household but was also greatly influenced by contracting scarlet fever followed by rheumatic fever when he was 10 years old. His illness led to a six month period of complete bed rest and regular visits from great doctors. That experience of how it feels to be a patient never left him. After passing the 11+ examination he went to King Edward VI Grammar School in Morpeth. He studied medicine at Newcastle Medical School, which was then the Medical School of Durham University in Newcastle. His younger sister Margaret (Meg) (1936–) also studied medicine and went on to become a child psychiatrist in London.

On qualifying he took his first house job at the Royal Victoria Infirmary (RVI) in Newcastle where he studied under Henry Miller (1913–1976), an internationally well-known neurologist who later became vice-chancellor of the University of Newcastle. His other hospital appointments included medicine, paediatrics and obstetrics.

In 1960, general practice was in a desperate state. Recruitment to the speciality was collapsing. *The Collings Report*, published in *The Lancet* in 1950, had painted a very dismal picture of general practice, highlighting the huge variations in quality and the lack of generally accepted professional standards at the time. Sir Donald's first week in practice made him realise that his basic medical education had not equipped him for his chosen career path. In his unpublished memoirs he noted that 'I had come to the conclusion that the people in the new College who were starting to talk about proper vocational training were dead right. I resolved to join them, to do my bit for the next generation of doctors and their patients'.

Sir Donald joined the College as an associate member in 1964, becoming a full member in 1965. The College has been of huge importance in his life. He described the early years of the College's history as a kind of 'protest movement' in which young, bright general practitioners wanted to change the nature of general practice from within. The College acted as the hub of the national network of the new trainers in general practice. Those doctors spearheaded the revival in general practice by bringing about needed change. He referred to his colleagues at that time as a 'band of brothers (and sisters)' sharing the same purpose. Sir Donald joined College Council in 1968. At that time he was one of the founders of vocational training in North East England. He went on to hold a number of key positions within the RCGP, most notably Honorary Secretary of College Council (1972–1978), chair of the Board of Censors (1979–1981) and chair of College Council (1982–1985). When chairman of College Council he launched The Quality Initiative, using clinical and medical audit to improve practice. He also delivered the William Pickles Lecture in 1975, which he titled 'The quiet revolution?', and was awarded both the Foundation Council Award and the RCGP President's Medal in 1979 and 1999 respectively.

Sir Donald, whilst juggling the demands of a young family and a busy practice, successfully completed his MD thesis on factors influencing the prevalence of cervical spondylosis in a general practice. The external examiner was none other than John Hunt, later Lord Hunt of Fawley (1905–1987), founder and former president of the College. The two remained good friends throughout Sir Donald's career. He was awarded FRCGP in 1972, as was his father who attended the same ceremony. Sir Donald held honorary degrees from seven universities in the United Kingdom and was an Honorary Fellow of six medical royal colleges in the United Kingdom.

In the early 1970s, the medical profession was in open revolt against the GMC. The government appointed an independent committee of Inquiry (The Merrison Committee) on which Sir Donald represented the RCGP. Far reaching reforms to the GMC followed, and, in 1979, the newly reconstituted GMC was formed. Because of his knowledge

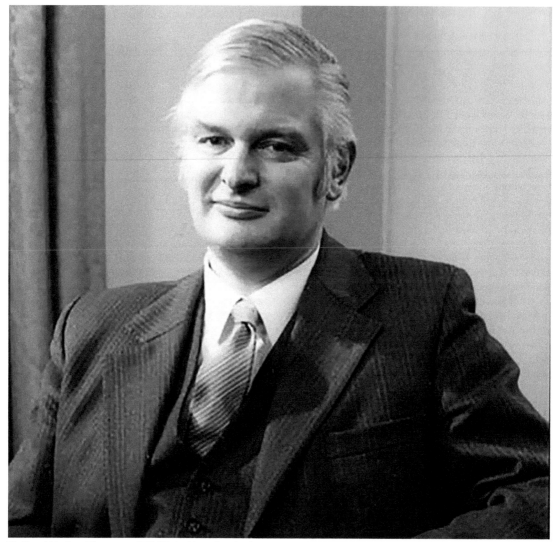

Sir Donald Irvine. (Courtesy of RCGP Archives, London.)

of medical regulation, the RCGP then asked Sir Donald to be its first representative on the new GMC. Sir Donald joined the Committee on Standards and Medical Ethics and, in 1984, he was elected chairman. He led the development of a new code of practice for the British medical profession. *Good Medical Practice* presented the profession with the principles of patient-centred practice, with the expectation that these principles would be upheld conscientiously by all doctors registered with the GMC. The guidance was first published in 1992. Today it underpins all medical practice, medical education and medical licensure in the United Kingdom and is in use by 12 other countries.

In 1995, Sir Donald was elected president of the GMC on a reform ticket. He knew that the public was losing confidence in the willingness and ability of the GMC and the wider profession to protect patients adequately from poorly performing doctors, manifest in several high profile cases culminating in the failure in paediatric cardiac surgery at the Bristol Royal Infirmary. Sir Donald put it to the leaders of the profession and government that the reactive system of medical regulation was no longer fit for purpose for twenty-first century medicine, and that it should be replaced by a proactive approach to licensing capable of assuring the quality of contemporary medical practice. The GMC adopted continuous relicensure through the process of revalidation so that patients and the public could be sure their doctor is currently up to date and fit to practise in his or her chosen field. It is still controversial with some doctors, but not with the public.

Following his time at the GMC, Sir Donald has had close work with several charities. The Picker Institute is a charity which works closely with government to ensure that patient experience remains at the heart of good medical care. It was established in the United States in the 1980s by Harvey Picker (1915–2008), a distinguished American scientist, manufacturer of x-ray machines and philanthropist. Picker was keen to try and understand why physicians in the United States were not particularly patient-centred, and thought that things could be changed by asking patients to record their experience of medical care and feeding the results back to clinicians. He established a sister organisation in the United Kingdom, Picker Institute Europe, and he asked Sir Donald, who had just retired from the GMC, to chair the Board of Trustees. Sir Donald subsequently joined the Board of Picker Institute Inc. in the United States. In promoting good care for patients Sir Donald was also a vice-president of the Patients Association, a role that he had held since 2002.

Furthermore, Sir Donald maintained a strong interest in and involvement with The Society for Cardiothoracic Surgeons in Great Britain and Ireland, particularly the leadership of Professor Ben Bridgewater (1963), Honorary Professor at Manchester Academic Health Science Centre. These surgeons have taken hands-on responsibility, individually and together, for setting and assuring their standards of practice. By publishing accurate results of their surgery, they have put into practice the essential data that should underpin revalidation. Sir Donald believed that they were already practising the kind of patient-centred professionalism that will become the norm in future.

Sir Donald was married three times and had three children, Alastair, Amanda and Angus all with his first wife, Margaret. In his spare time he enjoyed birdwatching, a legacy that stemmed from his time of bed rest as a child when he spent much time observing birds whilst convalescing. He was a Life Fellow of the Royal Society for the Protection of Birds and was a member of the British Ornithological Society. He enjoyed gardening and his beautiful garden contains a wonderful specimen of the Royal Horticultural Society's 'Caritas' rose that was commissioned and named by the RCGP to commemorate its 50th anniversary. He and Cynthia, his third wife, had 15 grandchildren.

In conclusion, Sir Donald's considerable contribution to developing quality and professionalism in general practice is best summed up in this statement: 'Patients want doctors who are technically excellent, honest and reliable, and who respect them and make them feel special. For them, the good doctor – the true professional – manages to combine scientific prowess with complete integrity and care for people'.

Sir Donald has devoted his entire career to this cause. He wrote and lectured extensively on general practice, medical education, patient-centred professionalism and quality themes in health. Over 133 papers and reports that he has edited or authored are deposited in the RCGP archives. He was appointed OBE in 1979 and CBE in 1986 for services to general practice, and was knighted in 1994 for services to medical ethics. His last two years were marred by ill health with cardiac and renal failure. Cynthia, a nurse, managed his home dialysis and looked after him with immense dedication and devotion. Sir Donald was born on 2 July 1935 and died at his home on 19 November 2018.

Further Reading

GMC. *Duties of a Doctor: Good Medical Practice*. London: GMC; 1995.

GMC. *Maintaining Good Medical Practice*. London: GMC; 1998.

Irvine D. *Teaching Practices: Report from General Practice No.15*. London: HMSO; 1972.

Irvine D. William Pickles Lecture 1975. 1984: The quiet revolution? *The Journal of the Royal College of General Practitioners* 1975;25(155):399–407.

Irvine DH. The performance of doctors I: Professionalism and self-regulation in a changing world. *British Medical Journal* 1997;314:1540–42.

Irvine DH. The performance of doctors II: Maintaining good practice, protecting patients from poor performance. *British Medical Journal* 1997;314:1613–15.

Irvine DH. *The Doctors' Tale: Professionalism and Public Trust*. Oxford: Radcliffe Medical Press; 2003.

Irvine DH. A short history of the General Medical Council. *Medical Education* 2006;40; 202–11.

Irvine DH. Memoirs of my career in medicine. Unpublished Memoir, RCGP Archives.

Irvine DH. *American Osler Society. John P. McGovern Award Lectureship. Patients, Their Doctors and the Politics of Medical Professionalism*. Dover: The American Osler Society; 2014.

Irvine DH, Hafferty F. Every patient should have a good doctor. In: Bridgewater B, Cooper G, Livesey S, Kinsman R (eds.). *Maintaining Patients' Trust: Modern Medical Professionalism*. Oxford: Dendrite Clinical Systems; 2011.

RCGP. *The Future General Practitioner: Learning and Teaching*. London: RCGP; 1972.

RCGP. *Quality in General Practice. Policy Statement No. 2*. London: RCGP; 1985.

70 MARSHALL MARINKER (1930–)
Sharon Messenger

In the 1960s, Marshall Marinker was a general practitioner in Grays, Essex. He went on to become one of the most innovative thinkers and writers about general practice as an academic discipline. John Horder (1919–2012), former President of the RCGP in his nomination of Marinker for FRCGP in 1971, wrote: 'What has impressed me most, working very closely with him in the last three years, has been the breadth of his approach to medicine, his exceptional gifts for abstract thought, for speaking and writing…'

Marinker published and lectured widely, contributing to the development of general practice theory, the methods and quality of clinical teaching and the shaping of health care policy. This led, in 1972, to his appointment as Foundation professor of community health at the newly established University of Leicester Medical School.

Marinker's parents were Polish Jewish immigrants from Warsaw. In 1914, they settled in Stepney, in London's East End. His sister, Ros Marinker (1910–), and brother, Simon Marinker (1912–), did not see a further sibling for some time. Eighteen years after Simon's arrival, and alarmed at the cessation of her menses, his mother consulted a Dr Marshall who diagnosed an early menopause. Marinker likes to point out that he was named in celebration of this misdiagnosis.

At the outbreak of the Second World War (1939–1945), Marinker was despatched to live in Bath, Somerset. He returned to live in North London in 1946. He attended the City of Bath School, and later Haberdashers' Aske's School in Hampstead, London, where he joined the Arts sixth form, hoping to study English at the University of Cambridge. He wanted to be a poet. His brother had been an outstanding prize-winning medical student. Not daring to compete with him, initially he refused to consider a medical career, but later changed his mind. Following national service in the Royal Artillery, he was accepted at the Middlesex Hospital Medical School and qualified in 1956. After house jobs in medicine, surgery and obstetrics and gynaecology at the Bedford General Hospital, and with no other preparation for general practice, let alone any formal training, he became an assistant to a general practitioner in Debden, Essex.

Debden was a post-war London Country Council housing estate, built to re-house London's East Enders whose homes had been destroyed in the Blitz. Utterly unprepared, Marinker now found himself with almost sole round-the-clock responsibility for some 4000 people who had qualified for this scarce housing by dint of major and multiple health problems. The workload was consequently prodigious.

Following this, Marinker then secured a junior partnership in one of the Nuffield Health Centres in Harlow. These showpieces were the creation of Lord Stephen Taylor (1910–1988), a public health physician and advisor to the then Labour Government. Taylor had attracted the support of the Nuffield Foundation in building these state-of-the-art health centres, richly equipped and staffed, and with the full participation of Local Authority nursing, midwifery, health visiting and social care services. The senior partners, Herbert Bach (1913–1971) and Mildred Gordon, were excellent doctors deeply committed to the highest standards. Nonetheless, restless to develop and implement his own ideas, he moved to a three-man partnership in Grays, Essex. Here, following the untimely death of the senior partner, he was able to leave and set up his own practice.

Two developments at this crucial stage shaped Marinker's future life in medicine. In January 1965, he applied for a place to one of the psychoanalyst Michael Balint's (1896–1970) teaching-cum research seminars. In Balint, Marinker found an inspirational father figure, an intellectual challenge and a cultural icon. Participation in this work revolutionised his understanding of clinical medicine, and determined his future approach to teaching and research. The second life-changing event was his encounter with the College. He had telephoned to ask for help in developing a research idea and spoke to the College General Administrator, Eileen Philips. Within days he was contacted by many of the College's leaders and research luminaries: Robin Pinsent (1916–1987), Donald Crombie (1922–2000), Ekke Kuenssberg (1913–2001), Basil Slater (1928–2017) and others, who invited him to visit them and were, in his own words, beyond generous in the support, advice and practical help that they now gave him.

Later, Marinker was elected to The Northern Home Counties Faculty Board. Soon he was appointed its Honorary Secretary. It was here that he met Paul Freeling (1928–2002) who was to become his close lifelong friend, confidante and intellectual sparring partner.

In Horder, then Chair of the College's Vocational Training Sub-committee, Marinker found a champion for his ideas, and another lifelong friend. Marinker had written a report on his Jephcott Fellowship, suggesting how the Balint approach to clinical research could be incorporated into a new style of clinical training and this was published in the College *Journal*. Its philosophy would inform much of his future work. Horder recruited him onto the working party charged with charting the future of specialist training for practice. Its published report was called *The Future General Practitioner: Learning and Teaching* (1972) and set the RCGP's academic agenda for the next decade and beyond.

Marinker now convened the *London Teacher's Workshop*, a group of experienced general practitioner tutors who over the next three years developed models of the trainer–trainee interaction and the content, methods and style of teaching from the general practice consultation.

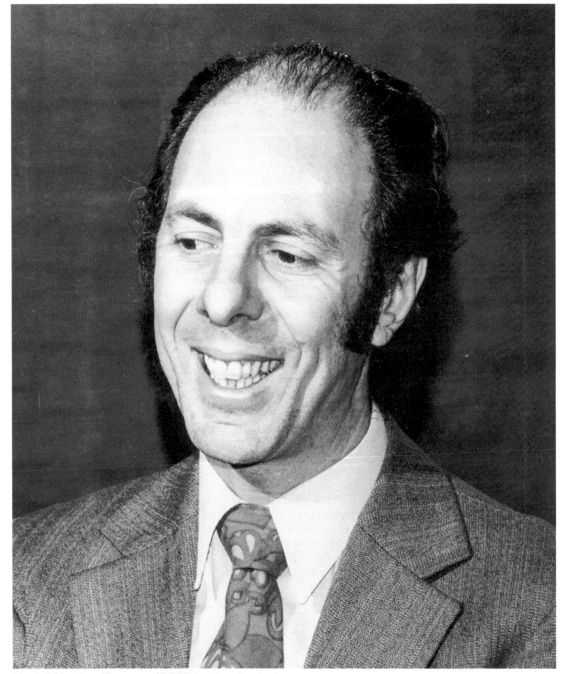

Marshall Marinker. (Courtesy of RCGP Archives, London.)

Marinker went on to become further involved with the RCGP. He was a member of the College Council (1974–1989) and served on its research committee (1966–1970) as registrar; the College Education Committee (chair 1974–1978 and 1981–1983) and later as chair of the Committee on Medical Ethics (1987–1989). He was for some years an examiner for the MRCGP, and he gave the 1974 William Pickles Lecture, 'Medical education and human values'.

In 1991, he was awarded the RCGP George Abercrombie Prize for contributions to literature. His approach to writing was summed up in his claim that 'I write not to tell you what I know but to find out what I think'. Communicating his ideas in a number of similar epigrammatic utterances, a few gained some traction:

There is a hidden curriculum in medical education that is based not on the medical school's declared intentions, but on the clinical behaviour of its teachers.

If the imagination of the academic general practitioner does not reflect his own clinical experience but only the clinical expectation of others he will contribute nothing to medicine but the dry rustling of a career bibliography.

I've listened to your story, Mrs Smith, and you are a clear case of Librium. You had better have some anxiety. In the face of illness which the doctor recognises well but cannot respectably name, the diagnosis is no longer the rationale for the treatment. It has become the alibi for the treatment.

The diagnostic task of the specialist is to reduce uncertainty, to explore possibility and to marginalise error. This contrasts sharply with the diagnostic task of the general practitioner. This is to accept uncertainty, to explore probability and to marginalise danger.

With regards to Marinker's university career, this began in 1971 when he was appointed tutor, and soon after, senior lecturer, in general practice at St Mary's Hospital Medical School, London. Here he was supported and championed by Professor Geoffrey Rose (1926–1993), whom he greatly admired. In 1974, he became the Foundation Professor of community health at the University of Leicester Medical School and later, between 1991 and 2006, he was Honorary Professor at Guy's, King's & St Thomas' Medical School. He was chair of the Council of Europe's Working Party on *The Future of General Practice in Europe* (1975–1977) and author of its report to the constituent parliaments. This and similar work was acknowledged in the award of an honorary MD from the University of Tampere, Finland in 1982, and honorary membership of the Finnish Association of General Practice in 1993. Similarly, for work in Portugal with Horder, John Walker (1928–) and Julian Tudor Hart (1927–2018), he was made an Honorary Member of the Portuguese College in 1994. He was appointed OBE in 1991.

Established in the 1980s, and funded by the multinational pharmaceutical company Merck, Sharp and Dohme, The MSD Foundation was an independent charitable trust concerned with medical education: its first chairman was Sir Douglas Black, and its first director the television documentary maker Karl Sabbagh. Marinker was recruited onto its Board of Governors and when Sabbagh resigned, Donald Irvine (1935–2018), a close personal friend and now Board Chair, persuaded him to leave Leicester and take over. Here he developed a seminal programme of Professional Leadership Workshops, year-long exercises designed to encourage and explore the ideas of the brightest and best young doctors in practice. Commissioned by Regional Health Authorities throughout England, Scotland and Wales, they were designed and carried out with some of his most talented colleagues and friends.

Marinker came late and quite by accident to an interest in health service policy. It began in 1983 when he was invited to take part in a workshop, chaired by the economist Lord Vaizey, and including the chief medical officer and similar leaders of the profession. They were asked to consider future reforms to the NHS and their deliberations were published in *A New NHS Act for 1996*. In his chapter, Marinker had suggested a cautious experiment in transferring the commissioning of hospital services to general practice control. Eventually something along similar lines was introduced by government as *Fund Holding* and not as an experiment. Initially this innovation was vehemently opposed by the BMA, the RCGP and the profession at large, and he was widely criticised for having suggested it.

Away from medicine he has enjoyed his family life and various hobbies. He married Sheila Harris in 1954 and they have three children and seven grandchildren between them. Divorced in 1978, he then married Jeanette Miller. In active retirement and deep contentment they live in a deconsecrated Victorian Gothic church in North London, where he lists his interests as 'conversation, theatre, reading, creative writing, classical music and my dog Lizzie'. He was awarded a masters degree in creative writing from City University. He has a somewhat flamboyant dress style and a collection of over a hundred bow ties.

Further Reading

Marinker M. On the boundary. *The Journal of the Royal College of General Practitioners* 1973;23(127):83–94.

Marinker M. William Pickles Lecture 1974: Medical education and human values. *The Journal of the Royal College of General Practitioners* 1974;24(144):445–62.

Marinker M. *The Doctor and his Patient*. Leicester: Leicester University Press; 1975.

Marinker M. *Teaching General Practice*. London: Kluwer; 1981.

Marinker M. What is wrong and how do we know it? In: Louden I, Horder J and Webster C (eds.). *General Practice under the National Health Service 1948–1997*. Oxford: Clarendon Press; 1998.

RCGP. *Oral History interview with Robert MacGibbon*, 16 March 2015.

RCGP. *The Future General Practitioner: Learning and Teaching*. London: RCGP; 1972.

71 JAMES MCCORMICK (1926–2007)
Tadhg J.G. Blunt and Neil Metcalfe

James Stevenson McCormick was born in County Dublin, Ireland, on 9 May 1926. He attended Avoca School in Dublin, and later studied in The Leys School in Cambridge.

McCormick qualified as a doctor when he was awarded MB from Clare College, University of Cambridge in June 1950. Following this he spent two years with the RAMC in India and Malaysia. He then went on to begin his training as a house surgeon at the Royal Sussex County Hospital in 1953, before, in 1954, becoming a house physician at St. Mary's Hospital in London. On reflecting on this time, he reported that '[my] newly acquired MB entitled me, without any further experience of any kind, to embark on a career in general practice.... in 1950, by comparison of today, therapeutic impotence was the norm.... we did silly things, but no more than today. As a house physician I carried out autohaemotherapy as a remedy for psoriasis. This involved taking 10ccs, as they were then, of blood from the antecubital fossa and injecting it into the buttock of the unfortunate. This I am sure did as much good as homeopathy and was thought to stimulate the phagocytes. I was not a skilful house surgeon but there was one operation which was delegated to me and which I carried out with skill and 100% success. This was to relieve the pain of intermittent claudication by cutting the Achilles tendon, which got rid of the pain, but at what a price!'

McCormick's first foray into general practice was as an assistant in Leicestershire, from 1954 to 1955. However, in 1955, he moved to Greystones, County Wicklow, a small seaside town on the east coast of Ireland south of Dublin, where he practised as a full-time general practitioner.

In the 1960s, McCormick became involved with the College, later the RCGP. The RCGP is arranged around regional faculties within the United Kingdom and Ireland. At the time, there were four in Ireland, one for each province. General practitioners in the Republic of Ireland did not have an independent council; they were linked to the RCGP in the United Kingdom. During this time, McCormick became the East of Ireland Faculty representative on College Council. He remained on the Council as vice-chairman into the 1970s. He delivered the 21st James Mackenzie Lecture in 1974 entitled 'Fifty years of progress'. In 1985, he was awarded the Foundation Council Award.

McCormick's interest in medical education started early, setting up Ireland's first general practice student attachment scheme in 1967. He put general practice into political discussions, and changed the way general practitioners learned and operated in Ireland. In 1971, the then Minister of Health, Erskine Childers (1905–1974) established the Consultative Council on General Medical Practice under the chairmanship of McCormick. Its purpose was to examine general practice in Ireland, focusing on training, numbers of general practitioners required, nursing staff and the overall effectiveness of general practice in relation to other branches of medicine. A report followed in 1974, *The General Practitioner in Ireland*, which recognised general practice in Ireland as inadequate. It found a stark distinction between different socio-economic groups, which reflected a difference in quality of care delivered. The report, which later became known as the *McCormick Report*, produced 107 recommendations: a sizable amount for a report of its kind. It took many aspects from the NHS such as the encouragement to improve teamwork within practice, stemming from McCormick's work in the NHS and his extensive links with the RCGP. This encompassed the development of a group partnership of three to six doctors and to attach public health nurses to group practices. Contemporaneously in the Republic of Ireland, the vast majority of general practitioners worked very much single-handedly, and practice nurses were extremely rare. The *McCormick Report* made it a huge impact on traditional attitudes and social deprivation. A substantial part of the *McCormick Report* looked at postgraduate training in general practice. It recommended a three year training of general practitioners in a combination of community and hospital settings. This was an improvement on the then standards but he was still unsatisfied, citing the need for more relevant training. The *McCormick Report* provided a catalyst for changes in general practitioner training that has helped general practice to the modern day.

In July 1973, McCormick was elected to professor in the Department of Social Medicine at Trinity College Dublin (TCD), later becoming the Department of Community Health in 1977. For this he left full-time general practice. McCormick was also the dean of the medical school at TCD from 1974 to 1979. He was hailed by Davis Coakley in his 2014 book, *Medicine in Trinity College Dublin*, as someone to 'encourage students to think critically and to question everything'. In this book he also quotes McCormick as saying 'Science without caring is inhuman; care without science is dangerous'. McCormick disagreed with the state of medical education, rejecting the overvalue on training and undervalue of education.

In 1984, the Irish College of General Practitioners (ICGP) was established. The RCGP was no longer capable of covering the academic needs of general practice in Ireland. Up until 1978, the GMC (UK) retained responsibility for medical education in Ireland. The governing of general practice in Ireland needed a more direct influence from within. McCormick was one of the creators and founding presidents along with John Mason (1931–2005) and Cormac MacNamara (1944–2004), with McCormick undertaking the presidency from 1986 to 1987. It became

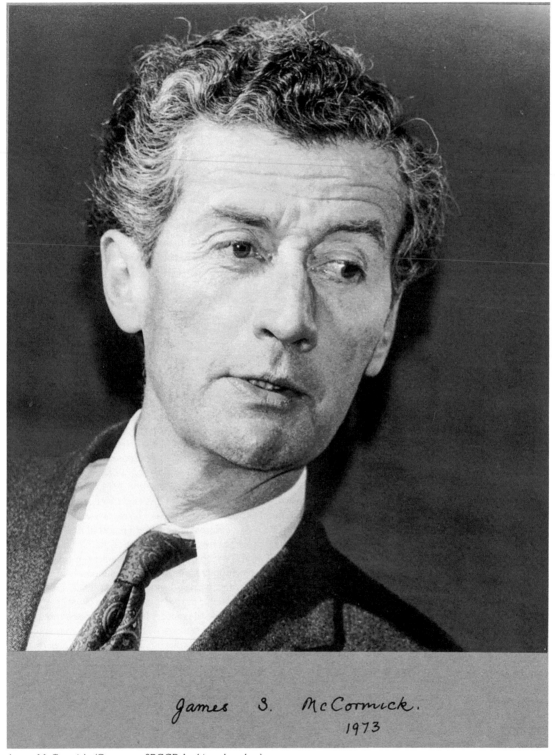

James S. McCormick.
1973

James McCormick. (Courtesy of RCGP Archives, London.)

the representative organisation for education, training and standards in general practice, just as McCormick had envisaged.

Alongside his academic work, McCormick was actively involved in Trust, a charitable body that provides health and social service to homeless people. He was chairman for many years and in this role challenged the norms of society and fought for the rights of the misfortunate.

The first of McCormick's books was *The Doctor: Father Figure or Plumber* (1979). It covered the duty of care that doctors have to their patients. It suggested that knowledge, skills and statistics are only part of the role of the general practitioner. This overarching theme is reflected in the title choice. His background in social medicine allowed him to scrutinise the principal issues that doctors and patients face within general practice. Throughout the blossoming of his academic career he maintained frequent patient contact, treating patients in his practice in Greystones despite his academic responsibilities.

McCormick developed an important relationship with Professor Petr Skrabanek (1940–1994) in the 1980s. This would go on to define a great deal of his future work. McCormick and Skrabanek wrote a book called *Follies and Fallacies in Medicine* (1989). McCormick's education in liberal Cambridge was a far cry from Skrabanek's communist upbringing in Czechoslovakia. This difference resulted in an expertly written piece of work. The book challenged the orthodoxy of public health and existing medical issues. The most controversial aspect of the book was its defiance of the decisions made by medical authorities interpreting research data. It questioned the strict adherence they have to evidence-based medicine. In a review by emeritus professor, Philip Steer (Imperial College London) in 2008, he states, 'our understanding of risk is universally poor. Allowing yourself to be disproportionately influenced by a single bad (or good) outcome can deny hundreds of patients appropriate treatment'. Steer harmonises with large aspects of the book and acclaimed it as a 'medical classic' that 'encourages an appropriate scepticism about medical dogma'.

McCormick wanted to be known as a sceptic, but not the synonym of cynic. His aim was to discourage health professionals from blindly believing all research data conclusions, and that evidence can only prove so much. He described himself as suffering from *scepticaemia*, wittily defining it as 'an uncommon generalised disorder of low infectivity. Medical School education is likely to confer lifelong immunity'. He viewed it as a positive for progress in health.

McCormick was very much for the individual, against the population approach to health, particularly in the use of health screening. He championed the personal relationship between the patient and the family doctor, which he successfully maintained even throughout his prosperous academic career as an internationally renowned scholar. In 2005, he reported at the 30th anniversary of the Eastern Regional General Practice Training Programme, 'I have been lucky to have practised medicine when it was relatively easy and I am glad not to be now doing my career. General practice is not easy, it was not easy when I was practising, and it has become more difficult. More difficult because of the change in patients' expectations, the possibility of litigation and the complexity of advancing knowledge. Nevertheless general practice is a marvellous job. Go well! And enjoy it!' He died on 2 January 2007 and was survived by his wife Biddy, whom he met when she was a charge nurse at St. Mary's.

Further Reading

Coakley D. *Medicine in Trinity College Dublin – An Illustrated History*. Dublin: Trinity College Dublin; 2014.

McCormick J. In the beginning. In: O'Dowd T (Chmn.). Department of Public Health in Primary Care. *Specialist Training Programme in General Practice: Celebrating our 30th Anniversary*. Dublin: Health Service Executive; 2005.

McCormick J. The Irish College of General Practitioners. *The Journal of the Royal College of General Practitioners* 1984;34(268):586–88.

McCormick JS. Fifty years of progress. *The Journal of the Royal College of General Practitioners* 1975;25(150):9–19.

O'Dowd T. James McCormick. *British Journal of General Practice* 2007;57(536):249.

Skrabanek P, McCormick J. *Follies and Fallacies in Medicine*. Glasgow: Tarragon Press; 1989.

The Consultative Council of General Medical Practice. *The General Practitioner in Ireland*. Dublin: The Stationery Office; 1974.

72 SIR DENIS PEREIRA GRAY (1935–)
Neil Metcalfe

Denis Pereira Gray was born at his father Sydney's (1899–1975) family practice house in Exeter on 2 October 1935. He attended Exeter School where he became a chess enthusiast. He was captain of the British Boys chess team that toured the Netherlands in 1954. He went to St. John's College, University of Cambridge, where he admitted he spent as much time on chess as on medicine. He played for the Combined British Universities' chess team in 1957 and was captain of the British team for the World Student Team Championship in Hungary in 1959. The United Kingdom team was crushed by the chess machines of Eastern Europe, but he reported it 'was a wonderful experience'.

Sir Denis studied at the Medical College of St Bartholomew's Hospital, qualifying in 1960, and after house jobs in Bournemouth and Hastings, joined his father as an assistant, becoming a partner in 1962. This practice had been started by his grandfather, Joseph Wenceslaus Pereira Gray (1869–1937), in 1895 and when he retired in 2000 there had been only three senior partners in 105 years, from three generations of one family. He initially found general practice difficult as patients rarely had the classic diseases he had been taught and did have different problems and behaved in ways which he did not understand. He learnt how general practitioner training was needed. He gained much from his father. In 1969, he wrote that it had taken him seven years to learn to split the body up into systems and it took him another seven years to put them back together and be a doctor relating to the patient as a person. From the RCGP he was awarded MRCGP in 1967, and then, in 1973, FRCGP.

Sir Denis had been picked up by the College leadership after winning the Hunterian Society Gold Medal twice and the Sir Charles Hastings Clinical Prize twice. The Founding Editor of the *College Journal* Richard McConaghey (1906–1975) put him on the Editorial Board in 1968 and steered him saying that he could not 'ride two horses at once' being then on both the Councils of the BMA and the RCGP. He gave up the BMA and committed himself to the RCGP. A big event was when the RCGP appointed him as honorary editor of the *Journal of the Royal College of General Practitioners* (*Journal*).

Sir Denis edited the *Journal*, from 1972, unpaid, from his home supported by one secretary. He started this role when 35 years old, without a higher university degree, so he had to learn his craft on the job reading statistics books at home and checking proofs on Cornish beaches. He improved the quality of articles adding methodological rigour and tackled controversial issues. In 1976, the RCGP appointed his wife, Jill (1937–), as assistant editor and she greatly professionalised the *Journal*. He introduced the RCGP *Occasional Paper* series, editing and publishing 78 of them, as well as several *Reports from General Practice*. The RCGP republished several classic books. He also took over what had previously been the College's *Annual Report*, editing it for 15 years as the *RCGP Members' Reference Book*, all from the Exeter office. In 1978, he was awarded the George Abercrombie Award and in 2013, the Rose Prize for original work in the history of general practice in the British Isles.

McConaghey's great achievement was to establish the *Journal* as the first scientific journal of general practice in the world, included in *Index Medicus* in Washington. Sir Denis, when retiring as editor in 1980, handed over the *Journal* as the world number one journal of general practice.

When chairman of the Communications Division in 1981, Sir Denis established the first patient group in any British medical institution. Away from the RCGP, he and his wife edited the *Medical Annual* for five years, from 1983 to 1987.

The University of Exeter was established in 1955 and local doctors initiated the first Postgraduate Medical Institute (PGMI) outside London in 1963, within it. In the mid-1960s, Sir Denis wrote a paper proposing a postgraduate university department of general practice within the PGMI. The idea was welcomed but there was no money, so the University of Exeter bid to the Department of Health and Social Security (DHSS) for funding.

The timing was perfect because the Royal Commission on Medical Education (1968) had recommended postgraduate training for general practice like those in hospital based specialties. The DHSS was wondering how to achieve this when the Exeter bid arrived. It agreed to fund the first postgraduate university department of general practice in Europe in 1973, for five years, as a pilot, and the post of senior lecturer in charge was advertised. Sir Denis was appointed with, a year later, three other part-time senior lecturers in general practice. These four senior lecturers worked together so closely they were nicknamed 'the gang of four'. They threw themselves into developing vocational training. Exeter was not the first to start these as vocational training schemes started to be formed all over the United Kindom but Exeter was unique with four general practitioners with senior university posts developing vocational training rigorously. They introduced academic study of the consultation, used video-recordings and drama students doing role play. Interactive small group work was developed and research projects encouraged. Sir Denis's *A System of Training for General Practice* (1977) became an international blueprint. In its heyday the department received over 100 applications for four to six places on its training scheme. A partnership with the general practitioner regional adviser service was formed in 1975, which lasted for 25 years. All the senior lecturers first authored books on practice

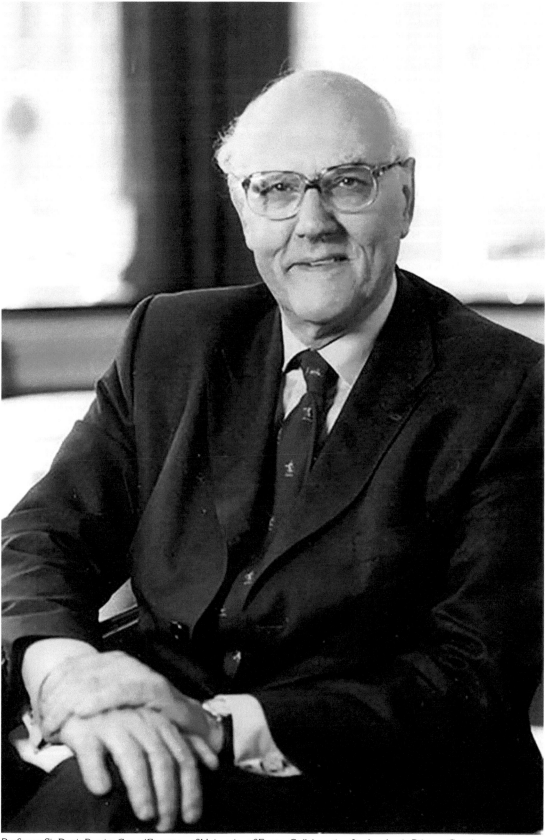

Professor Sir Denis Pereira Gray. (Courtesy of University of Exeter Collaboration for Academic Primary Care.)

management, general practitioner training and practice nursing. International visitors arrived with numerous invitations to lecture abroad. *The Lancet* published two editorials on Exeter, the first on 'GP training – Exeter style' in 1978 and the second on personal doctoring in 1980. Several WHO consultancies followed.

Strong links were built with the general practices in which the four lecturers worked clinically, especially the St. Leonard's Practice where Sir Denis had developed new data-recording systems and internal audits run from a 'quality assurance room'. Visitors included several Government Ministers like Sir Geoffrey Finsburg and Lord Glenarthur and four Chief Medical Officers. This included from England Sir Donald Acheson and Sir Kenneth Calman, later whom was awarded *fellowship ad eundem gradum*, from Scotland Sir John Reid and from Wales Dame Deidre Hine. Other visitors included the President of the GMC, Sir Donald Irvine (1935–2018), a director of NHS Research and Development (Professor Swales) and numerous regional professional and NHS leaders. St. Leonard's quietly showcased British General Practice.

In 1983, the WHO selected the University of Exeter Department of General Practice to host a seminar on the future of medical schools in Europe. WHO brought 12 deans of European medical schools to Exeter with national figures like Sir John Reid. Sir Denis became the first general practitioner ever to chair a week-long WHO seminar. Ironically, the future of undergraduate medical teaching in Europe's mainly specialist orientated medical schools was planned in a postgraduate university general practice department at a university then without an undergraduate medical school.

The intense energy displayed by Sir Denis resulted in a high output. His four books include *Training for General Practice* (1982), *A History of the RCGP* (1992) and he has published over 50 chapters and almost 200 publications in peer-reviewed journals. His 20 eponymous lectures in three countries include the 24th James Mackenzie Lecture in 1977 on home visiting, prevention and behavioural medicine entitled 'Feeling at home'.

Sir Denis was appointed professor of general practice in 1986, the first general practitioner professor in the South-Western region. Six months later the University of Exeter also appointed him director of what had become the Exeter Postgraduate Medical School, with predominantly specialist, consultant staff. He switched from teaching to research, leading a higher degree programme which enabled many colleagues in general practice and the allied professions to obtain Master of Philosophy (MPhils)/Doctor of Philosophy (PhD)/MDs. Exeter established the first multi-professional Master of Science (MSc), tailored for general practice. Sir Denis supervised three of his own partners in the practice, who obtained MPhils (Exon). His most cited research was with a postgraduate student on symptom attribution, explaining why general practitioners with good patient relationships may miss diagnosing depression.

A crisis in the RCGP led to Sir Denis being elected chairman of Council at only 10 days notice. He held this post from February 1987 to November 1990, longer than any other RCGP chairman. As chairman, he led on the introduction of Fellowship by Assessment (1989), the leading quality assurance programme for general practitioners in Europe, later achieved by over 300 doctors.

In 1994, Sir Denis was elected by registered medical practitioners in England to the GMC. His interest in general practitioner training culminated in his election as chairman of the Joint Committee of Postgraduate Training for General Practice (1994–1997), the national regulator. The theme of this chairmanship was the introduction of summative assessment for general practice, so that for the first time in the United Kingdom every doctor entering general practice was individually assessed outside the practice, as in specialist medicine. This three-year chairmanship finished in May 1997 and the same year he was elected, unopposed, as president of the RCGP (1997–2000).

Sir Denis received numerous awards and honours. He was awarded the Foundation Council Award in 1980. A year later he was appointed OBE and was then knighted in 1999, whilst president, for services to quality assurance in general practice. In 1998, he was awarded fellowship of the Academy of Medical Sciences and, in 2000, was the first British general practitioner elected to the Institute of Medicine of the National Academy of Sciences, Washington DC, in the United States.

The Academy of Medical Royal Colleges comprises the Presidents of all the Medical Royal Colleges and Faculties and Sir Denis was elected vice-chairman (1998–2000) and then chairman (2000–2002), the only general practitioner ever. He steered the Royal Colleges to develop systems of standard setting for revalidation, suitable for each specialty. The Trustees of the Nuffield Trust then elected him the first medical chairman of the Trustee Board (2003–2006).

Sir Denis retired clinically from general practice in 2000, but maintained good working relationships with the partners and was appointed consultant to the practice, where he continues research and teaching. Today he continues to be incredibly active. He has a long-standing interest in continuity of care coining the term 'Personal Lists' in general practice. He joined an international research collaboration to study it, which revealed that patients receiving continuity develop more trust in their family doctors. The paper that he and his team published in *BMJ Open* in 2018 was the first to bring together international evidence from nine countries, including from the United Kingdom, about the relationship between regular appointments with the same doctors and death rates. About it, he explained 'arranging for patients to see the doctor of their choice has been considered a matter of convenience or courtesy: now it is clear it is about the quality of medical practice and is literally a matter of life and death.'

Sir Denis is president of the children's charity What About the Children? and patron of the National Association for Patient Participation, usually chairing their national conferences. He has been awarded honorary doctorates by three British universities and seven honorary memberships or fellowships of medical Colleges or Faculties, two abroad.

Sir Denis is happy that he got two things right in his life. The first was marrying his wife and they have four children, including two qualified as general practitioners, and 13 grandchildren. The other was choosing general practice, when it was unpopular. He says: 'It's the best job in the world...very challenging intellectually and emotionally. I don't think there is a job to touch it'.

Further Reading

Editorial. Comment on *A System of Training for General Practice. Occasional Paper 4*. London: RCGP. *The Lancet* 1978;311(8056):134–35.

Kessler D, Lloyd K, Lewis G and Pereira Gray D. Cross-sectional study of symptom attribution and recognition of depression and anxiety in primary care. *British Medical Journal* 1999;318:436–40.

Mainous AG III, Baker R, Love M, Pereira Gray D and Gill JM. Continuity of care and trust in one's physician: Evidence from primary care in the United States and the United Kingdom. *Family Medicine* 2001;33:22–27.

Pereira Gray D, Evans P, Sweeney K, Lings P, Seamark D, Seamark C, Dixon M and Bradley N. Towards a theory of continuity of care. *Journal of the Royal Society of Medicine* 2003;96(4):160–66.

Pereira Gray DJ. *A System of Training for General Practice: Occasional Paper 4*. London: RCGP; 1977.

Pereira Gray DJ. Feeling at home. *The Journal of the Royal College of General Practitioners* 1978;28:6–17.

Pereira Gray DJ. The key to personal care. *The Journal of the Royal College of General Practitioners* 1979;29:666–78.

Pereira Gray DJ (ed.). *Forty Years On: The Story of the First Forty Years of The Royal College of General Practitioners*. London: Atalink; 1992.

Pereira Gray DJ, Sidaway-Lee K, White E, Thorne A, Evans PH. Continuity of care with doctors – A matter of life and death? A systematic review of continuity of care and mortality. *BMJ Open* 2018; 8(6):e021161.

73 ALASTAIR GEOFFREY DONALD (1926–2005)
Julia Humphreys

Alastair Geoffrey Donald was born on 24 November 1926 in his father's Leith Mount surgery, Edinburgh, to Henrietta Mary Laidlaw and Pollok Donald (1881–1955, a general practitioner and graduate of the University of Edinburgh). His formal education began at Edinburgh Academy, where he attended for primary and secondary schooling. He studied medicine at Corpus Christi College, University of Cambridge, graduating in 1948. He later attended the University of Edinburgh where he completed his medical training in 1951. He continued the family tradition of general practice as the third generation to work in this field.

Donald showed early prowess as both a formidable academic, as well as a talented athlete. His abilities secured him a scholarship at Edinburgh Academy, where he was awarded the honour of being Head Ephor. As a talented sportsman, he went on to represent both the universities of Cambridge and Edinburgh for the quarter mile dash, and received Blues at both institutions.

After graduation and working as a house officer, Donald joined the family practice founded in 1883 by his grandfather George Donald (1849–1933, a graduate of the University of Glasgow). He continued to practise as a general practitioner and served the community of Leith and Cramond until he retired in 1991. He married Patricia Ireland in 1952 and they had three children, Tricia, Ian and Bill. His daughter, Patricia Donald MBE (1953–, a graduate of the University of Edinburgh), is the fourth generation within the Donald family to work as a general practitioner in the family practice. His first marriage ended in 1998 and he later married Gladys Leslie.

In 1954, Donald became a founder associate of the newly established College, working as an advocate for medical education within general practice, and ultimately elevating the status and profile of the specialty. Graham Buckley (1945–) said of Donald: 'The key role Alastair played was to harness the disparate and sometimes mercurial talents of others to create and establish high quality postgraduate training programmes for General Practice across the country'. At the by now named RCGP, Donald was South East Scotland Faculty chairman (1970–1972) and provost (1973–1974), chairman of the Board of Censors (1978–1979). He then became one of only four other individuals to have held the post of both chairman (1979–1982) and president (1992–1994) of the RCGP. During this time, he also deputised as president for one year in 1995 for HRH the Prince of Wales. In between these roles, he was also appointed chairman of the JCPTGP (1982–1985). This role afforded Donald the opportunity to further shape medical education.

His time as chairman of the RCGP was marked by the 1980 siege of the Iranian Embassy next door in Princes Gate. The subsequent standoff between the terrorists and the SAS trapped him alone in the college building. He continued working and was amused to receive a phone call from a professor in Scotland who was having a particularly torrid time with his hospital colleagues and ended his diatribe with: 'I feel under siege here, Alastair'. Donald was able to make his own escape under cover of darkness and the SAS used the RCGP as its base in preparing the storming of the embassy.

Donald's contribution and legacy to medical education both regionally and nationally continues to be seen. Whilst a general practitioner in his local community, he worked for over 20 years as the first appointed Regional adviser (1972–1991), contributing to the team that established postgraduate general practitioner training in the South-East of Scotland. He was later appointed to the role of lecturer at the University of Edinburgh at the world's first university department of general practice, which had been established in 1956.

At a time when general practice was considered to lack the intellectual gravity of other specialties, Donald acted as a mentor and inspiration to others to take up the mantle of a career in the speciality. Buckley, in his paper 'From Cullen to Calman. Medical education – Enlightenment to post-modernism' said a fitting tribute to the importance of Donald, his mentor for 25 years.

As an academic leader, Donald worked to publish numerous papers on the topic of anticipatory care, in which he showed himself an expert advocate for this forward-thinking model of preventative patient care. His theories helped to improve clinical outcomes and establish general practice as a proactive speciality, at the forefront of patient management. In 1985, he gave the 33rd James Mackenzie Lecture entitled 'Oasis or Beachhead'. His analysis of general practice supported the hypothesis that a balance must exist between 'old knowledge and new skills'. He also advised that the RCGP should exist as a sanctuary or 'oasis' from which general practitioners should 'return refreshed and revitalised'.

Alongside Donald's other roles, he established a further practice branch in neighbouring Cramond. He also returned to work at his previous school as president of the Edinburgh Academicals Club 1978 to 1981, and was chair of the Court of Directors of the Edinburgh Academy from 1985 to 1992. Following on from that, he also served as vice-chairman of the Medical and Dental Defence Union of Scotland (MDDUS) from 1992 to 1997. Whilst on the

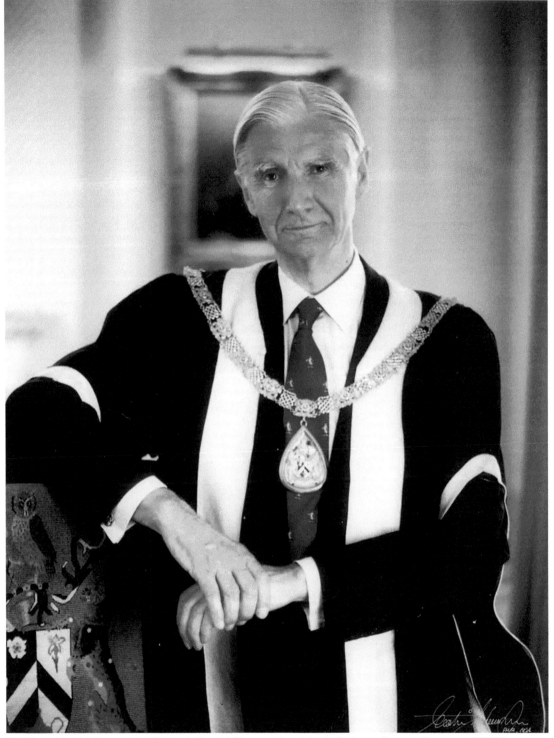

RCGP presidential photograph of Alastair Donald. Photographer: Martin Grahame-Dunne. (Courtesy of RCGP Archives, London.)

Armed Services General Practice Approval Board from 1987 to 1998, he particularly enjoyed his trips overseas to support the careers of serving doctors.

Donald's achievements were recognised by a variety of organisations. He was awarded FRCGP in 1971 and was appointed OBE in 1982 and CBE in 1992. He was also awarded the James Mackenzie Medal of the RCP, the Hippocrates Medal of the European Society of General Practice and, perhaps most poignantly, the Foundation Council Award of the RCGP in 1997, which recognised a lifetime contribution to patient care and to the specialty of general practice.

In his retirement Donald continued helping at the RCGP as he began a project that documented video recordings of the early years of the RCGP and those people whose tireless work helped to shape the future of the organisation. He remained a keen golfer and became captain of Edinburgh Academicals Golf Club. He was an elder at Cramond Kirk, and a member of Leith Rotary Club. Community and church remained important commitments throughout his life; as an active member of the local community he worked to help restore the historic Lamb's House. In recognition of this work he was awarded the Paul Harris Fellowship by Rotary International.

Donald died suddenly on 5 June 2005 on the golf course at Luffness. The obituaries and biographical accounts of his life illustrate a much loved, respected and revered man, who left a significant legacy to his patients, community, colleagues and general practice. In his memory, the RCGP Scotland Alastair Donald Award is fittingly awarded to individuals in recognition of outstanding contribution to service delivery, education, research and community.

Further Reading

Anon. Dr Alastair G Donald. *The Scotsman: Scotland on Sunday* 2005; 7 July.

Buckley EG. From Cullen to Calman. Medical education – Enlightenment to post-modernism. *British Journal of General Practice* 1994;44(384):326–30.

Donald AG. Integration of patient care. *The Journal of Royal College of General Practitioners* 1977;27(174):54–55.

Donald AG. James Mackenzie Lecture 1985. Oasis or beachhead. *The Journal of the Royal College of General Practitioners* 1985;35(281):558–64.

Donald AG, Garvie D. The MRCGP International. *British Journal of General Practice* 1998;48(428):1092.

Horder J, Howie J. Alastair Donald. *The British Journal of General Practice* 2005;55(516):564–65.

Thomson DM. General practice and the Edinburgh Medical School: 200 years of teaching, care and research. *British Journal of General Practice* 1984;34:9–12.

4 IAN GIBB BOGLE (1938–2014)

Katherine Moor, Stuart Pinder and Neil Metcalfe

Born in Liverpool in 1938, Ian Bogle went to study medicine at the University of Liverpool. He graduated in 1961 and later, in 1999, was awarded an honorary MD. In 1962, he joined an inner-city general practice called Priory Medical Centre in Belmont Grove, Liverpool, where his father, John Bogle (1912–1991), was a partner, and which was founded in 1911 by his grandfather George Bogle (1879–1964). It was this same practice, with a cohort of 12,000 patients, in which he stayed throughout his career in general practice.

Bogle had a keen interest in medical politics and throughout his lifetime was involved in both local and national medical politics. He was elected onto the local medical committee (LMC) in 1969, served as secretary of the Liverpool LMC (1973–1990), and was vice-chair of Liverpool LMC (1979–1981). During his time as the LMC secretary, he sat on the Liverpool Executive Committee in July 1973 and subsequently the Liverpool Family Practitioner Committee in September 1984. He was also on the Liverpool Area Health Authority (Teaching) in 1979. All of these roles were aided by his emotional sense of fair play and work in general practice in Liverpool. This was summarised by David Pickersgill (1946–), a former general practitioner and BMA treasurer (2002–2011), who on recalling his first memory of Bogle speaking at an LMC conference revealed that 'Ian told the tale of a colleague going for a pee at the end of morning surgery, only to find that the entire loo had been stolen'.

In July 1979, Bogle was elected onto the GMSC of the BMA now known as the GPC. It was on this committee that he became a GMSC negotiator and subsequently chairman in 1990, a role which he carried out until 1997.

In what could be seen as the pinnacle of Bogle's career he was elected, in 1998, in a four-way contest as BMA Council Chairman (1998–2004). He succeeded Sir Alexander Macara (1932–2012) and had a noticeable difference in his approach to the role. Bogle was more of an introvert than Macara and once commented that public speaking 'screws me up completely'. The former chairman of the GPC, John Chisholm (1950–), described him as a 'magnificent team leader and team builder' whose advice was never foisted upon others but always sought. Bogle was elected into the role at a time when the NHS was radically changing. NHS walk-in-centres and NHS Direct were new introductions and junior doctors were working more than 100 hours a week. It was from his role as chairman that Bogle negotiated with the Labour government new contracts for doctors, at a time when the introduction of the European Time Directive limited the number of working hours. During his time as BMA Council chairman Bogle continued to work in his Liverpool practice part-time, believing that he could not advise appropriately without continuing to be a practising doctor.

Bogle was seen throughout his years of service to be critical of the NHS's increasing use of target setting. According to Bogle such target setting 'left little room for professional accepted national judgement'. He felt that the NHS was becoming managed by computers and targets via tick boxes and spreadsheets and that instead doctors and patients should have a larger say. He overlooked the call for revalidation and suggested a simple system based on appraisals, audits and the idea of continual professional development as a doctor. He was chairman at the time that regulation of patient data was being discussed and saw the introduction of named doctors who were responsible for the protection of patient and service-user information known as Caldecott guardians. This being at a time of an ever-increasing computerisation of the NHS.

What did seem to be key in Bogle's approach as both the general practitioner and BMA chairman was the importance of the patient. One particular example of this was a story he told frequently of an eight-year-old girl he met as a junior doctor. She was dying of renal failure but could not be treated with dialysis due to the dialysis unit not yet being installed in Liverpool and, therefore, nothing could be done for her. He felt it was a huge injustice to cut this young life short, and said this experience taught him the importance of making connections with patients, and, as a general practitioner, particularly thought this was important when seeing patients throughout their entire life.

Bogle was highly revered by friends and colleagues. In 2014, BMA Council chairman Mark Porter (1962–) spoke highly of Bogle and noted his patience, how he conducted himself with good humour and that 'for Ian the interests of the BMA and the doctors were paramount'. Former BMA Council chair Hamish Meldrum (1948–) stated that 'I, along with doctors and patients throughout the United Kingdom, owe Ian a huge debt of gratitude and, those of us who did so, are privileged to have known and worked with him'.

Other awards and recognition were given to Bogle. In 1991 he was awarded Fellowships of both the BMA and the RCGP. He was awarded an honorary MD from the University of Liverpool in 1999. In recognition of his service to Liverpool general practitioners, and to the LMC, he was awarded honorary life membership of Liverpool LMC in April 2000. He was appointed CBE for services to the medical profession during the Queen's Birthday honours in June 2003. A year later, he received the BMA gold medal for distinguished merit.

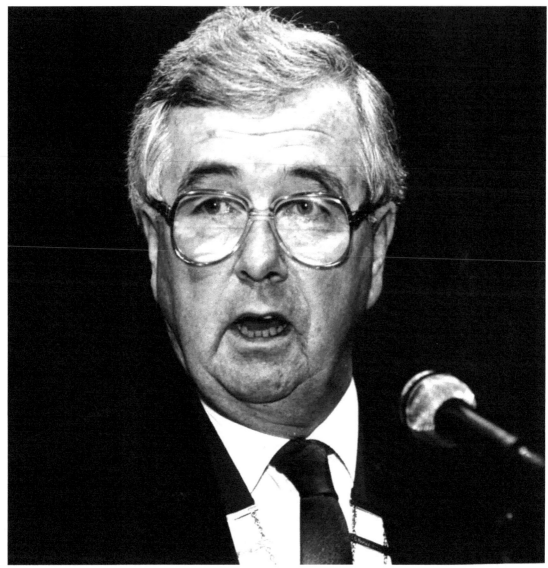

Ian Bogle. (Courtesy of BMA Archive.)

Away from medicine, Bogle was a known to be a keen golfer and true to his roots was as an avid supporter of Liverpool Football Club. He died on 21 June 2014 leaving his wife and two daughters, three grandchildren and one great grandchild. The following was written in his obituary in the *BMJ*: 'During his medicopolitical career, he fought to improve general practice, equality of access to services, and the standard of care delivered to patients. He was a true friend to Liverpool, and even in his retirement, he kept a very happy interest in what was happening to the health service, both locally and nationally'.

Further Reading

Barnett R. Obituary: Ian Gibb Bogle. *British Medical Journal* 2014;349:5362.

Beecham L. Doctors will meet PM's challenges, Dr Bogle declares. *British Medical Journal* 2000;321(7252):56.

Bogle I. The joy of health. *The Lancet* 2001;357(9252):316.

Harling R. A new chairman for the BMA. *British Medical Journal* 1998;317:166.

75 IAN RICHARDSON (1922–2010)

Zahra Ramzan

Ian Milne Richardson was born on 3 April 1922. In pursuit of his ambition to be a surgeon, he attended the University of Edinburgh and qualified with honours in 1944. However, a severe skin allergy prevented him from persuing his chosen speciality. Therefore, he instead went down a different path, first being awarded MRCP, in 1946, before taking a year out from hospital medicine to work as an assistant in a general practice in Dunfermline. He later completed a diploma in Public Health in 1948, before working as an occupational health physician in Glasgow for the next four years at the iron and steel tube manufacturers Stewards and Lloyds.

Richardson's main passion was educating the next generation of medical professionals. He continuously strived to improve his teaching methods, which he commented on when delivering the William Pickles Lecture in 1981 entitled 'Verities yet in their chaos':

> For most, but not all whole-time academics, teaching is their raison-d'être, and it remains my own priority. I am aware, at times acutely, of the poor quality of much university teaching... I used to attend inaugural lectures, no matter the faculty... because I wanted to learn more about successful teaching methods.

In 1952, Richardson relocated to Aberdeen where he worked as a senior lecturer in social medicine. Whilst at Aberdeen, he organised optional student attachments to general practice as he felt students did not witness the reality of general practice often enough. He believed that teaching should incorporate more community based teaching.

Public health and social medicine were the subjects Richardson undertook further at higher education level and he was awarded an MD in 1953. This was followed up by him receiving a PhD at the University of Aberdeen in 1956 on the subject 'health of men in heavy industry'. He concluded that although the reduction in heavy work may be beneficial as workers age, it must be a gradual process, specific to each individual. Employers have the duty of making sure the workers do not feel psychologically unhappy or feel that their skills are not utilised adequately. He then continued his work as an educator at the University of Aberdeen, alongside other research projects including, in 1965, analysing student opinions on general practice attachments. He realised that the current schemes were not sufficient to give insight into general practice. This built the foundation for his later work in creating general practice attachments.

In 1967, the University of Aberdeen acquired funding from the Nuffield Provincial Hospitals Trust which was used to fund the creation of a General Practice Teaching Unit. Richardson applied for the post of reader against 43 other applicants, most of whom were general practitioners with little to no academic teaching experience. When he was awarded the post of reader it caused discontent amongst those who preferred to have appointed a senior practising general practitioner. Three years later, in 1970, he became professor of general practice.

Throughout his lifetime, Richardson engaged in many research projects, some of which focused on the effectiveness of clinical placements at general practices during university. The results of these studies, along with the influences of Michael Balint (1896–1970) and Richardson's own position as reader allowed him to develop a vocational training scheme involving practices in North East Scotland. He also campaigned for general practice to be held in as high a regard as much as other specialities resulting in the creation of the University of Aberdeen's Department of General Practice in 1970. He urged the University of Aberdeen to form a partnership with the RCGP. He stated that experience in general practice would allow students the following: to view a wider range of illnesses; experience continuity of care to understand why patients are referred to hospital; gain tolerance by observing multiple patients with the same diagnosis; witness patients that refuse treatment and advice as they believe they are not severely ill; to gain insight into patient's lives by way of home visits or shadowing family doctors and being able to experience general practice as 'an alive, a changing, challenging, and satisfying discipline'.

In 1970, Richardson published an article in the *Journal of the Royal College of General Practitioners* entitled 'Patients and students in general practice'. This study was discernible to others at the time due to focusing on patient reactions rather than placement effectiveness. He suggested patients may not have full autonomy when asked whether students could observe their appointment. The system in place was to ask the patient for permission within the consulting room just before their appointment. Richardson concluded several methods would be more efficient in ensuring an autonomous decision. These methods included giving the patient more time to make the decision such as when they first enter the waiting room. Additionally, he recommended replacing the leading question of 'are you okay with someone observing' instead sending out letters to patients explaining the programme with an optional consent form giving the option to opt in rather than opt out. This study resulted in two practices requesting advanced consent, a method which is now implemented in practices internationally.

In regards to research on consultations Richardson co-authored, with Ian Buchan (1941–), the *Time and Motion Study* which was published as part of the Scottish Health Service Studies No. 27. They observed 124 general

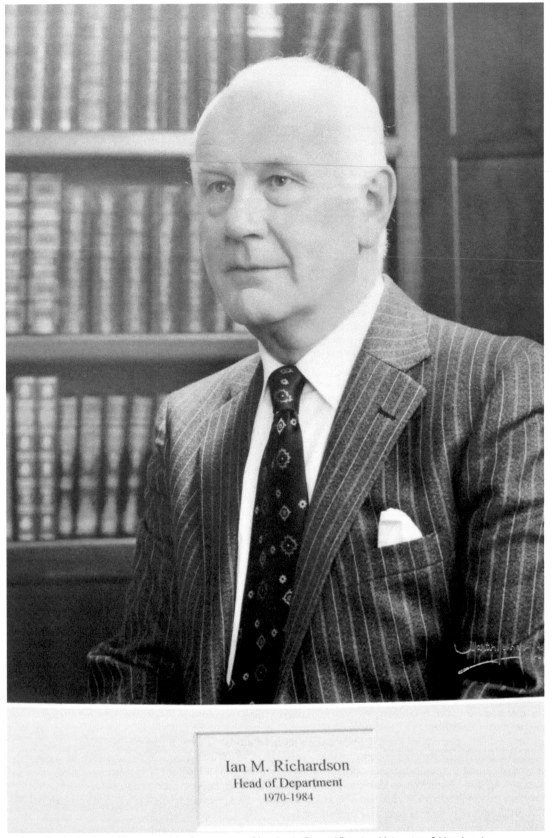

Ian M. Richardson
Head of Department
1970-1984

Professor Ian Richardson. (Courtesy of the Department of Academic General Practice, University of Aberdeen.)

practitioner consultations and found that there was an average time of 5.3 minutes per consultation. This was a revolutionary study whereby Buchan and Richardson promoted the idea of a 10-minute long consultation. This is now used as a framework for booking appointments in most general practices within the NHS.

The Department of General Practice at the University of Aberdeen became independent in 1970 after receiving a grant from the James Mackenzie Fund. This made it the first department that did not have to rely on NHS funding, instead receiving funding from the University Grants Committee. This allowed independent appointments of several general practitioners including, in 1976, John Howie (1937–). This allowed more time for Richardson to engage in further research projects, which included the creation of the Foresterhill Health Centre in 1977. This centre was designed to act as a teaching health centre. The centre included three functioning practices and various community services. These successfully served to ensure students gained more experience of working with patients throughout the year, unlike the previous vocational scheme which took place during the holidays, gaining interpersonal skills alongside their normal academic studies.

Richardson became dean of the University of Aberdeen Faculty of Medicine in 1980, and in doing so became the first general practitioner to ever hold such a title there. However, this coincided with required budget cuts of 24 per cent, which meant that instead of implementing improvements he instead had to focus on making cuts.

Richardson retired from his position as dean in 1984. He relocated to Auchterarder, Scotland, where he worked to improve local practices' efficiency by summarising patient notes. He was a family man and preferred to separate his personal and professional life. He spent his retirement surrounded by his wife and two daughters, one of whom followed in his footsteps and became a general practitioner, as well as his five grandchildren and his labradors. He enjoyed playing golf, was an avid gardener and a sports car enthusiast. He died on 16 December 2010 aged 88 years old. His memory is honoured via the creation of the Richardson Prize in General Practice at the University of Aberdeen funded by his friends and colleagues and is awarded to its best student in clinical general practice.

Further Reading

Buchan IC, Richardson IM. *Scottish Health Services Statistics, No 27: Time Study of Consultations in General Practice*. Edinburgh: Scottish Home and Health Department; 1973.

Howie J, Whitfield M (eds.). *Academic General Practice in the UK Medical Schools, 1948–2000: A Short History.* Edinburgh: Edinburgh University Press; 2011.

Richardson IM. Retirement: A sociomedical study of 244 men. *Scottish Medical Journal* 1956;1(12):381–91.

Richardson IM. Patients and students in general practice. *The Journal of the Royal College of General Practitioners* 1970;20(100): 285–87.

Richardson IM. William Pickles Lecture 1981: 'Verities yet in their chaos'. *The Journal of the Royal College of General Practitioners* 1981;31(227):328–33.

76 SIR MICHAEL DRURY (1926–2014)

Rebecca Kingston

Victor William Michael Drury was born on 5 August 1926 in Bromsgrove, Worcestershire. He was the youngest of George and Trixie Drury's three sons but his father died when Drury was nine years old. He was educated at Bromsgrove School, having received a foundation scholarship. Much of his thirteenth year was spent in hospital due to a bicycle accident but this experience inspired him to study medicine.

Drury began studying medicine at the University of Birmingham in 1943. His contemporaries noted his hard-working attitude but it also seemed that he spent a lot of time in the Student Guild. He became politically active and an accomplished public speaker, taking on the role as vice-chairman of the University Conservative Association in 1948 where he opposed the BMA's rejection of the NHS. Drury graduated from Birmingham with Honours in 1949.

Drury met his wife Joan (née Williamson, 1926–2015) in 1944 whilst both were studying at Birmingham. They married in 1950 and had four children together. She played an important role in support for his career and was even known to occasionally scrub up in the operating theatre to help him when they were short-staffed at Kidderminster Hospital.

Drury's medical career began in surgery. After his house officer post at Birmingham's General Hospital, he became resident surgical officer at Kidderminster Hospital. He remembered this job as horrendous, having to deal with stresses and responsibilities far above his station and training. Before his career as a general practitioner, he was called to do national service in the RAMC when he was sent to Singapore and Kuala Lumpur (1951–1953). He returned from the military to work with Brian Gaunt (1909–1998) at his general practice in Bromsgrove, where he was to remain a general practitioner for 38 years. He continued his work in general surgery at the local hospital where he assisted Mike Doran (1911–1995). One of his first forays into research was a co-published paper in 1963 with Doran in the *British Journal of Surgery* in 1964 on deep vein thrombosis. Published work by general practitioners was unusual at the time but this paved the way for an academic career. Much of his later research involved drugs and their interactions but he also studied the role of practice nurses.

Against the backdrop of low morale in general practice in the 1960s, Drury worked hard to help improve aspects of general practice. One area that he identified as important to the success of general practice was well-trained medical secretaries and receptionists. He helped set up relevant courses and produced the first edition of *The Medical Secretaries Handbook* in 1965, which went on to be very successful. He later designed courses for practice nurses and practice receptionists in the 1980s. He was a passionate advocate of the multidisciplinary team in general practice and his beliefs were further strengthened after a seven month trip to general practices in Europe, the United States and Canada, funded by the Nuffield Foundation in 1966.

In 1973, Drury became part-time senior clinical tutor in general practice at the University of Birmingham. It was in this role that he was able to lay the foundations for better teaching in general practice for medical students, helping it gain greater respect as an academic discipline and raise its status as a career choice. Working together with Robin Hull (b.1931) they enabled general practice attachments to become a mandatory part of the medical curriculum, emphasised the holistic approach to medicine and created a number of educational videos which were sold throughout the world. In 1979, Drury and Hull published *Introduction to General Practice*, a book designed for medical students. Despite its success, the book became known as 'Dreary and Dull' by the students much to the delight of its good-humoured authors. This was all achieved whilst still working part-time as a partner at his practice, demonstrating his dedication to his clinical work.

Early on in his career, Drury had become involved with the RCGP. In 1970, he was awarded FRCGP and in the same year he became chairman of the Midlands Faculty, later provost (1977–1979). Nationally he held several committee roles including chairman of the Practice Organisation Committee, the Research Committee and Education Committee. He was also a MRCGP examiner. This was before holding the title of president of the RCGP (1985–1988).

Aside from his work with the RCGP, Drury was also busy on other committees. This included the Regional Research Committee, visitor for Joint Committee on Higher Professional Training (from 1975) and chairman of the Executive Committee of the Association of University Teachers of General Practice (1979–1980). His stature in the medical profession was such that he was elected as the first general practitioner to be vice-chairman of the Conference of medical Royal Colleges and their Faculties by the presidents of the specialist medical Royal Colleges. He served from 1987 to 1988.

There was further acknowledgement for Drury's dedication to general practice. He had been appointed OBE in 1978 but from 1980 to 1991, he became the first professor in general practice at the University of Birmingham. Further academic recognition came in 1983 when he was asked to give the James Mackenzie Lecture. His speech about adverse drug reactions and prescribing was entitled 'Foxglove and chips'. In 1983, he became civilian advisor in general practice to the army and was elected to the GMC in 1984. Later, when undertaking the aforementioned role of RCGP president, he had to deal with increasing tensions between the examiners and members of the RCGP as a result of the examiners criticising the training of general practitioners. This culminated in the dismissal of the Chief Examiner and

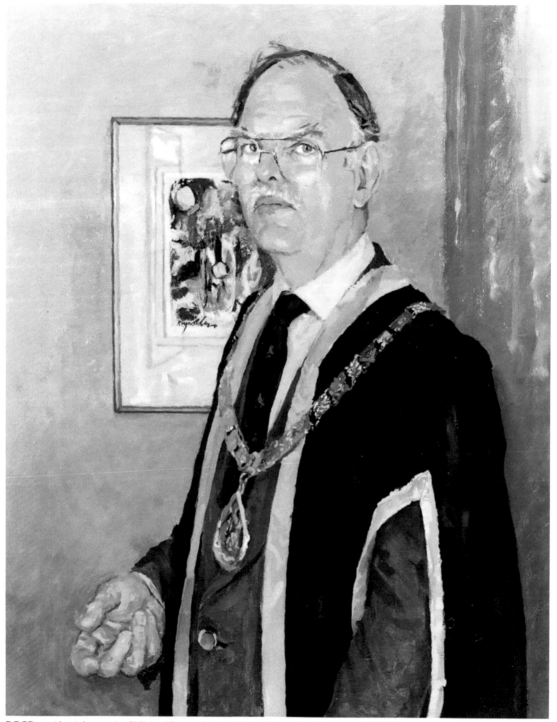

RCGP presidential portrait of Michael Drury. Artist: Michael Reynolds. (Courtesy of RCGP Archives, London.)

bad press coverage. This could have seen an end to the RCGP but Drury is often credited with playing a key role in preserving it due to his tact and diplomacy. In his role, he also stressed the importance of general practitioner out-of-hours care. Following his successful term as president and for his services to medicine, he was given a Knighthood in 1989. He later was awarded the Foundation Council Award in 2001.

Drury was known for his jovial and relaxed personality. He was described in his obituary in the *British Journal of General Practice* as 'unassuming, approachable, patient, a superb listener, unflappable, and interested, all combined with a wonderful wit and sense of humour'. His partners at work were supportive of his many enterprises, marvelling and laughing at his stories when he returned. Drury's phenomenal memory was often praised and the partners found his knowledge so impressive that it was often easier to ask him than look up the answer in a book. There are also many stories of his kindness and welcoming nature, including his custom to visit new partners at the surgery with a bottle of champagne.

Drury retired in 1991. In retirement he was chair of Age Concern and the Muscular Dystrophy Campaign. His outstanding achievements and commitment to general practice have helped construct a much-improved system with better trained doctors. Ever since June 2013, the RCGP have given an award named after Drury that was established to recognise contributions from staff members based in the faculties of devolved councils. He died on 11 June 2014, aged 87 years old.

Further Reading

Anon. Obituary: Sir Michael Drury. *The Times*. 2014; 11 November.

Doran FS, Drury M, Sivyer A. A simple way to combat the venous stasis which occurs in the lower limbs during surgical operations. *British Journal of Surgery* 1964;51:486–92.

Drury M. *The Medical Secretary's Handbook*. London: Baillière Tindall and Cassell; 1965.

Drury M, Hull R. *Introduction to General Practice*. London: Baillière Tindall and Cassell; 1979.

Drury VW. James Mackenzie Lecture. Foxglove and chips. *The Journal of the Royal College of General Practitioners* 1984;34(260): 129–39.

Hull R. *Just a GP*. Oxford: Radcliffe Medical Press; 1994.

Thomas K, Hobbs R. Sir Michael Drury: An appreciation. *British Journal of General Practice* 2014;64(625):410.

77 JOHN GARVIE ROBERTSON HOWIE (1937–)

Anna-Marie Dale

John Howie was born in Glasgow on 23 January 1937, son of Sir James Howie (1907–1995), formerly director of the Public Health Laboratory Service of England and Wales. He was educated in Aberdeen and Glasgow aspiring to be a teacher. However, during his final year, whilst in hospital with appendicitis, he decided to study medicine. In 1961, he graduated from the University of Glasgow.

During his first year as a house officer, Howie looked after a friend from medical school who had been admitted to his ward with acute leukaemia. Now meaning to work as a haematologist, he spent four years in pathology, bacteriology and haematology despite having originally wanted to become a general practitioner. During his final two years in pathology he worked two evenings a week at the practice of his friend James Wright, who he joined as a partner in 1966. Soon after, they amalgamated with Fred Christie to become a three-man group.

Howie's research career started in his first year in pathology. Based on his personal experience, his research focused on the diagnosis and management of appendicitis and abdominal pain. This was an area of considerable doubt and uncertainty at the time. He published work on iron staining as a diagnostic marker for recurring appendicitis, and calculated morbidity and mortality rates for different treatment approaches to abdominal pain where appendicitis was a possible diagnosis. Other work, published in the *BMJ* and in *Cancer*, distinguished different types of mesenteric adenitis and disproved a possible link between appendectomy and bowel cancer.

In his practice in Partick, Glasgow, Howie became interested in how decisions to prescribe antibiotics during winter respiratory epidemics were made. Along with Angus Clark from a neighbouring practice, they carried out a randomised study of antibiotic against placebo for flu-like illnesses, finding no benefit for normally-fit antibiotic takers. This was his first step in a career-long effort to help to provide an evidence base for the discipline of general practice and to help understand the different ways in which clinical decisions were made in hospital and in general practice.

In 1970, Howie moved to a lectureship in general practice at the University of Aberdeen where his research into antibiotic prescribing and respiratory tract infections developed further. His many research projects around the subject showed that antibiotic prescribing did not affect the outcome of minor respiratory infections; in due course he showed that not prescribing antibiotics for minor respiratory infections (in this example, sore throats) did not increase the likelihood of subsequent glomerulonephritis or rheumatic fever. He hypothesised (and later confirmed) that general practitioners often carry out their diagnostic and treatment decisions backwards, the diagnostic labels they record being rationalisations of the treatment decision they have already made.

In 1976, Howie published a landmark study in the *BMJ* involving a series of pictures of sore throats with clinical histories attached. The histories remained the same but patients' personal circumstances were varied. He showed that general practitioners' treatment decisions were often affected by the patient's 'social and psychological history'. This included showing that more antibiotics were prescribed to children whose mothers were prescribed psychotropic drugs. This provided evidence that the biomedical decision-making process taught in medical school fits hospital settings more comfortably than in general practice where social determinants are more influential.

However, against this Howie had also shown that in the hospital setting, appendectomies were more likely if the patient was related to a member of the medical profession, or that there was a family history of appendicectomy, although not necessarily of appendicitis. This confirmed that decision-making in hospital practice had more similarities to general practice than was often taught. His research goal then was to produce a model explaining how clinical decisions are made at consultations that would apply to general practice and hospital settings.

In 1980, Howie moved to the University of Edinburgh to be professor of general practice. Over the years that followed, he published widely about the nature and outcome of consultations in general practice. His next research centred round the determinants of stress in general practitioners and how stress adversely affected the care of patients such as with more prescribing and less attention to co-morbidity, particularly in the area of psychological and social problems. Then, given the opportunity to evaluate a trial of fund-holding in Scottish practices in the early 1990s, his team developed an outcome measure (enablement) as an alternative to patient satisfaction, and showed that patients with incentivised conditions fared better in terms of consultation length and outcome than did patients with non-incentivised conditions, the commonest of which were also those with high levels of psychosocial co-morbidity. A later four-centre study in the United Kingdom showed that doctors who spent longer at consultation and whose patients knew them better enabled more patients than did other colleagues. That work also drew attention to the need to include a measure of the ethnic backgrounds of both doctor and patient when making judgements about the quality of outcomes. In 2006, Howie and Stewart Mercer (1957–) proposed the CQI-2 (Consultation Quality Index – 2) as a quality care measure of general practice consultation based upon four main factors: patient enablement, continuity of care, consultation length and empathy.

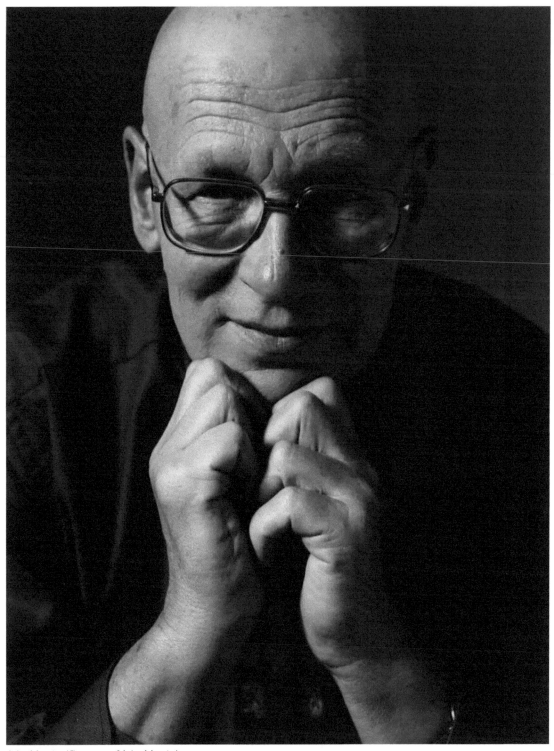

John Howie. (Courtesy of John Howie.)

In 1996, Howie first described his consultation model encompassing the factors that influence diagnostic and management decisions, modifying it twice in later years. The model shows how 'patient needs', the 'Values' of both doctors and patients and the 'context' within which the consultation takes place relate and interact to form 'outcomes'. He concluded that although general practice and hospital medicine are different, they remain on a spectrum which differs by how much they are influenced by patient factors and by disease factors. He also concluded that the complexity of any comprehensive descriptive model of consultations explains why guidelines and targets are so hard to apply to the day-to-day work of general practitioners.

A key but quite different contribution that Howie made to general practice was his lead involvement in negotiations for the funding of academic general practice. In 1981, Howie and John Walker (1928–), the then professor of general practice at the University of Newcastle, began a 10-year campaign to provide an analogue to Service Increment for Teaching (SIFT) monies through which the NHS supplemented teaching hospital budgets in England and Wales and Additional Cost of Teaching (ACT) budgets in Scotland. Eventually, in 1992, £2.3 million was allocated towards 'Academic General Practice', a fund which has revolutionised the ability of general practice to provide sustained high-quality teaching within medical schools in the United Kingdom, and helped confirm the importance of general practice as a discipline in its own right and its importance within medical schools.

Since 1978, Howie has received numerous awards and delivered many guest lectures. He delivered the 34th James Mackenzie Lecture in 1986 entitled 'Quality of caring: Landscapes and curtains'. A decade later, he was appointed CBE in the 1996 New Year Honours List. In 2002, he was awarded an honorary DSc degree by the University of Aberdeen in acknowledgment of 'advancing the cause of research in the general practice context'. Finally, he was presented with the RCGP Discovery Prize in 2012.

After 1970, when Howie moved to Aberdeen, his clinical sessions reduced to three a week. There he worked as an assistant with James Gauld and Iain Ross. In Edinburgh, he became a full partner in the Mackenzie Medical Centre Practice run by the staff of the University Department of General Practice, again working three sessions in clinical practice. Until recently he continued to publish articles related to general practice consultations.

Howie was supported and greatly influenced by his wife, Margot, herself a practice nurse, and by their experiences bringing up their three children. In his spare time he plays golf, bridge, gardens and helps manage a local community café.

Further Reading

Howie J. Diagnosis in general practice and its implications for quality of care. *Journal of Health Service Research and Policy* 2010;15:120–22.

Howie JG. James Mackenzie Lecture 1986. Quality of caring: Landscapes and curtains. *The Journal of the Royal College of General Practitioners* 1987;37(294):4–10.

Howie JGR. Mesenteric adenitis. *British Medical Journal* 1969;2:449–50.

Howie JGR. Clinical judgement and antibiotic use in general practice. *British Medical Journal* 1976;2:1061–64.

Howie JGR. Addressing the credibility gap in general practice research: Better theory; more feeling; less strategy. *British Journal of General Practice* 1996;46:479–87.

Howie JGR. *Patient-Centredness and the Politics of Change. A Day in the Life of Academic General Practice*. London: The Nuffield Trust; 1999.

Howie JGR. In retrospect – A reflection on a 50 year research journey. *Family Practice* 2014;31:1–6.

Howie JGR, Bigg AR. Family trends in psychotropic and antibiotic prescribing in general practice. *British Medical Journal* 1980;280:836–38.

Howie JGR, Clark GA. Double-blind trial of early demethylchlortetracycline in minor illness in general practice. *Lancet* 1970;ii:1099–102.

Howie JGR, Timperly WR. Cancer and appendectomy. *Cancer* 1966;19:1138–42.

Mercer SW, Howie JGR. CQI-2 – A new measure of holistic interpersonal care in primary care consultations. *British Journal of General Practice* 2006;56:262–68.

78 JULIAN TUDOR HART (1927–2018)

Olivia Owen

Julian Tudor Hart was born in London on 9 March 1927 to Alison Macbeth (1896–1952), an endocrinologist, and Alexander Tudor Hart (1901–1992), an army surgeon and general practitioner. His father represented the South Wales Miners' Federation in a dispute with their local general practitioners over medical care. Tudor Hart had a middle-class upbringing and was educated privately at King Alfred and Dartington Hall Schools in England and at Pickering College, Ontario, Canada. During his formative years, it was his aspiration to become a general practitioner in a coal-mining village despite his parents desire for him to enter a different profession. Both his parents were politically active: his mother a member of the Labour Party and his father the Communist Party, and Tudor Hart developed his Socialist beliefs at an early age. His Marxist values would remain at the centre of his work during his long career in the medical profession.

Tudor Hart commenced his medical education at the University of Cambridge in 1947 and completed his clinical training at St George's Hospital Medical School, London. He graduated in 1952. Whilst he was a house officer, he worked at Kettering and Watford General Hospitals. He then went on to work as a general practitioner in North Kensington, London, until 1957 when he returned to work in hospital posts for a further two years to gain more experience.

With an enthusiasm for epidemiology and support from his friend, former patient and Honorary fellow of the RCGP, Sir Richard Doll (1912–2005), Tudor Hart embarked on a two-year period of epidemiological research. He initially worked under Doll and later under Archie Cochrane (1909–1988). Tudor Hart joined the MRC in 1960 and worked in their Pneumoconiosis Research Unit (PRU) in Llandough, South Wales. This is where he gained exposure to the poor health experienced by residents of coal-mining communities. Although Tudor Hart had great respect and admiration for the work of Cochrane, he disagreed with the unit's 'detached observational role' and saw the need for research-based practices and so left the PRU after only one year.

The treatment of patients was something that Tudor Hart missed and so, in 1961, he relocated to Glyncorrwg, a small mining village in West Glamorgan, South Wales. This is where he would settle as a general practitioner for the next 30 years with his wife Mary Thomas, together with whom they had three children. From 1968 onwards, Tudor Hart would use his previous epidemiological research experience combined with the expertise of his wife, who had also worked under Cochrane, and the support of the MRC to examine the population from his own practice. The approximate 2000 patient number were all studied meticulously. He screened them for treatable disease risk factors. Through this population-based approach, he reduced age standardised mortality rates, achieving rates nearly 30 per cent lower than equivalent coal-mining communities. His work emphasised the importance of continuity of care and of doctors getting to know their patients well.

Since his early days as a general practitioner, Tudor Hart had a keen interest in hypertension and how it should best be managed in general practice. It was whilst working as a general practitioner in London that he started to measure the blood pressure of all his adult patients on a routine basis, becoming the first doctor to make it part of their regular practice. He wrote his prize winning Butterworth Gold Medal Essay in 1975, an award presented by the RCGP, which covered a number of points on diagnosis and management including the fact that blood pressure readings should be repeated at least three times. He was also the first general practitioner to publish a book on hypertension, which was titled *Hypertension: Community Control of High Blood Pressure* (1980). Building on his opportunistic blood pressure screening as a general practitioner in London, hypertension was one of the most important treatable risk factors that he screened for at his rural South Wales practice. He screened 100 per cent of the male and 98 per cent of the female population and followed them up, doubling his treated caseload. He identified that general practitioners need to possess the qualities of enthusiasm and commitment to make screening in general practice a success.

Tudor Hart's experience in the coal-mining community of Glyncorrwg led him to devise his 'inverse care law' which was published in *The Lancet* in 1971. The law proposed that 'the availability of good medical care tends to vary inversely with the need for it in the population served'. He was awarded an Honorary MRCP for this development and later was awarded FRCP.

The education of medical students was an area where Tudor Hart was forward thinking. During his George Swift Lecture in 1984, delivered to the Wessex Faculty at the Royal United Hospital, Bath, he proposed that the majority of undergraduate teaching should occur in the community and in general practice. The lecture was titled 'The world turned upside down', which highlighted the radical nature of his proposal. The rationale for his suggestion was that medical students were being trained mainly by specialists, which he felt was an outdated approach as it did not adequately prepare them for a career in general practice, a common career path for them. He would later use these visionary ideas as a basis for his book, *A New Kind of Doctor* (1988).

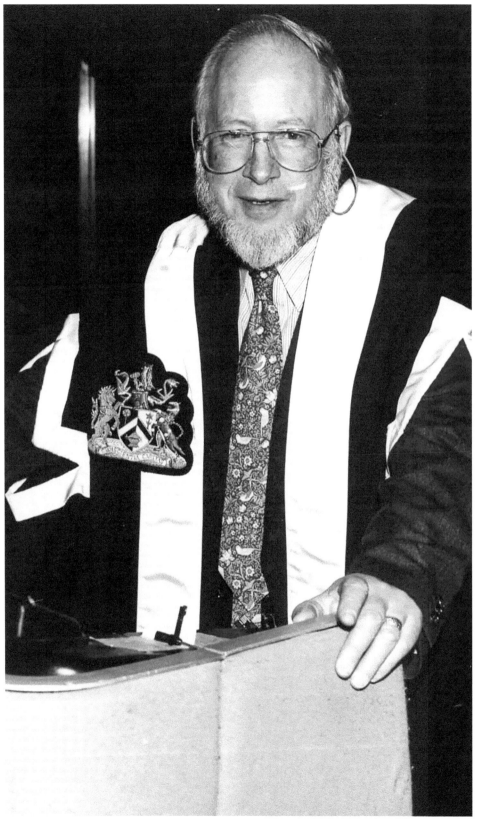

Julian Tudor Hart delivering the James Mackenzie Lecture in 1989. (Courtesy of RCGP Archives, London.)

During his career, Tudor Hart served as an elected member of the council of the RCGP for several years. He delivered the 37th James Mackenzie Lecture in 1989 entitled 'Reactive proactive care: A crisis'.

Throughout his life, Tudor Hart has remained politically active. He was known for his social line on health care but his political interest extended further than his career in medicine. He initially joined the Communist Party when 18 years old. Whilst in Glyncorrwg, he served two terms as a district councillor. He left the Communist Party in 1978 and joined the Labour Party in 1981.

After three decades as a general practitioner in South Wales, Tudor Hart retired. However, he remained academically active, continuing to publish papers in peer-reviewed journals and writing books, publishing his fifth, *The Political Economy of Health Care: A Clinical Perspective* (2006), as he was approaching his eighth decade of life. He was a Research Fellow at Swansea Medical School and occasionally worked as an external professor at the Wales Institute for Health Care, University of Glamorgan. He was also an Honorary Fellow of the University of Wales College of Medicine, Cardiff and of the University of Glasgow Medical School. He was president of the Socialist Health Association (SHA) from 1997 to 1999 and was also President of the SHA branch in Wales. He was awarded the George Abercrombie Award in 1987 for his contribution to medical literature and the RCGP Discovery Prize in 2006, celebrating his extensive contributions to research in general practice. He died on 1 July 2018 at the age of 91 years old. His health care innovation and groundbreaking research will continue to be a source of inspiration for generations to come.

Further Reading

Brindle D. Seeing red. *British Medical Journal* 2007;334:976–77.

Hart JT. The inverse care law. *The Lancet* 1971;297(7696):405–12.

Hart JT. James Mackenzie Lecture 1989. Reactive and proactive care: A crisis. *British Journal of General Practice* 1990;40 (330): 4–9.

Hart JT. Opportunities and risks of local population research in general practice. In: Pereira Gray DJ. *Forty Years On: The Story of the First Forty Years of the Royal College of General Practitioners*. London: Atalink; 1992.

Moorhead R. Hart of Glyncorrwg. *Journal of the Royal Society of Medicine* 2004;97:132–36.

79 ROBERT HARVARD DAVIS (1924–1999)
Matt Butler

Robert Harvard Davis was born in Llandaff, Wales, on 14 June 1924. His family were direct descendants of John Harvard (1607–1638), whose bequeathed fortune to a college established in Massachusetts in the early seventeenth century led to the university in the United States that bears his name. In his adolescence, he attended Marlborough College.

Davis studied medicine at Queen College, University of Oxford during the Second World War (1939–1945) as medical students were exempt from conscription. A keen cricketer, he was the opening batsman for the university from 1943. He earned his cricket Blue playing first-class matches including against the University of Cambridge at Lord's cricket ground. He graduated in 1947 after undertaking his clinical student years at Guy's Hospital in London. At this point, he suffered with a period of illness from pulmonary tuberculosis, which led to him being exempt from national service.

After qualification, Davis worked as a house officer, first in Farnborough and then back home in North Wales. His interest in academic medicine was catalysed during his role as a junior RMO in the North Wales sanatorium when he was encouraged to investigate the role of a novel drug, streptomycin, in the treatment of tuberculous sinuses. His review was published in *The Lancet* in 1949. After finishing his house jobs in 1950, he moved back to his hometown in Wales and assisted at his father's practice in Cardiff. His father was Henry Harvard Davis (1887–1961), a former major as Medical Officer in the First World War (1914–1918) and had set up his general practice in 1936.

In 1952, the College was founded with Davis as an inaugural member. He was selected to become the secretary of the research committee of the Welsh Faculty of the College. This research committee would ultimately develop into the *Journal of the College of General Practitioners*. As well as continuing as a full-time general practitioner, throughout the years 1960 to 1963 he studied under Paul Fourman (1918–1968) at the Royal Infirmary in Cardiff, working towards his MD, examining the incidence of hypoparathyroidism following thyroidectomy. This, as well as their investigation into parathyroid function through iatrogenic calcium deprivation, was published in *The Lancet*.

Davis was appointed, in 1967, as the senior lecturer and director of the General Practice Unit at the University of Wales College of Medicine with the remit of establishing general practice teaching and research. This was based upon a practice sited in a new housing complex in Llanedeyrn. He stated one of his primary aims upon appointment was to form coherent links between the university's department of general practice and general practitioners throughout Wales. The Professor of Medicine at the medical school is reported to have asked Davis on his appointment, 'What is it that you can teach medical students that I cannot?' Davis would go on to answer that question many times with his work and literature that he produced on medical education throughout his career.

Around the time of Davis' appointment, the Royal Commission on Medical Education published a report into undergraduate training which recommended that dedicated teaching time in general practice with specifically appointed senior staff should be given to medical students. This report was reinforced by efforts from the RCGP who were encouraging universities to create general practice teaching departments in the medical schools. In his career, Davis was influential in making these recommendations a reality.

Davis was also at the forefront of establishing general practice as a scrupulous academic discipline. He travelled across Wales with his colleague Derek Llewellyn (1928–2007) to establish a range of undergraduate and postgraduate teaching and training practices. Throughout this time he refined his research and teaching activities and was present on many general practice advisory bodies. His efforts were richly rewarded and by the 1980s academic general practice was a discipline commended by students and researchers alike.

Thoughts on the organisation of general practice from the BMA, the RCGP and the Department of Health and Social Security were pulled together by Davis when chairing the Standing Medical Advisory Committee's subcommittee. The report, known as the *Harvard Davis Report* and published in 1971, formed numerous conclusions on how general practice should be organised. Recommendations included continuing the trajectory of increasing staff numbers and practice sizes, and prudently limiting patient capacity to 2500 per general practitioner.

Davis was instrumental in raising charitable funds and with the support of the Welsh NHS he used these to create a new general practice in the Llanedeyrn Health Centre site. This practice was officially opened by HRH the Prince of Wales in 1972. In the same year, Davis was given the title of Honorary Director of the General Practice Teaching Unit. The establishment of the centre allowed for the creation of a multidisciplinary environment which was conducive to progress in the field of academic general practice. He constantly developed the diagnostic coding systems, utilising the computers at the medical school to assist with a database, a visionary idea at the time. Further royal visits occurred in 1973 when HRH Prince Phillip, the then chairman of the RCGP, was shown around the General Practice Unit at Llanedeyrn by Davis. Davis became reader in general practice in 1973 and foundation professor in 1979.

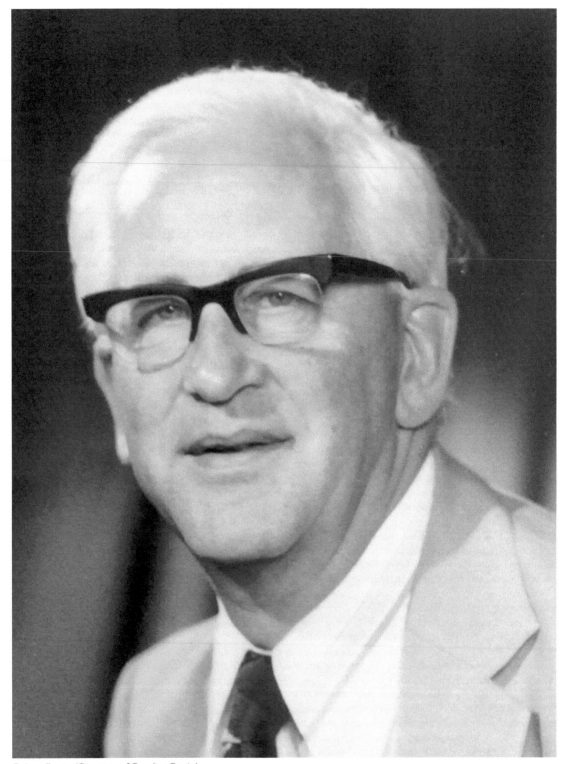

Robert Davis. (Courtesy of Caroline Davis.)

Davis chaired the RCGP Welsh Council from 1977 to 1980. In 1979, he produced an influential model of the general practice consultation alongside his colleague Nigel Stott (1939–). The model described four aspects of the doctor-patient relationship: management of presenting problems, modification of help-seeking behaviour, management of continuing problems and opportunistic health promotion. This model was to be a fundamental aspect in the teaching of general practice. He served on many other committees including the Medicines Commission and the Child Health Services Committee, and wrote papers and textbooks including *General Practice for Students of Medicine* (1975).

Between 1979 and 1986 Davis was Professor of General Practice at the University of Wales College of Medicine. When he retired that year, the RCGP Welsh Council founded the annual Harvard Davis Lecture, with Davis himself providing the inaugural eponymous lecture on 'General practice and the unity of clinical medicine'. He left a thriving multidisciplinary department of general practice at the University of Wales, situated around the enlarged Llanedeyrn Health Centre. Undergraduate students were now being taught at the centre as well as in a network of teaching practices throughout the area. Collaboration with postgraduate training courses had always been encouraged by Davis.

Upon retirement Davis resumed his interests in golf, gardening, birdwatching and fishing. He died on 16 January 1999 as professor emeritus, leaving his wife, Valerie, and a son and daughter. He was described by Llewellyn and Stott, two of his closest professional colleagues as a 'genial companion, journeys [passing] quickly in his company'.

Further Reading

Davis R. Streptomycin in the treatment of tuberculous sinuses. *The Lancet* 1949;254(6587):982–84.

Davis RH. Harvard Davis Lecture 1986. General practice and the unity of clinical medicine. *The Journal of the Royal College of General Practitioners* 1987;37(298):196–98.

Davis RH (Chmn.). *The Organisation of Group Practice. A Report of a Sub-Committee of the Standing Medical Advisory Committee*. London: HMSO; 1971.

Howie J, Whitfield M (eds.). *Academic General Practice in the UK Medical Schools, 1948–2000*. Edinburgh: Edinburgh University Press; 2011.

Llewellyn D, Stott N. Robert Harvard Davis. *British Medical Journal* 1999;318:878.

Stott NCH, Davis RH. The exceptional potential of each primary care consultation. *The Journal of the Royal College of General Practitioners* 1979;29(201):201–5.

80 NIGEL CH STOTT (1939–)
Sabrina Samuels and Paula Tebay

Nigel Clement Halley Stott is one of the towering figures of academic generalist medicine. Committed to active clinical practice for most of his career, his work integrated multidisciplinary thinking, dedicated, intuitive patient care and principled rigour in pioneering research and teaching. He was born in Durban, South Africa, on 27 November 1939. His physician father, Halley Harwin Stott (1910–2004), founded the Valley Trust in KwaZulu-Natal, South Africa, an innovative socio-medical project promoting an integrated approach to health care, combining curative services with initiatives to develop sustainable soil quality, the growth of fresh food, healthy diet, employment and effective leadership in an area of significant social deprivation. This influenced his focus on the health of whole general practice populations and anticipatory care.

Leaving the University of Cape Town in 1961, Stott continued his studies at the University of Edinburgh, attaining a first-class BSc (Hons) in pathology and graduating in medicine in 1966. He returned to South Africa to complete six months as a pre-registrar at King Edward VIII Hospital in Durban, followed by a surgical placement at Edinburgh Royal Infirmary. As a senior house officer, he worked at the Western General Hospital in Edinburgh, where he was awarded MRCP. As a registrar he worked for the MRC Clinical Population and Cytogenetics Unit in Edinburgh from 1968 to 1970. As a trainee general practitioner, he completed postgraduate courses in epidemiology, statistics and demography. In 1971, his developing interest in general practice brought him back to his roots in South Africa. As physician in charge at St. Lucy's Mission Hospital in Tsolo, Transkei, he developed significant skills in organising and practising emergency medicine, general medicine, obstetrics, paediatrics and surgery in a context of limited medical resources.

Stott was appointed as senior lecturer for the University of Wales College of Medicine (UWCM) in 1972. An early research interest in the management of common infections in general practice led to the development of his first major publication in 1976, in collaboration with epidemiologist Robert West. Stott and West are widely recognised for one of the first randomised controlled trials that rigorously evaluated the hypothesis that antibiotics do not speed the recovery of uncomplicated lower respiratory tract infections. This influential research has had significant long-term impact on the way in which antibiotics are now prescribed. Several other landmark studies followed, including a key study published in 1979 on children with winter upper respiratory tract infections, which highlighted the over-prescription of antibiotics and the need for improved parent education.

Stott worked closely with Robert Harvard Davis (1924–1999) to develop one of their first conceptual publications that outlined a framework for encouraging clinicians to explore and use the 'exceptional potential in each primary care consultation' to address co-morbidity, offer health promotion and to negotiate help-seeking behaviour with patients. Together they produced the Stott and Davis model (1979), or the Cardiff Framework, as Stott modestly called it. This framework for managing the general practice consultation still enjoys wide currency, and is taught in undergraduate and graduate curricula around the world.

Stott is well known for his clear-sighted integration of academia and clinical practice. In 1979, he moved to Southampton for a year to work as professor of primary medical care, and in the same year he was awarded FRCP for his outstanding contributions to medicine. His seminal book *Primary Health Care: Bridging the Gap Between Theory and Practice* (1983) promoted integration between disciplines, whole systems thinking and horizontal integration, and drew on third world examples of good practice.

In 1986, Stott succeeded Davis as professor of general practice and Head of Department at UWCM. During this period of continued clinical practice and integrated work with the health centre team, he led the multidisciplinary academic department at Llanedeyrn Health Centre, and worked closely with social anthropologist Professor Roisin Pill. Together, their research contributed greatly to improve general practice and understanding, including studies on diabetes, the views of working-class women and health promotion. He influenced and inspired academics in his department to generate an outpouring of innovative research publications. Under his leadership, the department performed successfully in National Research Assessment Exercises and Teaching Quality Assessment Exercises.

Stott was an active member of several academic committees and as the appointed Foundation chairman from 1983 to 1988, he oversaw the establishment of the George Thomas Trust for Palliative Care in South Wales. Now renamed as George Thomas Hospice Care, this centre remains the major provider of Cardiff's specialist palliative care. From his department in 1988, he steered the establishment of the first postgraduate diploma in Palliative Care course in the United Kingdom. He chaired the local medical committee's ethics committee (1987–1991) and was a member, then chair, of the research committee of UWCM from 1994 to 1999. In 1996, he chaired a RCGP working party, which produced an important report concluding that as the size of a general practice team grows arithmetically, the lines of communication grow geometrically.

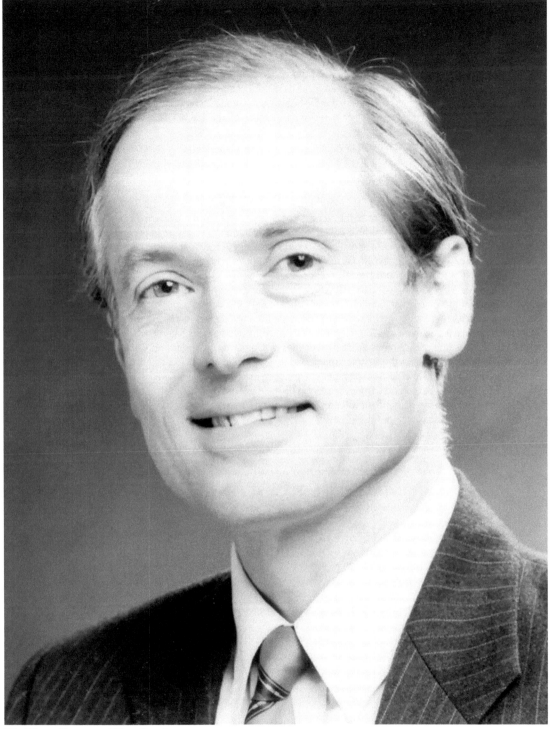

Nigel Stott. (Courtesy of Mary Stott.)

Stott chaired a landmark *MRC Topic Review: Primary Health Care* (1997) that heralded a significant change in attitude in the MRC towards the funding of general practice based research and capacity development. This was at a time when the MRC was specifically specialist and biomedically orientated. This report had significant impact on the status of general practice as an academic discipline during the mid-1990s.

From 1999 to 2004, Stott served at the GMC. This was an exciting and challenging time of transition when the GMC was exposed to pressure from the media and the public to an unprecedented extent, whilst undergoing rigorous assessment by independent consultants. He served as deputy chair on the GMC Professional Performance Committee (2000–2004) and notably he chaired the GMC's Investigation Committee between 2004 and 2008. From 2006 to 2008, Stott was the only medically qualified member of the Higher Education Funding Council for Wales.

Stott developed key reports and documents in general practice to inform policies of the National Welsh Assembly in 2001. Furthermore, he worked widely as an external examiner for university medical departments in the United Kingdom, and held visiting appointments in New Zealand, South Africa, Hong Kong and Singapore. A popular speaker at conferences and training events, he was known for speaking lucidly, without pomposity.

Stott was awarded MRCGP in 1969 and FRCGP in 1987. For many years he chaired the RCGP Welsh Council. He delivered 'When something is good, more of the same is not always better' as the William Pickles Lecture in 1993 and was honoured with the George Abercrombie Award for his contribution to literature in general practice in 1997. In recognition of his services to primary care and general practice medicine, he was appointed CBE in 2001. He was later awarded an honorary fellowship at the University of Cardiff in 2007. In his address, he spoke of the importance of integrity in the context of scholarship and clinical practice, and the need for graduates to protect freedom of speech.

Stott married Eleanor Mary Collingwood (née Townroe) in 1965 and together they have a daughter and two sons. He served as chairman of the local Parish Church Council (1999–2004). His interests include gardening, conservation studies and sailing. His work continues to inspire and influenced many conditions, clinicians and academics alike. Retiring from the academic department in 2000, he continued active involvement in chairing trial steering committees, contributing to major research programmes at the universities of Cambridge, Cardiff and Oxford, including a key 10-year study on diabetes. He paved the way for many budding general practitioners to encourage and motivate others, to strive for best practice and to champion general practice in academic and medical circles. He has been a great mentor, and continues to be a friend to many leaders in the field of academic general practice around the world. He is recognised as a distinguished emeritus professor of general practice who brought immense rigour, creativity and stature to his academic discipline.

Further Reading

Stott N (Chmn.). *The Nature of General Medical Practice: Report from General Practice No. 27*. London: RCGP; 1996.

Stott N (Chmn.). *MRC Topic Review: Primary Health Care*. London: MRC; 1997.

Stott NC. William Pickles Lecture 1993: When something is good, more of the same is not always better. *British Journal of General Practice* 1993;43(371):254–58.

Stott NCH. Management and outcome of winter respiratory tract infections in children aged 0–9 years. *British Medical Journal* 1979;1(6155):29–31.

Stott NCH. *Primary Health Care – Bridging the Gap Between Theory and Practice*. Berlin: Springer-Verlag; 1983.

Stott NCH, Davis RH. The exceptional potential of each primary care consultation. *The Journal of the Royal College of General Practitioners* 1979;29(201):201–5.

Stott NCH, Pill RM. 'Advise yes, dictate no': Patients' views on health promotion in the consultation. *Family Practice* 1990;7: 125–31.

Stott NCH, Pill RM. *Making Changes: A Study of Working Class Mothers and Changes in their Health-Related Behaviour over 5 Years*. Cardiff: University of Wales College of Medicine; 1990.

Stott NCH, West RR. Randomised controlled trial of antibiotics in patients with cough and purulent sputum. *British Medical Journal* 1976;2(6035):556–59.

31 MARTIN ROLAND (1951–)

George Higginbotham

Martin Roland was born on 7 August 1951. He attended Rugby School in Warwickshire from 1962 to 1968. Following in the footsteps of both his father, Peter Roland (1912–2013), and grandfather, Josef Rosenbaum (1895–1963), he considered his choice of a medical career a natural one, and made the decision at a young age to pursue it.

Roland began his medical studies at Merton College, University of Oxford, in 1969. He was awarded a first-class honours degree in Physiological Sciences in 1972. During these preclinical years, he enjoyed the weekly supervisions more than the lectures or practicals, and it was the independent learning and enquiry necessary for these supervisions that he found most inspiring. During his clinical training at university, he was dissuaded by the impersonality of many medical specialities. He found himself drawn to specialities requiring more humane contact with patients, particularly general practice and paediatrics. A week with a rural general practitioner in Pembrokeshire served as further inspiration, especially the relationship that the general practitioner had with their patients and community. On completing studies at medical school, Roland had decided upon a career in general practice.

Following medical school and house officer jobs in Oxford and Bath, Roland, in 1975, entered into a vocational training scheme in Cambridge. As a general practitioner trainee, his enquiring mind led him to undertake research projects. However, it was personal reasons that influenced his decision to apply for an academic post. Such a post would allow him to spend a few years working in London without requiring a permanent commitment to a particular practice and it was London where his wife, Rosalind Roland (1948–), was a lecturer in paediatrics at University College. He took up an academic general practice post in 1979, and subsequently began his doctorate, looking at predictors of outcome for lower back pain. As a result, the Roland Morris Disability Questionnaire (RMDQ) was created and it aimed to assess patients' self-rated physical disability. The RMDQ was initially intended for use as a measure of clinical trial outcome but has since been considered useful in the monitoring of patients in clinical practice.

In 1983, Roland returned to the Newmarket Road practice in Cambridge, taking up a position as a partner. Initially, he continued teaching at St Thomas' Hospital for two sessions a week, before instead taking up the part-time position as director of studies at the University of Cambridge School of Clinical Medicine, where he worked until 1992.

Roland found the biomedical-oriented environment in Cambridge a challenging one to conduct research and development in general practice. Consequently, in 1992, he made the decision to move to the University of Manchester to take up the position of chair in general practice. He would remain in this position for the next 18 years. During this time he delivered the 46th James Mackenzie Lecture in 1998 titled 'Quality and efficiency: Enemies or partners?'.

Following completion of his doctorate, Roland's research interests changed to focus more on understanding and improving the delivery of primary care within the NHS. His research was split into two distinct phases: the initial one looking at the interface between primary and secondary care in terms of hospital referrals; the second one researching quality of care. This latter interest led to his landmark achievement, helping to lay the groundwork for a system of clinical targets in general practice. Due to his position as director of the National Primary Care Research and Development Centre (1999–2009), he was invited to join the BMA negotiating teams as one of five expert advisors, working within the Quality and Outcomes Framework (QOF) subgroup towards a new General Medical Services contract. As with his fellow advisor colleagues, he had not previously been involved in political negotiation before the development of QOF. However, as a team, they were committed to the idea that quality within general practice was measurable, and should be rewarded.

After nine months of regular meetings, the resulting framework was introduced on 1 April 2004. It took the form of a voluntary annual reward and incentive programme, providing financial reward to general practices for the provision of 'quality care', including the management of common chronic diseases, management of public health concerns, and the implementation of preventative measures. The financial impact was so great, that some practices generated 25 per cent of their income through QOF incentives. The QOF encouraged general practices to improve on their management of chronic diseases, and to engage with secondary prevention.

Once QOF had started Roland took on an analytical role. He contributed to a review of the QOF system and noted, as he had during the initial negotiations, that the framework was limited in that it was lacking in areas such as mental health and cancer. In this review, he also questioned the efficacy of financial incentives in general practice, and proposed that the proportion of a practice's income from incentives should be reduced. In addition to the reduction in scale of the QOF, he also suggested the need for it to become more flexible.

Roland has had further roles following his work with QOF. He became professor of health services research at the University of Cambridge in 2009. In 2014, he chaired a commission into the current and future primary care workforce, instructed by the Secretary of State for Health, Jeremy Hunt. The Commission's final report, *The Future of Primary*

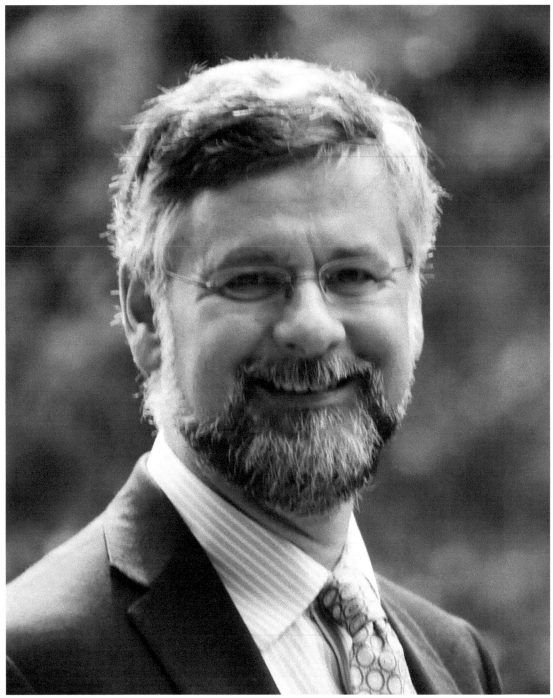

Martin Roland. (Courtesy of Martin Roland.)

Care: Creating Teams for Tomorrow, was published in July 2015. Included within this report were recommendations for an expanded multidisciplinary team within primary care, closer relationships with specialists and improved information technology links between community care, primary care and hospital specialists. These recommendations were largely taken up in NHS England's *General Practice Forward View* published in April 2016.

In 2003, Roland was appointed CBE for Services to Medicine, in recognition of his longstanding input into health policy. Six years later, in 2009, he received the George Abercrombie Award for special meritorious literary work in general practice. Outside the world of medicine, he enjoys hill walking in the Lake District, listening to classical music (particularly opera) and playing golf.

Further Reading

Roland M. General practitioner referral rates. *British Medical Journal* 1988;297:437–38.

Roland M. James MacKenzie Lecture 1998. Quality and efficiency: Enemies or partners? *British Journal of General Practice* 1999;49(439):140–43.

Roland M (Chmn.). *Future of Primary Care: Creating Teams for Tomorrow. A Report of the Primary Care Workforce Commission*. London: Health Education England; 2015.

Roland M, Campbell S. Successes and failures of the United Kingdom's Pay for Performance Program. *New England Journal of Medicine* 2014;370:1944–49.

Roland M, Morris R. A study of the natural history of back pain. Part 1: Development of a reliable and sensitive measure of disability in low-back pain. *Spine* 1983;8(2):141–44.

Roland M, Morris R. A study of the natural history of back pain. Part 2: Development of guidelines for trials of treatment in primary care. *Spine* 1983;8(2):145–50.

82 JOHN ALEXANDER REID LAWSON (1920–2001)
Emily Brown

John Alexander Reid Lawson was born in Dundee in 1920. The son of a rope maker was educated at the high school of Dundee before going onto attend the University of St Andrews, qualifying as a doctor in 1943. During his time at the University of St Andrews, he was a keen sportsman, representing the university at hockey and cricket, and achieving a single figure golf handicap whilst a member of the Royal and Ancient Golf Club of St Andrews. Following their marriage in 1944, he and his wife Pat had two sons, two daughters and later ten grandchildren. Their home in Dundee, 'The Ridges', had a wonderful garden with a hill down towards the sea, which he loved. The Lawson family were close and happy and Pat would often accompanied him on work trips. Friends and colleagues enjoyed spending time with them and speak very highly of him, remembering him as a wonderful dinner companion with a brilliant sense of humour.

Lawson enjoyed a long and distinguished medical career. In 1944, he joined the RAMC and was initially posted to the Burmese Jungle as Regimental Medical Officer in The Queen's Own Cameron Highlanders. He also spent time serving in Japan and witnessed the aftermath of the nuclear bomb at Hiroshima. By the time of his demobilisation he had reached the rank of Major. He went on to have a number of hospital posts, and then, in 1948, just months before the establishment of the NHS, he became a general practitioner in Dundee, where he practised until 1986. He stated that he was drawn to become a general practitioner because 'it was to do with people'.

Lawson had an extensive and fruitful involvement with the College. This started when, shocked by the findings of the *Collings Report*, he became a foundation member in May 1953. He became heavily involved with RCGP Scotland, holding offices of Provost, chairing the East Scotland Faculty (1960–1964) and chairing the Scottish Council (1966–1968). In 1964, he became a member of College Council and proceeded to hold numerous offices, including chairman of the Publications Committee and chairman of the Joint Committee for Postgraduate Training in General Practice. He became chairman of the RCGP Council in 1973 and held this position until 1976.

In 1982, Lawson was appointed president of the RCGP, a post he held until 1985. During this time, in 1984, he gave the Victor Johnston Memorial Oration to the Canadian College of General Practitioners. He also visited Australia, Finland, Kuwait and New Zealand on RCGP business. Alongside these roles he continued to work tirelessly as a general practitioner and also as a popular trainer and he served as a regional adviser in general practice from 1972 to 1982. Throughout his presidency, RCGP affairs were run well and without trouble. Whilst he made no significant changes to the RCGP nor its development plan, he allowed the organisation to run smoothly and to mature. The chairman of the RCGP Council at the time was Donald Irvine (1935–2018), with whom Lawson worked well. Lawson also enjoyed good relationships with the heads of the other Royal Colleges. Colleagues felt that as president, Lawson inspired 'the trust and confidence of his colleagues' through 'his equanimity, his balance and his judgement'. He was whole-heartedly dedicated to the RCGP, as illustrated by the countless positions he held, as well as in making the regular long journeys from Dundee to the RCGP's headquarters at Princes Gate in Knightsbridge, London.

A defining act in Lawson's career was his involvement in the 'What Sort of Doctor' initiative. Instigated by the Board of Censors in September 1980, it aimed to develop 'a method of assessing the performance of general practitioners in the setting of their own practices'. This would become a salient theme at the RCGP throughout the 1980s. He was chairman of the first working group from 1980 to 1981, which looked at the assessment of quality of care in general practice. He continued his work as a member of the second working group from 1982 to 1984. Following a third working group and five years of work, this initiative led to the publication, in 1985, of the *What Sort of Doctor: Report of General Practice No. 23: Assessing Quality of Care in General Practice*. It was the first published analysis of what defined good general practice. This work developed a framework for assessing quality in general practice through four areas: values, accessibility, competence and communication skills. The report had three key areas of significance. Firstly, it redirected RCGP thinking away from educational process and towards outcome. Secondly, it produced a framework for performance review which remains largely unchanged today. Thirdly, it led the RCGP to start visiting and assessing general practices overall. Consequently, the 'What Sort of Doctor' initiative is considered to have had a huge impact and is linked to the later establishment of Fellowship by Assessment.

A number of awards were given to Lawson. He was awarded FRCGP in 1967. Later, in 1979, he was appointed OBE in recognition of his dedication and extensive contribution to general practice. Later, in 1999 and two years before he died, he received the RCGP Foundation Council Award for special meritorious work in collection with the RCGP. He is remembered fondly and with admiration for his wide ranging contributions to the College and RCGP and to general practice as a whole. Today he is remembered by the East Scotland Faculty of the RCGP when they award the annual Lawson Prize to a final year medical student, based on excellence in general practice, and also host the annual John Lawson Lecture, which highlights a current topic of interest.

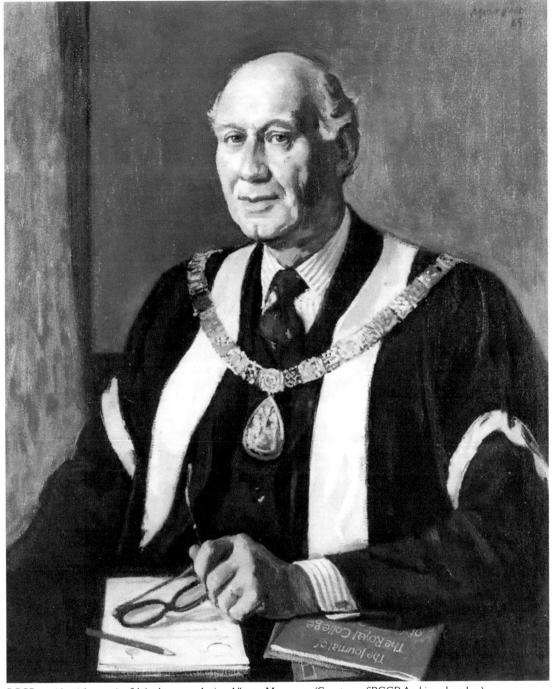

RCGP presidential portrait of John Lawson. Artist: Alberto Morrocco. (Courtesy of RCGP Archives, London.)

Further Reading

McCormick J. John Lawson: An appreciation. *British Journal of General Practice* 2003;53:422.

RCGP. *What Sort of Doctor: Report of General Practice No. 23*. London: RCGP; 1985.

RCGP Archive. John Lawson, interview by Alastair Donald, filmed by William Fulton, in Dundee, 1996. Video reference C-AV-C1-12.

83 SIR BRIAN JARMAN (1933–)

Sophie Joyce Brotherton

Brian Jarman was born on 9 July 1933 in London, the eldest of two sons. His mother was a housewife and his father was an engineer. He attended Barking Abbey School and, in 1951, he obtained an exhibition at the University of Cambridge. Whilst at Cambridge, he enjoyed rock climbing and was captain of the tennis team. He graduated with BA in Natural Sciences in 1954 which became MA in Natural Sciences in 1957.

In 1954, Jarman undertook national military service and, in 1956, spent a year working for the Army Operational Research Group. In 1960, he began working as a geophysicist after obtaining a PhD in Geophysics at Imperial College. He spent two years in the Sahara Desert in Libya and a year in Holland. He married in 1963 and had three sons.

At the age of 31 years old, Sir Brian decided to pursue a career in medicine. He did not think he would enjoy a long-term career as a geophysicist and had been vaguely interested in medicine since he was a young man. In 1964, he enrolled at St Mary's Hospital Medical School. He was offered a place provided that he passed an intelligence test and obtained a Biology A level. He admits that his decision to study medicine created a significant financial strain. His father disapproved. As an undergraduate he won prizes in seven medical subjects and, in 1969, was awarded a first-class Honours Degree in Medicine.

Jarman's first medical role was as a house physician at St Mary's Hospital, London. In 1970, he worked as a surgical house officer at St. Bernard's Hospital, Gibraltar. After completing an elective at Harvard Medical School, he returned to work as a resident in medicine at Beth Israel Hospital where he worked under Professor Howard Hiatt (1925–) who is renowned for his involvement in the discovery of messenger RNA and his role as the dean of the Harvard School of Public Health.

Jarman's time at Beth Israel Hospital was cut short when one of his sons was diagnosed with acute lymphoblastic leukaemia (ALL). At the time there was no cure. Jarman became aware of a clinical trial with curative intent at the Royal Marsden Hospital, London. He took time out of training to care for his son, administering most of the chemotherapy medication himself. The treatment was successful and his son became one of the first survivors of ALL in the United Kingdom.

General practice was entered into by Jarman when he began working at Lisson Grove, London. General practice appealed to him because he enjoyed patient contact. He remained there until 1998. As a general practitioner, he became interested in epidemiological research as a general practitioner trainee. His breakthrough was the development of the Underprivileged Area Score which allowed general practitioners to be paid different amounts according to the level of deprivation within their area.

Between 1974 and 1978, Jarman became a member of the Community Health Council, a patient representative body, an unusual step for a doctor at that time. In 1976, he was elected to the Kensington, Chelsea and Westminster local medical committee and, in 1978, became the general practitioner member of the Bloomsbury District Management Team. Later, in 1983, he became professor of general practice at Imperial College.

As a general practitioner, Jarman designed the Lisson Grove Benefits Program. This is a computer program which calculates the distribution of social security benefits. He invited workers from social services to use the program at Lisson Grove Health Centre in an attempt to integrate health and social care. The program later became adopted at citizen advice bureaus and social services across the country.

Sir Brian also became involved in mortality data research. In the late 1980s he became involved in NHS Resource Allocation and had to sign the Official Secrets Act in order to access the confidential Hospital Episode Statistic (HES) data. He later used the HES data to develop the Hospital Standardised Mortality Ratio (HSMR) which compares the number of hospital observed deaths to the number of expected deaths over a period of time after accounting for patient factors such as age, sex and diagnosis. In 1999, he published a groundbreaking paper in the *BMJ* 'Explaining differences in English hospital death rates using routinely collected data'. Using the HSMR, he highlighted significant variation in adjusted mortality between hospitals in England. The main adjustment factors were the patients' age, diagnoses and the proportion of emergency admissions. The number of hospital clinicians per hospital bed and general practitioners per head of population best accounted for this variation in HSMRs. However, as his calculations were based on confidential data, the individual hospitals could not be named alongside their HSMRs. In 2000, after an initial refusal by Frank Dobson, the former Secretary of State for Health, Jarman was granted permission to publish the hospital names by Simon Stevens who was special advisor to Alan Milburn, the Secretary of State for Health.

Jarman served on the panel for the Royal Bristol Inquiry from 1999 until 2001. He was approached by Sir Ian Kennedy, Chair of the Inquiry, but was initially reluctant as he had just retired. He eventually agreed after receiving a phone call from the Deputy Chief Medical Officer. The inquiry investigated paediatric cardiac surgical mortality for open heart operations in children under one year old at the Royal Bristol Infirmary from April 1991 until March 1995.

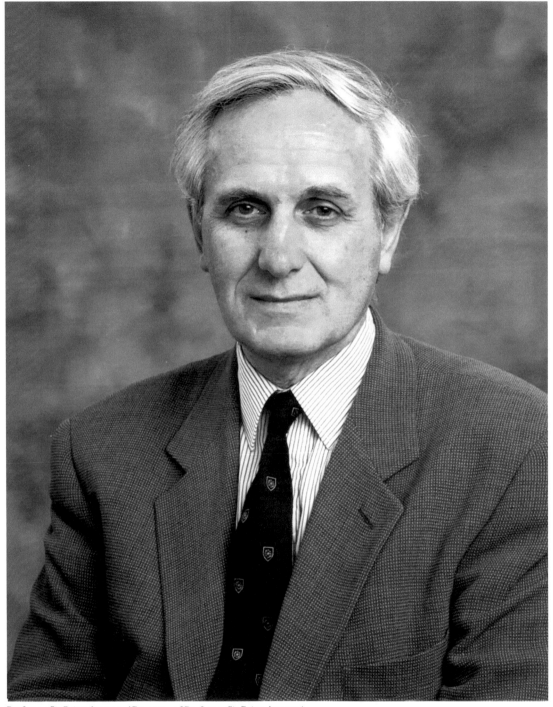

Professor Sir Brian Jarman. (Courtesy of Professor Sir Brian Jarman.)

The data concluded that mortality in Bristol was significantly higher than at other centres. Furthermore, the inquiry exposed a culture of deep-rooted inadequacy in monitoring patient safety. This led to several important changes within the NHS as part of the NHS Reform and Health Care Professions Act 2002, which included measures for increased patient involvement and greater regulation of health care professionals. In light of the events at Bristol, in 2002 he helped to establish the Dr Foster Unit at Imperial College which uses the HSMR to analyse United Kingdom hospital mortality data on a monthly basis. The HSMR is used in countries around the world.

Various inquiries into the events at the Mid Staffordshire NHS Foundation Trust took place between 2008 and 2013. In 2013, the Mid Staffordshire Public Inquiry, chaired by Robert Francis QC, was published. Several concerns were raised over the significantly high mortality rate as indicated by the monthly mortality alerts sent by Imperial College. Staffing levels, patient concerns and surgical performance also raised alarm bells. The inquiry received much media attention and those high up within the NHS were criticised for stating they were unaware of the extent of the problem.

The Dr Foster Unit played an important role in the inquiry. They sent letters to the Chief Executive of the Mid Staffordshire NHS Foundation Trust regarding significantly high mortality rates for certain procedures and diagnoses. In 2001, Dr Foster Intelligence, a separate organisation, started to publish yearly HSMRs produced by Imperial College for Acute English hospitals including Mid Staffordshire NHS Foundation Trust.

The HSMR came under scrutiny when the West Midlands Strategic Health Authority asked the University of Birmingham to perform an independent review in 2007. The Mid Staffordshire Independent Inquiry concluded that the Dr Foster Unit had correctly identified a problem which was consistent with other lines of inquiry and that it would have been irresponsible not to investigate further.

There have been various notable awards and honours for Jarman. In 1988, he was appointed OBE. Two years later he delivered the 38th James Mackenzie Lecture entitled 'General Practice, the NHS review and social deprivation'. He was knighted in 1998. In 2003, he became president of the BMA. He felt humbled that they were willing to accept someone who had criticised certain aspects of the medical profession. More recently, in 2014, he was awarded The President's Medal of the RCGP.

As an octogenarian, Jarman continues to work on data analysis as co-director of the Dr Foster Unit and is an emeritus professor at Imperial College.

Further Reading

Aylin P, Bottle A, Jarman B, Elliott P. Paediatric cardiac surgical mortality in England after Bristol: Descriptive analysis of hospital episode statistics 1991–2002. *British Medical Journal* 2004;329(7470):825.

Jarman B. James Mackenzie Lecture 1990. General Practice, the NHS review and social deprivation. *British Journal of General Practice* 1991;41(343):76–79.

Jarman B. *Mid Staffordshire Public Inquiry Brian Jarman Witness Statements and Oral Hearing.* In: Francis R (Chmn.). *The Mid Staffordshire NHS Foundation Trust Public Inquiry: Report of the Mid Staffordshire NHS Foundation Trust Public Inquiry.* London: HMSO;2013.

Jarman B, Gault S, Alves B, Hider A, Dolan S, Cook A et al. Explaining differences in English hospital death rates using routinely collected data. *British Medical Journal* 1999;318(7197):1515–20.

34 MICHAEL PRINGLE (1950–)

Sarah K. Taylor

Mike Pringle was born on 14 May 1950 in Aylesbury in Buckinghamshire and was inspired to study medicine by his local general practitioner, whom he admired for both his rapport with his patients and his academic astuteness. He was educated at St. Edward's School in Oxford before attending Guy's Hospital Medical School in 1968.

After graduation, Pringle worked as a house officer in the Royal Surrey County Hospital and Royal Hampshire County Hospital. He then spent seven months as a senior house officer in psychiatry before undertaking his general practitioner training in the rural village practice of Sonning Common, near Reading, where he worked under the supervision of Tom Stewart (1932–1991). Pringle himself has described Stewart as 'exactly the sort of role model that someone like myself would yearn for', citing Stewart responsible for strengthening his commitment to general practice. Whilst working at Sonning Common, he also worked with John Hasler (1937–), who has been described as 'significant [leader]…few people have been able equal' by Philippa Moreton in *The Very Stuff of General Practice* (1999).

Whilst at Sonning Common, Pringle was first exposed to the use of computers in general practice, with the practice being part of a pilot scheme in the mid-1970s to determine whether computers could be used to improve the delivery of general practice and whether they could be used to maintain the clinical records of patients. This early exposure to information technology in general practice so impressed him it became the subject of his early research, his MD thesis and of a chapter he also wrote for *The Very Stuff of General Practice*.

After completing his vocational training, Pringle joined a practice in Collingham near Newark in 1979, retiring as a partner in the practice in 2004. Since retirement, he has retained links with the practice through his role as education director at the Collingham Healthcare Education Centre. At Collingham, he worked as part of a team who were early adopters of computerisation, clinical audit and patient participation.

Whilst working in Collingham, Pringle started working as a senior lecturer at the University of Nottingham Medical School in 1989, becoming a professor in 1993. From 2002 to 2008, he was head of the School of Community Health Sciences and he retired as an emeritus professor of general practice in the summer of 2011. His academic interests span a range of subjects, in particular general practice information systems, quality of care and epidemiology.

It was whilst working at the School of Community Health Sciences that Pringle helped set up QRESEARCH in 2003, a database containing the anonymised general practice records of over 11 million patients, in over 1000 general practices in the United Kingdom. It is the largest database of its type worldwide and is used by clinical researchers to develop new risk prediction algorithms, which can be used by doctors to predict which patients are at risk of certain diseases so preventative interventions can be used. The most famous algorithm which has come out of QRESEARCH data is QRISK2: a cardiovascular disease risk predictor used daily by general practitioners today; other risk predictors using QRESEARCH data predict individuals risk of cancer, diabetes and fractures. Being able to identify high-risk patients allows doctors to treat their patients to reduce their chances of developing life-changing illnesses such as diabetes and cancer, as well as acute life-threatening events such as heart attacks. As well as being good for patients, it has had a real impact on public health interventions and enables better planning of health care spending, ensuring that over-stretched NHS budgets are being spent in the most appropriate ways.

Another important contribution Pringle has made to the field of health care informatics is his involvement with Primary Care Information Systems (PRIMIS), which he helped found in 2000. This is a system which gives general practitioners the tools to check their practice records for auditing purposes. Auditing tools from PRIMIS have successfully enabled practices to identify 'at-risk' patients who should be invited for flu jabs, it has helped clinicians balance the risk of bleeding in warfarin patients with the benefits of preventing strokes and has improved patient safety by flagging up patients who are at high-risk of prescribing errors.

Arguably one of Pringle's greatest contributions to general practice has been his development of significant event auditing. This is a form of auditing whereby a patient's care is reviewed to determine whether the outcomes have been beneficial or harmful to the individual. Following this a systematic and detailed analysis is performed to determine the overall level of care received and identify areas which could be changed to enable future improvements in health care. He was the first to describe this process of learning and reflecting from an individual patient's care, as opposed to the more traditional cohort study approach, whereby the care received by a group of patients was examined. This process now performs an integral role in the revalidation and appraisal processes for general practitioners and has been described as being a key part of the culture of general practice.

Pringle has had a strong involvement with the RCGP. He was awarded FRCGP in 1989 and six years later the John Fry Award. He became chairman of the RCGP Council from 1998 to 2001. He delivered the 50th James Mackenzie Lecture in 2002 entitled 'A dog's life'. In 2012, he was made the 23rd president of the RCGP and he completed his presidency in 2015.

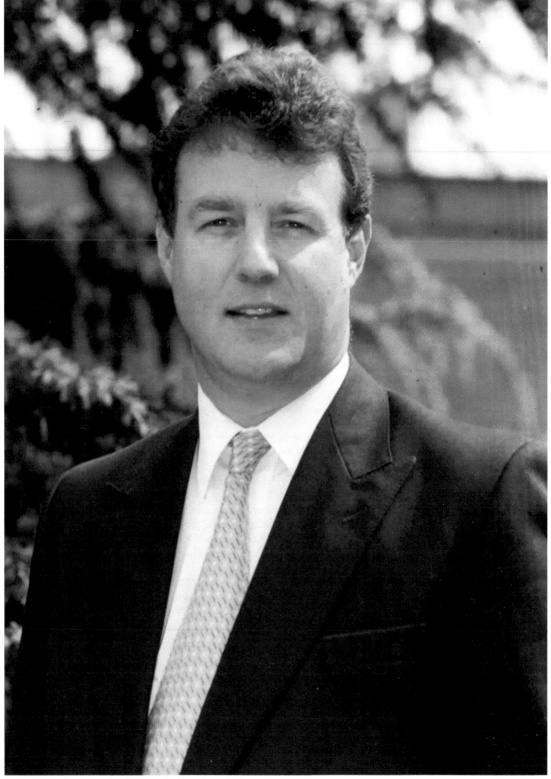

Michael Pringle. (Courtesy of RCGP Archives, London.)

In addition to his work with the RCGP, Pringle has held other significant roles. Firstly, he was an elected member of the GMC and one of his roles included being responsible for setting the regulations by which the fitness to practice of both practising general practitioners and students was assessed. Secondly, he has been a trustee for Arthritis Research UK since 2004 and was also made a trustee for the Picker Institute in 2009, a not-for-profit organisation which aims to use evidence gathered from patients to improve the care they receive. In 2011, he was appointed as a trustee for the Crime Reductions Initiatives which works in prisons and the community to help those affected by domestic abuse, alcohol and drugs. He was appointed CBE in 2001. Furthermore, he has given over 400 lectures in both English and Italian, across four continents.

Pringle has devoted a lifetime of work to general practice, working to improve care for patients nationwide through the widespread adoption of information technology in general practice, the process of revalidation and in the development of significant event auditing. In short, he is a general practitioner who, in his own words, has spent his career ensuring the 'delivery of health meets the aspirations of patients, societies and those of us who work in healthcare'. To help balance such work he enjoys gardening, chess and writing on both medical and non-medical topics. He lives with his wife, Nickie, with whom he has three daughters.

Further Reading

Cooper C. Interview: Listening carefully to all GPs. *GP* 2012; 5 October.

Moreton P. *The Very Stuff of General Practice*. Abingdon: Ratcliffe; 1999.

Pringle M. James Mackenzie Lecture. A dog's life. *British Journal of General Practice* 2003;53(497):963–67.

Pringle M, Bradley C, Carmichael C, Wallis H, Moore A. *Significant Event Auditing. Occasional Paper 70*. London: RCGP; 1995.

85 DAVID HASLAM (1949–)
Mariam Altheyab

David Antony Haslam was born in Birmingham on 4 July 1949. He is the son of a general practitioner, Norman Haslam (1904–1964), whose surgery at 1020 Bristol Road was part of the family house. This had a significant influence on him as he was introduced to medicine at a very early age and even spent his childhood occasionally playing in the waiting room surrounded by patients. He attended Monkton Combe School, a Somerset boarding school, between 1962 and 1967. Always wanting to follow his father and brother into medicine, he then went to study the subject at the University of Birmingham between 1967 and 1972. During his time at university he met his wife who was studying physiotherapy and today they have one daughter and one son who are a doctor and a writer respectively.

Haslam's children helped inspire him to pursue his passion for writing. During their early childhoods they had sleep difficulties that made him realise that there was a significant lack of literature on the subject. Consequently, he wrote a book entitled *Sleepless Children: A Handbook for Parents* (1984). This was a success and was subsequently translated into 13 languages. Furthermore, this led him to write over 1000 medical articles and publish 13 books for the general public on different health-related topics. Earlier achievements that testify to his talent in writing were seen when he won both the interfaculty studies essay prize and the pathological studies essay prize during his time at university.

After graduating from medical school in 1972, Haslam completed his junior hospital jobs in a number of different hospitals including Birmingham Children's Hospital and Birmingham General Hospital. Having always been interested in whole person medicine he became a general practitioner trainee in Stratford-upon-Avon before vocational training was mandatory. He subsequently spent the next 36 years working as a general practitioner in Ramsey, Cambridgeshire, much of it as a general practitioner trainer.

Haslam became involved with the RCGP after being invited to apply to be an examiner as he had been awarded MRCGP with distinction in 1978 and FRCGP in 1989. He served as chairman of the RCGP Examination Board between 1993 and 2001. His experience and interest in general practice, public health and medical politics all led to his appointment as chairman of the RCGP between 2001 and 2004. One of his key achievements in this role included increasing the number of general practitioners that applied for MRCGP. His ambition as chairman in 2001 was to increase the number of members of the RCGP to 20,000, something that has now been more than doubled. Furthermore, during his chairmanship he met with then Prime Minister Tony Blair, which led him to realise that there was limited understanding in the governmental sector on the importance of general practice and on its direct effects on secondary care. Hence, he came up with a short slogan, 'The risk sink of the NHS', with the aim that it would increase the government's awareness on the importance of general practice. In 2006, he delivered the 54th James Mackenzie Lecture entitled 'Who cares?' He later became president of the RCGP between 2006 and 2009 and between 2007 and 2009 he was elected as vice-chairman of the Academy of Medical Royal Colleges.

Haslam has also undertaken other roles with national organisations. This has included being a National Clinical advisor to the Care Quality Commission (2005–2009), and chair of the National Quality Board Quality Information Committee (2009–2010). After that he was appointed as president of the BMA between 2011 and 2012, becoming the only general practitioner to have ever been president of both the RCGP and BMA. He was a member of the Postgraduate Medical Education Training Board (PMETB) from 2003 to 2008 and of the NHS National Quality Board. He was a member of the NHS Modernisation Board, of Medical Education England (2009) and was co-chair of the Modernising Medical Careers Programme Board from 2006 to 2009.

Haslam has received a variety of awards. These include being appointed CBE in 2004 for his services and contributions to the medical and health care system. Moreover, in July 2014, he was awarded an honorary doctorate by the University of Birmingham, and in 2016 a Doctorate from the University of East Anglia. He is a Fellow of the Faculty of Public Health, a Fellow of the Academy of Medical Educators and has been awarded FRCP. Furthermore, in 2014, *Debretts* and the *Sunday Times* named Haslam as one of the 500 most influential and inspirational people in the United Kingdom.

Haslam has been the chairman of the National Institute for Health and Care Excellence (NICE); he was first appointed to this position in April 2013. This position allows him to oversee attempts at improving the contemporaneous health and social care of the population through producing evidence-based guidelines for health care professionals all over the United Kingdom. He is also visiting professor in primary health care at De Montfort University in Leicester, and professor of general practice at the University of Nicosia in Cyprus.

Finally, Haslam believes that one of the main reasons that he was able to take on so many positions of high responsibility was through considering opportunities using what he calls his deathbed test. This test he mentions is if when 99 years old, looking back on his life, would he regret not having given any new opportunity a shot? If he felt he

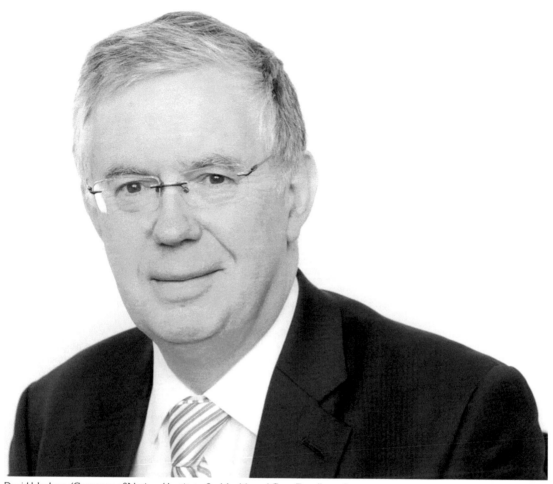

David Haslam. (Courtesy of National Institute for Health and Care Excellence.)

would have then he went for it. He is most proud of keeping true to his belief in high-quality general practice by being focused on patient centeredness, compassion and kindness. He also enjoys speaking to young general practitioners and to inspire them to always do the best that they can do for patients. Furthermore, he finds time to lead a balanced life and pursue some of his other interests that include music, travel, skiing, watching cricket, photography and running.

Further Reading

Anon. My working day: David Haslam. *Journal of the Royal Society of Medicine* 2010;103(4):162–63.

Haslam D. *Sleepless Children: A Handbook for Parents*. New York: Pocket Books; 1985.

Haslam D. Future directions for NICE. *Clinical Medicine* 2013;13(6):532–33.

Haslam D. Haslam's view: Try to put yourself in your patient's shoes. *The Practitioner* 2013;257(1762):39.

Haslam D. Communication skills are as important as diagnostic skills. *The Practitioner* 2016;260(1790):35.

Haslam DA. Who cares? The James Mackenzie Lecture 2006. *British Journal of General Practice* 2007;57(545):987–93.

86 ROGER HARVEY NEIGHBOUR (1947–)

Charmaine Carter

Roger Neighbour is an eminent retired general practitioner. An only child, he was born on 9 June 1947 in Berkhamsted, Hertfordship, into a non-medical family. His first awareness of the medical profession came when, aged five years old, he rode a tricycle whilst pretending to be an ambulance which led him to crash into the milkman simultaneously causing the milkman to break his leg. Later, at Watford Grammar School, he was further inspired by the enthusiasm and curiosity of his sixth form biology teacher. He went on to read Medical Sciences at King's College, University of Cambridge. There, unusually, he opted to study experimental psychology rather than biochemistry. This began a lifelong interest in psychological processes, particularly their role in the consulting behaviour of patients and the doctor-patient relationship. He finished his degree at St Thomas' Hospital, London, and after house jobs in Watford and Hitchin became one of the first three trainees appointed in 1972 to the newly established general practice vocational training scheme in Watford. During his general practice training he attended the Nuffield modular course for potential general practitioner trainers led by Paul Freeling (1928–2002), from which developed his interest in the methods and psychology of medical education.

From 1974 to 2003 Neighbour was a principal in general practice at his former training practice in Abbot's Langley, Hertfordshire. His special clinical interests were in psychotherapy, adolescent psychiatry, hypnosis and dermatology. He was a member of a Balint group for seven years, and undertook extensive training in Ericksonian hypnosis in the United States. He became first a trainer and then a course organiser with the Watford Vocational Training Scheme (1979–1986).

Neighbour has taken prominent roles with the RCGP. In 1984, he was appointed as an MRCGP examiner, later becoming convenor of the Panel of Examiners from 1997 to 2002. He was awarded FRCGP in 1987 and was elected president of the RCGP from 2003 to 2006. He is particularly proud of three things during his presidency: introducing new members awards ceremonies; setting up the Paul Freeling Award for meritorious work in the field of vocational training for general practice and establishing close relations between the RCGP and the pioneers of family medicine in Japan.

Neighbour is widely recognised for his writing and teaching about general practice. This is notably upon doctor–patient communication, the consultation, clinical generalism and medical education. In addition to numerous papers and articles, he is the author of *The Inner Consultation* (1987), *The Inner Apprentice* (1992) and *The Inner Physician* (2016). *The Inner Consultation* combined a simple 'five check-point' model of the consultation process with an array of techniques for directing a general practitioner's attention to significant cues in the patient's verbal and non-verbal communication. *The Inner Apprentice* extended the principle of 'focused attention' to the one-to-one relationship between trainers and trainees. *The Inner Physician* examined the contribution made by the general practitioner's own psychological mechanisms to the way they practise medicine, and included an in-depth account of the principles of clinical generalism. A collection of his medico-philosophical writings, *I'm Too Hot Now*, was published in 2005.

Neighbour has been given a number of other awards. He was awarded an honorary DSc degree from the University of Hertfordshire and honorary fellowships of the RCP and the Royal Australian College of General Practitioners. He received the RCGP's George Abercrombie Award for medical writing in 2001. In 2011, he was appointed OBE for his services to medical education. He is also entitled to use the post-nominals TTOM, having been awarded, when six years old, the *Tiny Tots* Order of Merit for writing a letter to the editor of that now defunct children's magazine.

Since his retirement from clinical practice in 2003, Neighbour has continued to lecture and teach extensively on the consultation, clinical generalism, medical education and allied topics. He is in demand as a speaker at conferences, and teaches consultation skills in masterclasses, workshops and seminars not just in the United Kingdom but abroad as well. Since 2005, he has been closely involved with the development of general practice in Japan through frequent visits there at the invitation of the Japan Primary Care Association.

Since his early twenties Neighbour has been a student and practitioner of Zen Buddhism. Zen's emphasis on surrendering the sense of self to the immediacy of the present moment chimes well with his fascination with the inner worlds of doctors and patients. He has also played the violin since four years of age, and plays to a semi-professional standard with orchestral and chamber music groups. He is particularly fond of the music of Schubert, and has proposed and published a controversial theory about the possibility that the composer was the singleton survivor of a twin pregnancy. On a sporting front, he enjoys golf, though ascertains that his golfing ability is an extremely un-professional standard. In 1996, he ran the London Marathon in a time of four hours, seven minutes. A fluent French speaker, he also enjoys spending time at his second home in Granville, Normandy.

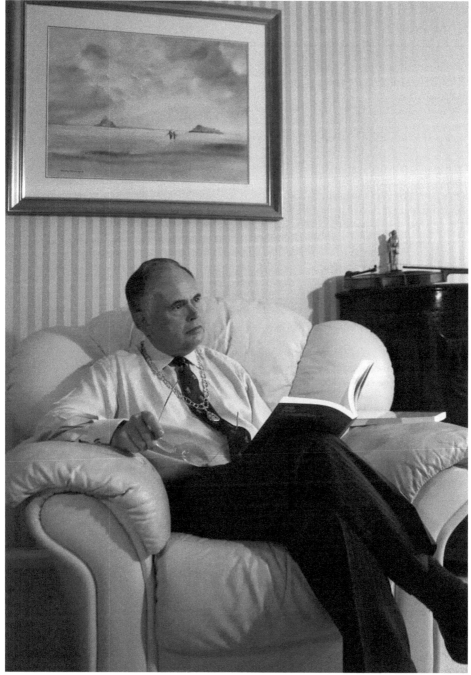

RCGP presidential photograph of Roger Neighbour. Photographer: Richard Keith Wolff. (Courtesy of RCGP Archives, London.)

Further Reading

Neighbour R. The doppelgänger revealed? In: Newbould B (ed.). *Schubert the Progressive*. Aldershot: Ashgate Publishing; 2003.

Neighbour R. *I'm Too Hot Now*. Oxford: Radcliffe Publishing; 2005.

Neighbour R. *The Inner Physician*. London: RCGP; 2016.

Neighbour RH. *The Inner Consultation*. Lancaster: MTP; 1987.

Neighbour RH. *The Inner Apprentice*. Oxford: Radcliffe Publishing; 1992.

87 IONA HEATH (1950–)

Amy L. Northall

Iona Caroline Heath was born on 7 January 1950, and grew up in Kent, where she attended Tonbridge County Grammar School for Girls. She studied the two-year biomedical science component of the medical degree, as well as the History of Art and Architecture, at New Hall College, University of Cambridge, before moving to the London Hospital in Whitechapel for the clinical component. She graduated in 1974 and worked in London for her house officer rotations.

Heath became a general practitioner trainee in 1975 at The Caversham Group Practice in Kentish Town, London. With regards to the RCGP, she sat the MRCGP in 1981, and was awarded the RCGP Fraser Rose Medal for achieving the highest mark that year. She was awarded FRCGP in 1992. Heath stayed on at the practice, becoming a partner when 27 years old and continued there for the following 35 years. When she first joined the practice, it had quite a left-wing approach, with members of staff related to members of the Communist Party. Various representatives from left-wing international embassies joined the already diverse and dynamic patient demographic. A social worker formed part of the practice team, as the partners all appreciated the influence of psychosocial factors on health and access to health care. This undoubtedly influenced her focus on tackling the inequalities in society and the importance of political analysis.

As a general practitioner trainer in 1989, and angered by the RCGP's decision to suspend general practitioner training in North London, Heath wrote her 100-word nomination statement and entered for ballot for sitting on RCGP Council. It was to her surprise that she topped the national ballot and continued to be elected year upon year (1989–2009), including for vice-chair (1996–1998). One of her first contributions whilst on the Council was to represent the RCGP in an enquiry into domestic violence organised by Victim Support, from which she produced a guide, aimed at general practitioners, with advice on recognising and managing domestic violence. This marked the beginning of a long involvement within RCGP management and policy.

Heath first chaired the Inner City Taskforce committee, hoping to increase the representation of general practitioners working in areas of deprivation on RCGP Council. She also chaired the Health Inequalities Group (1997–2003). As part of her ongoing interest in how ethics fits into health care, she chaired the RCGP's Medical Ethics Committee from 1998 to 2004.

Despite Heath feeling she had minimal experience in research, she was placed on the research committee when she first joined RCGP Council, which led to her attendance at her first international research seminar in Denmark. This event sparked her interest in international meetings, and led her to chair the RCGP's International Committee (2006–2009). She became heavily involved with WONCA, where she was an Executive (2007–2013), WHO liaison officer and also chair of Membership Committee (2010–2013). She also delivered a keynote lecture, 'The Art of Doing Nothing', at the WONCA Europe conference 2012. In 2006, she was awarded the Foundation Council Award in recognition of her work for the RCGP.

Heath was invited by Frank Dobson, Secretary of State for Health, to sit on the Royal Commission on Long-term Care of Older People (1997–1999). Along with the majority of the commissioners, she argued that elderly people should be deemed to have health issues when they can no longer care for themselves. However, the government instead accepted a proposal put forward in a minority report. For this reason, she described the CBE that she was appointed to in 2000 for Services to Older People as a 'second prize'. She also sat on the Human Genetics Commission from 2004 to 2007.

Heath undertook other roles. A colleague recommended her to Richard Smith (1952–), then the editor of the *BMJ*, as a member of the journal's primary care 'hanging committee' (1993–2001). As well as making recommendations on submitted papers, she began to write commentaries and editorials on specific interests. She was given a six-weekly 'Op-Ed' column in 2005, for which she continued to write until 2013. She was also Editor of the General Practice Series, published by Oxford University Press, between 1993 and 1999. In addition, she also chaired the *BMJ*'s Ethics Committee from 2005 to 2013.

Heath has delivered many lectures worldwide. She delivered the William Pickles Lecture in 1999 titled 'Uncertain clarity', in which she discussed the presence and roles of contradiction, meaning and hope in medical practice. Several years earlier, in 1995, she was awarded the Nuffield Trust's John Fry Fellowship, for which she delivered her lecture 'The mystery of general practice'. Here she delved into the often-misunderstood key roles of a general practitioner, which she argued are to: 'serve as interpreter and guardian at the interface between illness and disease… serve as a witness to the patient's experience of illness and disease'. 'The mystery of general practice' was published alongside 'Ways of dying' in her book, *Matters of Life and Death* (2007). She campaigned for the focus of medicine to move away from doctors being scared to face death and the dying patient and, in some cases, causing harm by unnecessarily

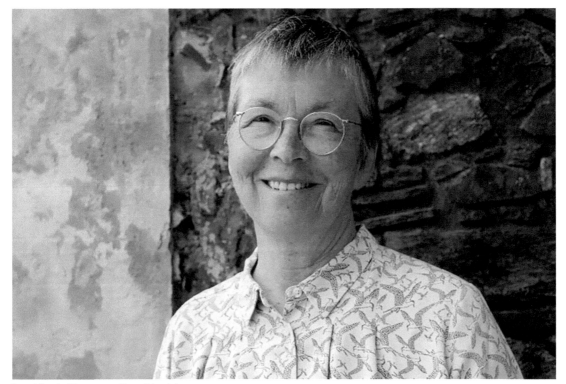

Iona Heath. (Courtesy of Iona Heath.)

prolonging life, towards a belief that death is an important and special process in the circle of life. She referred to novels and literature throughout these essays, proposing the idea that art helps us to understand the whole life of a person and the context in which illness presents: 'Doctors need both science and poetry and never more so than when caring for the dying'.

Heath was invited to deliver the RCP's 2011 Harveian Oration. This was titled 'Divided we fail'. Discussing the various forms of duality and dichotomy present within the medical profession, in ideas about the human body and throughout society in the form of inequalities, she argued that doctors have a wider responsibility than responding to illness and seeking signs of disease:

> Doctors should lobby much more strenuously to protect the vulnerable… we should treat those who are sick but this should be as well as attempting to minimise violence and abuse, and promoting a much more equitable distribution of wealth, hope and opportunity within society.

A further lecture of Heath's of note was when she presented 'Love's labours lost' at the Royal Society of Edinburgh's Michael Shea Memorial Lecture 2012. In it, she offered insight into how political and societal change has stifled professionals' creativity and the patient-sensitive practice of doctors, whilst favouring a more standardised set of behaviours. She ended by reminding the audience that: 'do everything possible not to lose the commitment, the courage, the openness, the willingness to keep thinking, that makes up the love in our professional labours'.

In an attempt to bridge the gap between clinical work and retirement, Heath was nominated two and then won the ballot to become the president of the RCGP in 2009. During her presidency a key aim was to support the RCGP Council members, especially Clare Gerada (1959–), then Chair of Council (2010–2013), in her opposition of the Health and Social Care Act 2012, and increase the number of fellowships awarded by the college so that more of the work done by so many general practitioners is properly acknowledged.

Since retirement, Heath has remained involved in the philosophical aspects of medicine. She mostly focused on her interest of overdiagnosis and overtreatment, and sits on the organising committee for the Preventing Overdiagnosis Conference. She has enjoyed maintaining her manual dexterity, which she relied upon in clinical medicine, by learning how to make sourdough bread and how to weave. This is following her own advice in *Matters of Life and Death: Key Writings:* 'The depth of time is more important than its duration'.

Further Reading

Heath I. *The Mystery of General Practice*. London: The Nuffield Provincial Hospitals Trust; 1995.

Heath I. *Domestic Violence: The General Practitioner's Role*. London: RCGP; 1998.

Heath I. William Pickles Lecture 1999. Uncertain clarity: Contradiction, meaning, and hope. *British Journal of General Practice* 1999;49:651–57.

Heath I. Combating disease mongering: Daunting but nonetheless essential. *Public Library of Science Medicine* 2006;3:e146.

Heath I. *Matters of Life and Death: Key Writings*. Oxford: Radcliffe Publishing; 2007.

Heath I. *Love's Labour Lost:* Why society is straightjacketing its professionals and how we might release them. Michael Shea Memorial Lecture. Edinburgh: International Futures Forum; 2012.

Heath I. Overdiagnosis: When good intentions meet vested interests. *British Medical Journal* 2013;347:f6361.

38 ANN MCPHERSON (1945–2011)

Georgie Patrick

Ann McPherson was born on 22 June 1945 in North London. She was the only child of Max and Sadie Egelnick, both of whom were secular Jewish communists. Her father's profession was a tailor. She was raised in Golders Green and attended Copthall County Grammar School in Mill Hill.

After leaving school, McPherson went on to study medicine at St George's Hospital Medical School where she graduated amongst the top of her class with distinction in 1968. Whilst at university she was known for her involvement in social and political activities as well as her academia. In the same year of her graduation she married Klim McPherson, a public health epidemiologist; together they lived in North London. They had three children, a son and two daughters: Sam, Tess and Beth.

Following graduation, McPherson trained at The Caversham Group Practice Kentish town and also in the United States where she was awarded an MA Harvard University. In 1978, she was awarded MRCGP with distinction, and a year later she began working at 19 Beaumont St. Practice in Oxford, where she became a partner and worked until she retired in 2007. She would also go on to become head of the RCGP Adolescent Health Group as well as establishing herself as a member of the government's Teenage Pregnancy Independent Advisory Group.

During her career as a general practitioner, McPherson became known amongst hospital consultants for her astute diagnostic skills. On one occasion she insisted that the hospital admit a lady whom she had correctly diagnosed with glucose-6-phosphate dehydrogenase deficiency. She was also known for her patient advocacy amongst both her colleagues and her patients. This was evident in her testimonials where one patient recalled 'She was a master at fighting on behalf of her patients, and the system soon learned to jump when she called'. She was available to her patients by telephone in the evenings and on weekends, paid home visits to her patients in the evenings and would rather run additional surgeries than turn patients away.

Alongside her accomplishments as a clinician, McPherson also earned a reputation for making medicine accessible. She published 30 books in total, including *The Diary of a Teenage Health Freak* (1987), which formed part of a series of books that she co-authored with the paediatrician Aidan Macfarlane (1939–) that aimed to address medical issues relevant to teenagers. The book sold over one million copies and has since been translated into 27 languages and serialised for Channel 4 TV in the United Kingdom. Her children provided the inspiration for her writing, as she desired to help them better understand their own health.

In addition to *The Diary of a Teenage Health Freak*, McPherson continued to make health accessible via her literary career. Further titles included *The Agony, the Ecstasy, the Answers: a Book for Parents* (1999); *Sex: the Truth* (2003); *Drugs: the Truth* (2003); *Bullying: the Truth* (2004); *Relationships: the Truth* (2004) and *The Truth: a Teenager's Survival Guide* (2007).

Following the success of their books, McPherson and Macfarlane devoted time to answering health questions online for 10–15 year olds in a virtual doctors surgery that could be found on their website *www.teenagehealthfreak.org*.

McPherson was also responsible for founding the charity Database of Individual Patient Experiences (DIPEx) with her friend Andrew Herxheimer, a clinical pharmacologist. The charity ran two websites, one aimed at adults (www.healthtalkonline.org) and one aimed at children (www.youthhealthtalk.org). The websites encourage users to share their own real-life experiences of a wide variety of disorders and illnesses. They include user-friendly information aimed at patients and their relatives, ranging from siblings to grandparents, to allow a better understanding of their condition. They also provide information to health care professionals, to enable them to better understand their patient's needs by exploring real-life accounts of patient experiences.

The research underlying the websites came from a health experiences research group that McPherson had established in the Department of Primary Health Care at the University of Oxford. In 2000, McPherson was appointed CBE for her work with women's and adolescent's health. During the same year McPherson also became a Fellow of Green Templeton College, University of Oxford, who have since established a Tribute Fund in her name with the intention of actualising her concept of the Oxford Health Experiences Institute. The organisation is currently called HEXI (Oxford Health Experiences Institute), and takes an interdisciplinary approach to transforming patient experiences of health care and illness into changes in policy and practice.

During her career there were times when McPherson encountered health problems of her own. In the late 1990s, she was diagnosed with breast cancer, which she managed to overcome. Subsequently, in 2007, she was diagnosed with pancreatic cancer for which she underwent a Whipple's procedure. In July 2009, she discovered that the pancreatic cancer had returned and this time it would prove terminal.

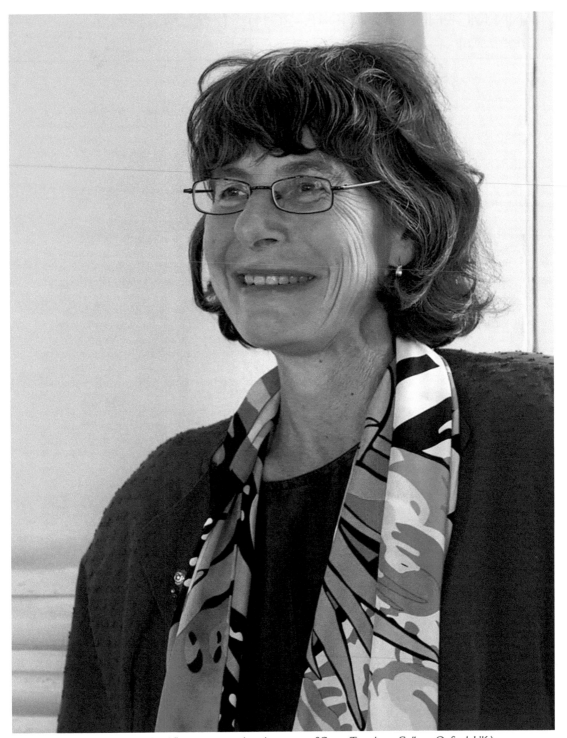

Ann McPherson. (Copyright Richard Seymour; reproduced courtesy of Green Templeton College, Oxford, UK.)

However, McPherson did not allow her battles with cancer go by without finding opportunities to better the experience for others. During an admission to hospital for breast cancer surgery, there was no bed for her on arrival and she was asked to wait in the patient's room. She found the room to be unclean and, after taking several photographs, went to inform the chief executive. Upon finding him to be absent, she insisted that his deputy went to see the room for himself.

Following her terminal diagnosis in 2009, McPherson initiated and chaired a project called Healthcare Professionals for Assisted Dying (HPAD). She referred to the project as happening 'by accident' as a result of an article she had written for the *BMJ* about assisted suicide that received much positive feedback from other doctors prompting McPherson to suggest they form a group. The mission of HPAD was to change the law such that 'terminally ill, mentally competent adults should have the choice of an assisted death, subject to legal safeguards'. The issue resonated with McPherson as in 2004 she had watched her own mother decline dialysis treatment when 95 years old. Her mother instead chose to stop her battle with kidney failure when she was ready, rather than receiving life-sustaining dialysis treatment as the hospital would have preferred. Linked to this in the same year McPherson became a patron of the campaigning organisation Dignity in Dying, an organisation that aims to achieve greater choice for individuals over end-of-life decisions, in order to alleviate suffering.

In 2011, McPherson was awarded the BMJ Group's communicator of the year award. At the ceremony she was represented by her husband and the actor Hugh Grant as she was too unwell to attend. She had previously persuaded Grant to support her website and he described her as 'part doctor, part campaigner, part stalker'.

McPherson continued her academic work in the Department of Primary Health Care until weeks before her death. Despite her work on HPAD during this time, she was angered that the law did not change prior to her death; she said on 19 May 2011, 'I can't understand why I have to carry on living like this, why I can't just die'. Nine days later she died from pancreatic cancer on 28 May 2011 aged 65 years old.

The RCGP now commemorates McPherson and her many contributions to health care with an annual Ann McPherson Annual Lecture.

Further Reading

Anon. Dr Ann McPherson. *The Telegraph* 2011; 31 May.

Laurance J. Dr Ann McPherson: The GP who believes she should be allowed help to end her life. *The Independent* 24 January 2011.

Macfarlane A, McPherson A. *The Diary of a Teenage Health Freak*. Oxford: Oxford University Press; 1987.

Macfarlane A, McPherson A. *The Agony, the Ecstasy, the Answers: a Book for Parents*. London: Little Brown and Company; 1999.

Macfarlane A, McPherson A. *Drugs: the Truth*. Oxford: Oxford University Press; 2003.

Macfarlane A, McPherson A. *Sex: the Truth*. Oxford: Oxford University Press; 2003.

Macfarlane A, McPherson A. *Bullying: the Truth*. Oxford: Oxford University Press; 2004.

Macfarlane A, McPherson A. *Relationships: the Truth*. Oxford: Oxford University Press; 2004.

Macfarlane A, McPherson A. *The Truth: a Teenager's Survival Guide*. Oxford: Oxford University Press; 2007.

McPherson A. An extremely interesting time to die. *British Medical Journal* 2009;339:b2827.

McPherson K. "Obituary – Ann McPherson". *The Lancet* 2011; 377: 2000.

Warlow C. Ann McPherson. *British Medical Journal* 2011;2;342:d3424.

JOHN CHISHOLM (1950–)
Saumil Shah, Stuart Pinder, James Parry-Reece, Atia Khan and Rizwan Akhtar

John William Chisholm was born on 29 December 1950. He is said to have a 'razor sharp' mind and a staggering memory, both of which were put to good use during his education. Chisholm attended Clifton College in Bristol before going on to study at Peterhouse College, University of Cambridge and Westminister Hospital Medical School. In 1974, he graduated with BChir from the University of Cambridge. A year later he received his MB. He is currently working as a general practitioner in Twyford, Berkshire. He is a non-executive director at Concordia Health.

Chisholm has always played an active role in trying to improve general practice. In 1977, he became a member of the GMSC at the BMA which was later renamed the GPC. In 1991, he was elected deputy chair for the GMSC. Six years later, in 1997, he was greeted with a standing ovation on election as chairman of the same committee. His election came during a time of growing unease amongst the general practitioner community, with recruitment and retention of general practitioners becoming an ever-worsening problem.

Since his appointment, Chisholm led the GPC who, together with representatives from the NHS, negotiated for the NHS Confederation on behalf of the Departments of Health in England and Northern Ireland and the devolved administrations in Wales and Scotland on issues ranging from general practitioner salaries to the structure of general practice services. Each topic has drastically reshaped the general practitioner contract in these countries. These negotiations meant he faced opposition from both the government and his own peers in hospitals, particularly for his demands which the *BMJ* described as a 'stonking' pay rise of 58.4% for general practitioners. Despite heavy opposition, he continued to negotiate a fair deal for general practitioners across the aforementioned countries. He understood that in negotiations there might be ill will. However, he commented, 'My wish is to move forward as much as possible by consensus, but there will be occasions when I and my negotiators have to cause ill feeling and if this is one of them, so be it'. This determination, coupled with many hours of negotiations and hard work, eventually led to the first constructive change to the national general practitioner contract since 1966. Over 79 per cent of the general practitioners, from a 70 per cent overall general practitioner turnout, voted that they wanted to implement the new contract (2003). The contract, known as 'Investing in General Practice: The New General Medical Services Contract', was enforced on 1 April 2004. This contract is commonly known as the 'First Blue Book'. Monitor, a regulator for health services in England, has described the contract both as a 'blessing and distraction'. It did bring in more investment and the right to opt out of out-of-hours responsibility, but since then there has been little progress and the contract has even been used to blame the increasing accident and emergency waiting times.

In 2004, Chisholm finished his six-year term as chair of the GPC, having overseen what he believed was the 'the turning point for General Practice'. The work that he had done was recognised when he was appointed CBE in 2000. Upon receiving this award he stated, 'I feel that it recognises not just my work but the work of the GPC and the support I have received from the staff and members of the Committee and the BMA'. During this time he also worked on trying to improve the standards of care by looking at the training of general practitioners by being part of the Joint Committee of Postgraduate Training.

Another subject that Chisholm has made an impact upon in is men's health. In April 2013, he was elected chair of the Trustees of the Men's Health Forum, an independent charity. He claimed 'we now know a lot about how to improve men's health but there is still a lot to do to put that knowledge into practice and make a real difference to men'. He has a particular interest in introducing education about self-care in schools and making sure that 'self-care aware' consultations become routine practice. He is also a trustee on the board of the self-care forum. He helped to form this through the NHS working in partnership programme (WiPP), a programme that stems from the Blue Book. He was a signatory to the self-care campaign that has eventually led to the formation of the self-care forum.

Chisholm has had roles with the RCGP. He has served on RCGP Council since 2007, represented RCGP Council for Work and Health, and chaired the RCGP Superannuation Trust Company Limited amongst a myriad of other posts. Currently, he is on the board of trustees of the RCGP. He has been awarded FRCGP. By 2010, his career had at that time been deemed by a panel of experts for *Pulse* to merit him being listed as the 11th most influential general practitioner of all time.

Having sat on the BMA Medical Ethics Committee (MEC) since 2004 and been deputy chair between 2012 and 2013, Chisholm was appointed chairman of the committee in 2014. He has a particular interest in 'patient rights, human rights, organ donation, the confidentiality and security of personal health information, professional standards, medical regulation, and criminal justice'. In his role as chair he has petitioned world leaders to respond to the increasing refugee crisis in the Middle East and Europe, commenting, 'All countries have obligations under international law to protect asylum seekers and refugees, and it is essential that Her Majesty's government meets those obligations and influences other countries by example'. He has also publicly condemned the Turkish government for the persecution of members of the Turkish Medical Association.

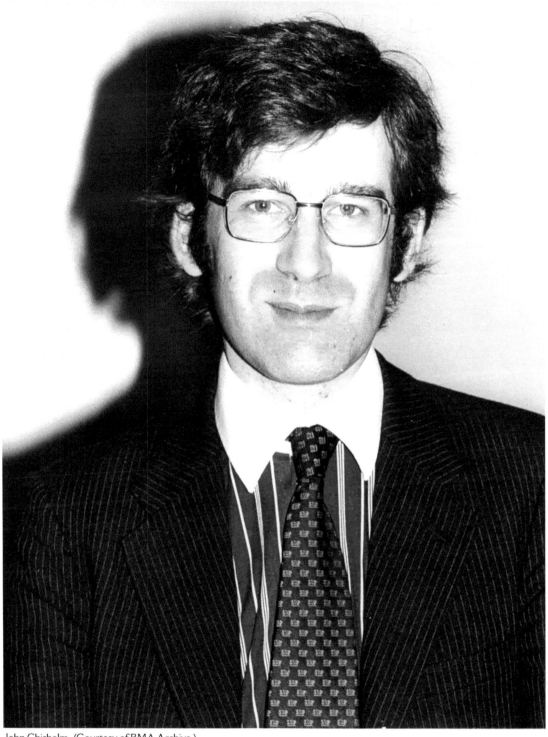

John Chisholm. (Courtesy of BMA Archive.)

During his term as chair, the MEC have lobbied Parliament on the Assisted Dying (no. 2) Bill and have called for the introduction of an opt-out system of organ donation throughout the United Kingdom. On the latter point he is quoted saying, 'As a doctor it is difficult to see your patients dying and suffering when their lives could be saved or dramatically improved by a transplant'.

Away from his medical career Chisholm is a keen musician. As an all-rounded person and dedicated general practitioner and he himself has recognised his need for continued self-development, and he continues to work tirelessly to make these improvements a reality.

Further Reading

Bogle I, Chisholm JW. Primary care: Restoring the jewel in the crown. *British Medical Journal* 1996;312:1624.

Department of Health. *Investing in General Practice, The New General Medical Contract*. London: Department of Health; 2003.

90 HAMISH ROBIN PETER MELDRUM (1948–)

Bernadette Wolff

Hamish Meldrum was born in Edinburgh on 14 April 1948. He was the younger of two boys born to Jim and May Meldrum. His father went on to become the director for education for Stirlingshire and his mother stopped working after the birth of their children. His decision to pursue a medical career was influenced by an interest in people and their ailments, an older brother already reading medicine as well as the varied career opportunities offered by the medical profession. He spent six years at the University of Edinburgh, from where he graduated MBChB in 1972. In addition to achieving his medical degree, sport was his primary interest and he represented his university at athletics, competing as a sprinter and as both a long and triple jumper. He also enjoyed golf, rugby, football, tennis and hockey.

Following graduation, Meldrum undertook house jobs at Edinburgh Royal Infirmary and Bangour Hospital before moving to Torquay in Devon. There, he worked in general medicine for three years as a medical senior house officer and medical registrar at Torbay Hospital. It was here that he also met his future wife, Mhairi a nurse, and had his first encounter with medical politics. He was the mess president in 1975, which was initially a social role. This role turned political when junior doctors nationally took industrial action over pay and conditions. Their issue concerned the 100-hour average working week and with overtime being paid at only one-third basic pay. He was involved in meetings throughout the South West of England trying to resolve matters, which he felt were wrong and in doing so got his first taste of medical politics. At that time strikes could be called after local meetings and Torbay Hospital narrowly voted against the strike action whilst Plymouth was one of the first hospitals to vote to strike.

It was around this time that Meldrum decided to leave hospital medicine and train as a general practitioner. Hospital medicine was not a happy work environment for him and he admitted he struggled trying to obtain MRCP. On the other hand, general practice had become a popular career choice but general practitioner posts were hard to come by with 50 to 60 applicants per post. He was accepted onto a general practitioner training scheme in Harrogate in Yorkshire where he completed his training with placements in obstetrics and gynaecology, paediatrics and a year as a general practitioner trainee. He moved with his wife and three children to the seaside town of Bridlington and joined the Bridlington Medical Centre on Station Avenue in 1978. This surgery provided a wide variety of services including maternity care, a minor injuries service and looking after the local hospitals. He enjoyed being a general practitioner for the long-term, holistic, whole family approach to medicine. Interestingly, it was during this time that he made it to the 1987 final of what was referred to then as 'televisions toughest quiz', *The Krypton Factor*, which tested participants' physical stamina and mental attributes. He finished third behind the show's first-ever female winner, Marian Chanter. He worked as a general practitioner in Bridlington for 33 years. However, with the demands of a medico-political career he retired from general practice in March 2011.

Meldrum had been involved in medical politics since the 1970s. He disliked the market reforms, particularly the concept of the purchaser–provider split introduced with the Community Care Act (1990) by the Conservative Health Secretary Kenneth Clarke under the then Prime Minister Margaret Thatcher. He felt that patients would see decisions made on financial reasons rather than health needs and it was these reforms that prompted his decision in 1991 to stand for the GMSC at the BMA, now known as the GPC. Since joining the GPC, he chaired the East Yorkshire local medical committee between 1996 and 1999 as well as becoming a GPC negotiator in 1997. In 1999, he was appointed as the joint deputy chairman of the GPC and elected to the position of GPC Chairman in 2004. A notable achievement during this time was as a member of the GPC team that negotiated the new general practitioner contracts which allowed general practitioners to opt out of out-of-hours work for only a six per cent pay cut which left many doctors pleasantly stunned. The new contract improved the pay and pensions for general practitioners, but more importantly helped combat the then recruitment problems into general practice.

Whilst chairman of the GPC he fought to protect the gains made in the new general practitioner contracts as well as leading and successfully winning a judicial review which allowed general practitioners' pensions to appropriately represent their earnings. Meldrum stood down from the GPC chairman role after being elected BMA Council chairman on 28 June 2007. Though reluctant to leave his GPC role, his new role was one he himself felt that he had the attributes to take on even though the BMA was going through an immensely difficult period. Junior doctors had lost a lot of confidence in the BMA over the Medical Training Application Service (MTAS) and the Modernising Medical Careers (MMC) problems. MMC was introduced to provide focused postgraduate training for medical staff in more defined timescales and thus deliver consultants following medical school graduation in seven to nine years and general practitioners in five years. However, there were a number of risks associated with this including the risk to service provision due to a loss of service input from trainees. Furthermore, the MTAS system on which the recruitment process depended upon had failed to allocate training places in a fair and transparent way and had failed to ensure that all places were allocated by 1 August 2007. To add to the challenge, at the same time there was uncertainty in the NHS with the new

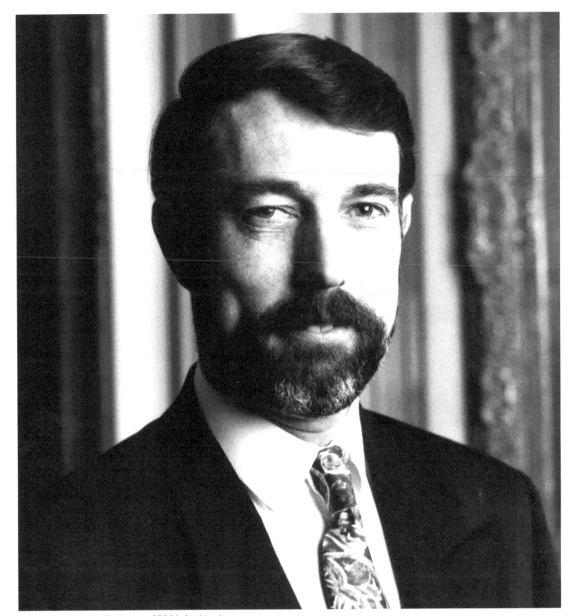

Hamish Meldrum. (Courtesy of BMA Archive.)

pension reforms and the implementation of the new Health and Social Care Bill which then became an Act in 2012. Meldrum's task was to rebuild trust within the organisation and ensure that doctors had the right working conditions to enable them to provide the best care for their patients. The government's new pension reforms, which would affect all doctors including general practitioners, called for an increase in contributions (up to 14 per cent for the highest earners) as well as requiring doctors to work up to the age of 68 years to draw a full pension. This led to an ongoing pensions dispute and ultimately Meldrum's reluctant co-ordination of doctors to take industrial action on 21 June 2012 for the first time in 37 years. This decision, he admitted, was one of the hardest things he had had to face. Despite minimal patient backlash, he had to counter the negative headlines in the national press and ultimately it was the BMA that was forced to back down.

The implementation of the new Health and Social Care Bill brought more challenges for Meldrum. He was accused by some members of the London Regional Council of the BMA for failing to promote members' views and for not taking a harder stance over the Health and Social Care Bill. It was a disagreement on tactics and they felt that the BMA should have opposed the Bill outright from the start. However, Meldrum, and the majority of BMA Council, believed that the best way forward was to keep communication open with the government and try to obtain a mutual resolution. Regardless of the challenges faced, some of his key achievements under his tenure included significantly increasing BMA membership, doubling profits in the BMJ group, negotiating a new staff and associate specialist (SAS) doctors' contract and achieving some beneficial changes to the Health and Social Care Bill. The significance of his role was highlighted when he was rated as the third-most influential person in the NHS and health care policy by *Health Service Journal* in 2010 (up from 32nd in 2009).

Meldrum ended his five-year BMA chairmanship in June 2012. He acknowledged that you cannot please everyone and urged doctors that nobody should be rushing to repeat or escalate industrial action. A year later, in 2013, he was awarded the BMA gold medal. He then semi-retired and he and his wife moved to Edinburgh. He has since joined the University of the Third Age, enjoys spending more time with his family, travelling and has resurrected his golf. He still has an active interest in medical politics and from 2014 is the deputy chairman of the BMJ Group, a member of the Audit Committee of the RCGP and works for a number of medical related boards.

Meldrum's emphasis on talking rather than a confrontational approach to politics has enabled him to achieve so much during very challenging times in his career. He has made countless personal sacrifices but his accomplishments have positively affected many of today's doctors. Finally, he has been awarded both FRCP and FRCGP and is one of only four people to have held the chairman positions of both BMA Council and the GPC.

Further Reading

Anon. 'Furious' Meldrum tells BMA: 'Back me or sack me'. *Pulse* 2011; 21 September.

Anon. BMA opts for outright opposition to health bill after knife-edge vote. *Pulse* 2011; 25 November.

Anon. Hamish, take a bow. *BMJ News* 2012; 26 July.

Gresham S, Jegatheesan M. 15 minutes with…The chairman of the BMA Council. *BMJ Careers* 2008; 2 February.

91 ELSIE ROSEMARY RUE (1928–2004)
Isabel Slark

Elsie Rosemary Rue (née Lawrence) was born in Hutton, Essex, on 14 June 1928. Her mother was a music teacher and her father worked as an accountant. When she was five years old the family moved to London, where she went on to win two scholarships to Sydenham High School. When she was 11 years old, she was evacuated to Devon during the Blitz. Whilst there she contracted tuberculosis and peritonitis. Subsequently, she spent a year in bed recovering after extensive surgery and did not attend school. It is believed this experience was key in her decision to pursue a career in medicine.

Rue attended the Royal Free Medical School for Women. She started when she was 17 years old and whilst there as a student, in 1950 married Roger Rue, an RAF pilot instructor. However, after informing the dean of the medical school that she wished to change her name, it was advised she should no longer study there as a married woman. Furious with the attitude of the dean, she resigned immediately. Determined to finish her training, she applied to the University of Oxford Medical School and completed her education in 1951 after taking the London University exams.

Being an extremely motivated woman Rue completed a year's hospital work, even though it was not compulsory to do so after qualifying from medical school at the time. Despite this passion for the profession, she encountered some difficulties once learning that none of the hospitals in Oxford would employ married female doctors. In 1951, after searching for employment, she took up work at Cowley Road Hospital, Oxford, and here was able to spend time completing a psychiatry course. Due to the attitudes at the time, she neglected to tell her employers that she was married with a child and when this information was later discovered they dismissed her immediately.

Kingsley Firth, a general practitioner whom Rue had met whilst completing the psychiatry course at Cowley Road Hospital, offered her a job in an industrial part of Oxford. Here she was one of only three doctors overseeing the care of 11,000 patients, many of whom were workers at the Cowley motor plant. However, even though polio was almost fully eradicated, Rue contracted polio from a patient, being the last person in Oxford to get it. Despite recognising her symptoms, she continued to work tirelessly throughout that day until she had finished her duties. She was left with one weakened leg and after months of rehabilitation she was able to walk with great difficulty and with the aid of crutches.

For a time, she taught Chemistry and Biology in various girls' schools and began to apply for medical jobs again. Whenever she arrived to an interview and was unable to climb the steps due to her leg, she would phone to say she had been accepted elsewhere.

Feeling defeated, by 1955 Rue had separated from her husband and had moved back to Hertfordshire to live with her parents. She found employment at a local general practitioner surgery and spent time as a medical officer for the RAF in Bovingdon. Life as a general practitioner was varied and involved a lot of home visits and assisting at births in the community and she enjoyed the diversity of the job.

Feeling it was time to move on, Rue became the Assistant County Medical Officer in 1960, working part-time as a Paediatrician in Watford. During this time, and to add to her many learned achievements, she spent an academic term in London at the Great Ormond Street Institute of Child Health.

Rue was a strong advocate for women within the profession. During the 1960s she developed a scheme which grew in popularity across the United Kingdom. It enabled women to train or work part-time and develop into specialists within their fields. It bettered the lives of many and addressed shortages within the specialities. She has received tremendous recognition for the scheme and its impact can still be seen within medicine today. She later became president of the Medical Women's Federation (1982–1983).

Rue became the assistant regional medical officer in 1965, then progressed in 1971 to senior assistant, finally becoming the regional medical officer in 1973. Amongst her many achievements, she helped to form the Faculty of Community Medicine in 1972, which is now the Faculty of Public Health and was its first female president. She then progressed to the regional general manager in 1984.

During this time, it was noted by the Health Minister that the country's hospitals were in dire condition. To help solve this, Rue argued for the withdrawal of full funding from the London hospitals. This was because of the area's decreasing population and she believed that these funds could be put to better use elsewhere. Due to this, she secured funds for the Oxford area and oversaw the development of new hospitals in Reading, Swindon and Milton Keynes. The hospital built in Milton Keynes was a particularly special achievement as it was the first hospital to be newly constructed rather than renovated from existing buildings like the rest. In 1988, she retired from clinical work and became the president of the BMA (1990–1991).

Rue had a successful career. Apart from writing many papers she was awarded an honorary MA from the University of Oxford. She was awarded *fellowship ad eundem gradum* by the RCGP in 1982. In 1991, she was awarded the Edward Jenner Medal of the Royal Society of Medicine. This is a medal established in 1896 by the Epidemiological Society of London and is awarded periodically by the Royal Society of Medicine to individuals who have undertaken distinguished work in epidemiological research. Her scheme allowing women to progress within the profession has had

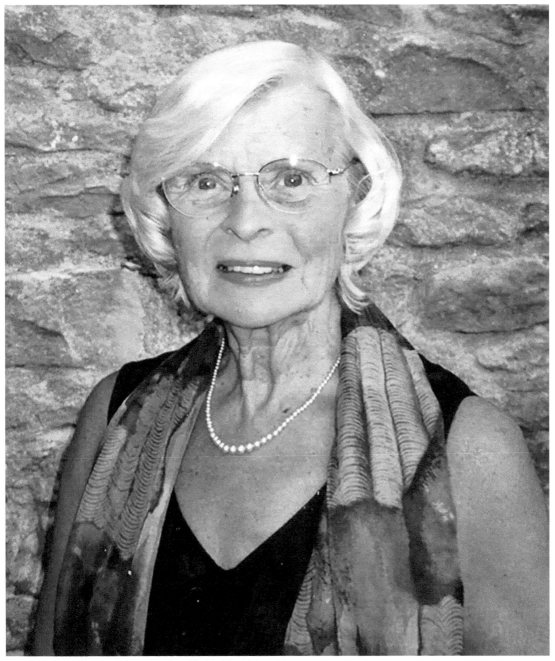

Rosemary Rue. (Courtesy of the Faculty of Public Health.)

a lasting effect and she was described by Terence Ryan (1932–), emeritus professor of dermatology at the University of Oxford, as 'a fighter for a health service, sometimes against governance, sometimes against entrenched views of a male dominated profession, but always as worthy representative and leader of the medical profession'. She died of bowel cancer on 24 December 2004 at her family home of forty years, in Stanton St. John. She was survived by her two sons, Randalph and Rolf.

Further Reading

Harding A. Obituary: Dame Rosemary Rue. *The Lancet* 2005;365(9459):566.

Morris PJ. Rue [*née* Laurence], Dame (Elsie) Rosemary (1928–2004). In: *Oxford Dictionary of National Biography 2001–2004*. Oxford: Oxford University Press; 2009.

Richmond C. Obituaries: Dame Rosemary Rue. *British Medical Journal* 2005;7484(330):199.

92 MARY 'MOLLIE' MCBRIDE (1931–2013)

Patricia Wilkie

Mary, always known as Mollie, McBride (née Gregson), was born in Bromborough, Wirral. She did not come from a medical family; her father was a commercial artist. Because of the war Mollie had a very interrupted education. She wished to study civil engineering. However, because she was under age, this required a signature from her mother, who refused to help but recommended medicine, a subject that had never occurred to McBride. She then applied to the University of Liverpool, where she qualified with honours in medicine in 1954 and where she was lady president of the Guild of Undergraduates. There were 90 students in her year but only nine women. At university she met her husband Louis, a dentist, and they married in 1956. Louis died in 1986.

McBride began her medical career as a house physician to Lord Cohen of Birkenhead (1900–1977) and then went straight into general practice as an assistant to a country doctor in Tarporley, Cheshire. 'If the patient had a fracture', she later wrote, 'you drove them to the hospital, took an x-ray, developed it yourself and then set it yourself with or without anaesthetic'. She then established the Lache Health Centre, the first modern health centre in Chester.

Everyone who knew McBride has described her energy and enthusiasm and this was very evident from early in her medical career. With an expansive career as a full-time general practitioner partner, a wife and a mother, she served as a general practitioner member of the then Mersey Regional Health Authority for six years. This was an unusual role for a woman and a general practitioner. She was also very active in the RCGP Faculties of Mersey, North Wales and East London; a RCGP examiner and for 18 years a member of the local medical committee of the BMA. She mentored many young doctors including one from Saudi Arabia who went on to be in charge of health care across the Middle East.

McBride's contribution to the RCGP was enormous. Together with her husband, they decided that they would spend the last two years of their professional lives working in developing countries as doctor and dentist. That was not to be. Following the death of Louis in 1986, she stood for election as Honorary Secretary of the RCGP in 1989. She tackled the election process, where prospective candidates give a short address to RCGP Council, with great skill, making very pertinent points combined with wit and humour. She won and was the first woman to hold the post, which she did from 1989 to 1994, and which was a time of major changes in the NHS. Denis Pereira Gray (1935–), past president of the RCGP, in his appreciation of McBride in the *British Journal of General Practice*, commented that she became Honorary Secretary at a very difficult time. The Margaret Thatcher and Kenneth Clarke reforms were the first of a major set of major changes for the NHS causing great anxiety at the RCGP. McBride took the trouble to contact members directly, had a calming influence and was always willing to listen. In the Nuffield Oral History Interview with Maureen Baker (1958–), who was then Honorary Secretary of the RCGP, McBride did comment with a twinkle that, as a female member of RCGP Council, there was a tendency in 1989 to expect her to pour the coffee.

In 1990, McBride made a very big decision and moved from her general practitioner practice in Chester to a small practice in the East End of London. As Pereira Gray said, 'many RCGP leaders have spoken about social deprivation but only Mollie McBride upped sticks and went to work where conditions were particularly difficult'. She was keen to show policymakers, government officials and NHS leaders how difficult things could be in socially-deprived areas. Several of these visitors were profoundly influenced, seeing at first hand the difficulties faced by general practitioners in the East End, often working in very under-resourced practices from very poor premises, but near multimillion pound NHS institutions. She was appointed to the Tomlison Committee (1993) in a personal capacity to report on health services in London.

McBride retired when she was 65 years old and returned to Chester where she applied her enormous energy, enthusiasm and compassion in her support for the Macular Society and for the Samaritans, where she was a listening volunteer regularly covering the difficult to fill Sunday morning dawn slot from 7 to 10am. She also became chairman of the Samaritans Friends Committee, where she helped to raise considerable funds through delightful persuasion and imagination. For example, she invited Jenny Joseph, author of the poem so often read at funerals 'When I am an old woman I shall wear purple' to give a talk. The charities supported by McBride refer to her catching enthusiasm and her outstanding support, kindness and friendship.

McBride's garden backed onto Chester croquet club where she became a very active member, described fondly by members as hitting a 'mean ball'. She introduced golf croquet to the club. This is a slightly easier game to play than the usual association croquet and particularly helpful for those whose sight is not so good including McBride who had developed macular degeneration. She also introduced a little social occasion, Boxing Day Plus 1, to help members who were on their own. They met on the day after Boxing Day to have a game if weather permitted, otherwise to simply enjoy a social occasion. She was delighted to be awarded a diploma as a croquet coach. The club named a trophy in her name for the person who has won the most games in golf croquet.

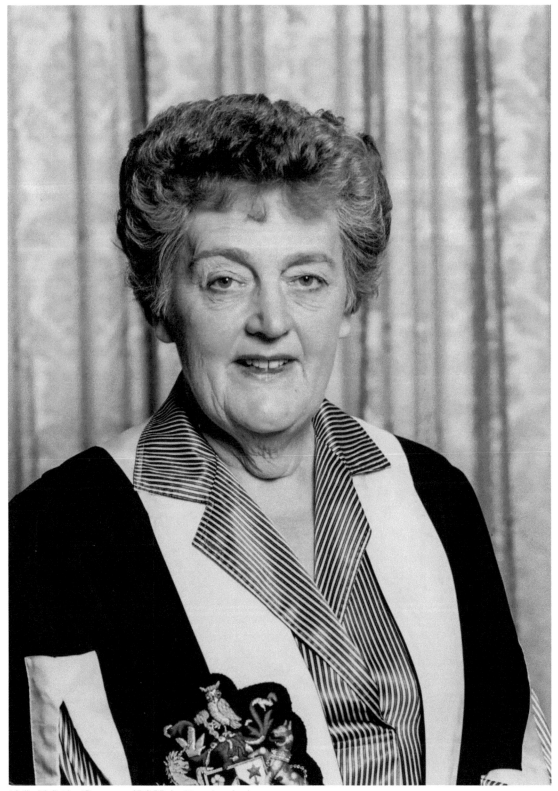

Mollie McBride. (Courtesy of RCGP Archives, London.)

In terms of other interests, McBride had several including bridge and the Chester Civic Society. She became Honorary Secretary of the Medical Women's Federation (MWF) from 1998 to 2000, and where she is remembered with respect and much affection. She was a member of the MWF for 32 years. The floral tribute on her coffin was in the MWF colours.

In December 1989, McBride was appointed MBE in the New Years Honours for services to medicine. She received other major awards including the Baron Dr ver Heyden de Lancey Award in 1986 and the Foundation Council Award in 1996.

McBride is survived by four sons and seven grandchildren. They have every reason to be very proud of a remarkable, brave, insightful and kindly woman who helped develop high standards in general practice.

Acknowledgements

I would like to thank all the members of the voluntary organisations supported by Mollie, who so enthusiastically gave their time and researched their records.

Further Reading

McBride M. Mary 'Mollie' McBride. *Medical Woman* 2014;3:36.

Pereira Gray D. Mollie McBride: An appreciation. *British Journal of General Practitioners* 2014;64(618):38.

RCGP. Dr Maureen Baker, Secretary of Council interviews Dr Mollie McBride, Honorary Secretary of Council (1989–1994) on 11 November 2008. Nuffield Oral History Interviews. RCGP Archives.

Watts G. Mollie Mary McBride. *The Lancet* 2014;383(9914):302.

93 DAME LESLEY SOUTHGATE (1943–)

Lucy Hamer

Lesley Jill Southgate was born on 25 September 1943. She completed her secondary education at Luton High School for Girls and proceeded to study for her degree in medicine at the University of Liverpool from 1962 to 1967. She was the first person in her family to attend university. After completing her pre-registration, she moved to Canada with her husband in order to undertake a residency programme in anaesthetics at McMaster University, Hamilton, Ontario. Whilst completing her residency programme, she had her first child and a year later moved back to England as her husband was still studying. In an interview with the Academy of Medical Educators (AoME) she noted that this was a particularly scary time filled with financial uncertainty, causing the family to move back in with her parents in Stevenage, Hertfordshire. Soon after returning, she joined a local general practice and later moved to work at a practice in Hoddesdon, Hertfordshire from 1971 to 1978.

Dame Lesley then decided to try and further her career. Firstly, in regards to the RCGP, she took the MRCGP and was surprised to learn that she passed with distinction. After eight years, the family decided to move back to Canada to pursue a two-year postgraduate programme in Family Medicine at the University of Western Ontario, London, Ontario. This is where her interest and passion for research and academic medicine arose. After completing the programme, she returned to the United Kingdom in 1979 and started work at the Barts and The London School of Medicine as a lecturer and ultimately, professor of general practice and primary care, the latter a role which she undertook between 1992 and 1995. Throughout these roles she balanced her clinical work at Well Street Surgery in South Hackney. In 1993, she delivered the 41st James Mackenzie Lecture entitled 'Freedom and discipline: Clinical practice and the assessment of clinical competence'. This paper explained her views on medical assessment and how this can serve to improve not only competence but also self-awareness, respect, honesty and empathy.

Dame Lesley's research interests were initially focused on the topic of sexually-transmitted infections, particularly chlamydial infections in women that she had encountered at her practice. One of her early research papers on chlamydial infections in women attending local general practices was dismissed as a reviewer did not agree that research data could be gathered in general practice. Dame Lesley appealed against the decision and the paper was eventually published in the BMJ in 1983. In the interview with AoME she noted that since this event she has published and reviewed many papers and always remembers to be 'fair and encouraging'.

In 1996, Dame Lesley became the chief examiner of the MRCGP. During her time in this role, she completed a three-year project with a team of experts to determine a way of getting a comprehensive insight into medical and clinical practice, and therefore how this could be assessed. At the same time, she undertook the role of chair of the GMC Development Programme for Performance Procedures. She stated that this is one of the defining moments of her career that she is proudest of. The aim of the scheme was to identify registered doctors whose clinical performance was a potential danger to patients. Some of those doctors had their licence to practice withdrawn. The approach has had an impact on subsequent developments in workplace-based assessment now used throughout the profession. She helped implement the programme up until 2004. Also in 1996, she became involved in leading a curriculum committee at The Royal Free and University College London Medical School which she undertook until 2004. She became professor of primary care and medical education between 1995 and 2004. This marked the beginning of a transition into the field of medical education for Southgate, an area that she would become renowned for.

On 12 June 1999, Dame Lesley was honoured with being appointed DBE for her services to standards of practice and Primary Care. Shortly afterwards, in 2000, when 57 years old, she ceased her part-time clinical practice when elected to become the president of the RCGP. She continued in this role until 2003. In the words of her successor, Roger Neighbour (1947–), she achieved 'great things as a personal doctor, an academic and an arbiter of high-quality practice'. In 2002, she was awarded an honorary doctorate [DSc (Hon)] by the University of Exeter. This was in recognition of several years of work preparing for the establishment of Peninsula Medical School. This was followed by another honorary doctorate awarded by the University of Keele in 2003.

After her time as president of the RCGP, Dame Lesley had a multitude of organisations reaching out to gain her expertise and advice. In June 2007, she started working with the Department of Health on a work-based assessment programme for health care scientists, which she continues to do today. From 2010 to 2015, she was a trustee for the Thalidomide Trust, a charity that aims to provide support and improve the quality of life for those affected by thalidomide. This has provided her the opportunity to work with senior members of the legal profession. In 2008, she formed, with others, the European Board of Medical Assessors (EBMA), a European non-profit organisation based at the University of Maastricht, to promote excellence in the assessment of clinical competence across the

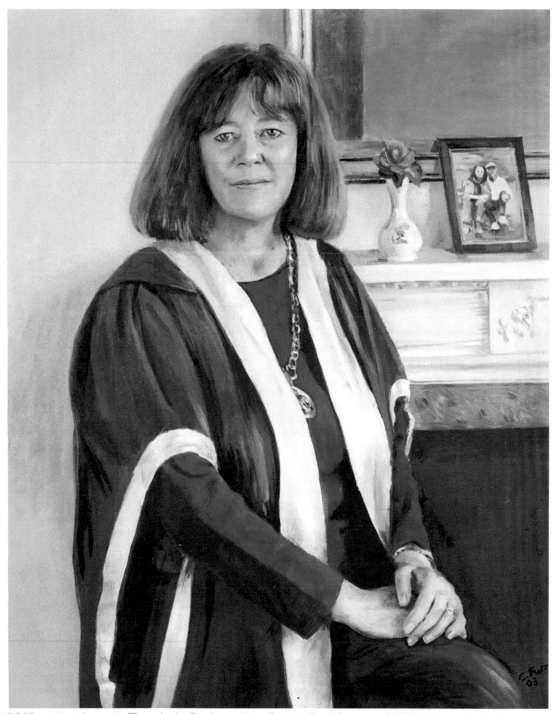

RCGP presidential portrait of Dame Lesley Southgate. Artist: Christian Furr. (Courtesy of RCGP Archives, London.)

European Union. The EBMA provides assessment for learning with detailed feedback for senior medical students and postgraduates in training. Dame Lesley's work with EBMA was an executive role and was the president of it from its creation until 15 November 2017. This is now an alliance of 14 medical schools committed to developing modern assessments for learning.

Dame Lesley's work in medical education and assessment has reached the furthest corners of the globe. In 2008, she was awarded the John P. Hubbard Award by the United States National Board of Medical Examiners (NBME) for her role in assessing competence and performance in physician practice. The Hubbard award is only given to individuals who have shown sustained, outstanding achievement. Shortly afterwards, in 2009, she was elected to be one of the very few international members on the board of the NBME. Other international work includes links with medical schools in Australia, Egypt, Ireland, Italy, the Netherlands and, where she plays a role supporting general practice assessment. In particular, she was given the title of Distinguished International Professor by the Medical Academy of St. Petersburg, Russia in 2002.

Dame Lesley states that one of her key roles and most unexpected experiences was her contribution as a curriculum lead in an European Union funded project based in Libya Civil War (2011). This project dealt with improving the quality of life for individuals affected by HIV, from the provision of drugs to the issue of stigma and lack of education. This project was stopped in 2011 due to the Libyan civil war. However, she has mentioned that one of her professional ambitions is to complete her work in Libya.

It is widely regarded that Dame Lesley is one of the modern-day greats of medical education, and has contributed to, and written, an abundance of papers and books over the years. This has been both as part of her various projects and individually. Some of these works include topics in the following: adolescent health, for example her work *Hot Topics in Adolescent Health: A Practical Manual for Working with Young People* (2001); peer assessment, for example her work on designing a peer feedback tool to assess Foundation Year doctors in the United Kingdom; professionalism, for example she has written many papers on professionalism in medical practice and how it should be assessed. She continues her work in these fields today and focuses her attentions on carrying out several roles. In 2016, she retired from her position as professor of medical education at St George's University of London (2004–2016), and now advises on assessment for the United Kingdom programme Modernising Scientific Careers. She is currently president of the EBMA, which she notes is her favourite role so far in the medical education field. In her spare time, she enjoys gardening, travelling and visiting her family in Calgary, Canada, where she now has two great grandchildren.

Further Reading

Archer J, Norcini J, Southgate L, Heard S, Davies H. Mini-PAT (Peer Assessment Tool): A valid component of a National Assessment Programme in the UK? *Advances in Health Sciences Education* 2006;13(2):181–92.

Bekaert S, Southgate L. *Hot Topics in Adolescent Health*. London: CRC Press; 2011.

Hilton S, Wiltsher C, Bligh J, Walsh K, Worthington R, Piele E et al. *Excellence in Medical Education: Values of Medical Educators*. London: Academy of Medical Educators; 2011.

Southgate L. James Mackenzie Lecture 1993. Freedom and discipline: Clinical practice and the assessment of clinical competence. *British Journal of General Practice* 1994;44(379):87–92.

Southgate L. Professional competence in medicine. *Hospital Medicine* 1999;60(3):203–5.

Southgate L, Cox J, David T, Hatch D, Howes A, Johnson N et al. The assessment of poorly performing doctors: The development of the assessment programmes for the General Medical Council's performance procedures. *Medical Education* 2001;35(s1):2–8.

Southgate L, Cox J, David T, Hatch D, Howes A, Johnson N et al. (2001). The General Medical Council's performance procedures: Peer review of performance in the workplace. *Medical Education* 2001;35(s1):9–19.

Southgate L, Dauphinee D. Continuing medical education: Maintaining standards in British and Canadian medicine: The developing role of the regulatory body. *British Medical Journal* 1998;316(7132):697–700.

Southgate L, Hays R, Norcini J, Mulholland H, Ayers B, Woolliscroft J et al. Setting performance standards for medical practice: A theoretical framework. *Medical Education* 2001;35(5):474–81.

Southgate L, Treharne J, Forsey T. Chlamydia trachomatis and Neisseria gonorrhoeae infections in women attending inner city general practices. *British Medical Journal* 1983;287(6396):879–81.

94 STUART CARNE (1926–)

Katherine Halford

Stuart John Carne was born on 19 June 1926 in London to Bernard and Millicent Carne, a bank manager and milliner respectively. He was educated at Willesden County Grammar School, North West London, in the Borough of Brent. He went on to study medicine at Middlesex Hospital Medical School, now a part of University College London, from where he graduated in 1950.

Carne's working career began as a house surgeon at Middlesex Hospital and he went on to become house physician, house surgeon and casualty officer at the Queen Elizabeth Hospital for Children in Bethnal Green. Before his career as a general practitioner, he became a Flight Lieutenant in the medical branch of the RAF (1952–1954), and it was there that he did his national service. His links with the RAF were maintained throughout his career, as he served a Civilian Medical Advisor.

Carne practised as a general practitioner in West London from 1954 to 1991. In 1957, he succeeded Aston Ridley Dale (1882–1957) in a single-handed practice at Goldhawk Road, West London. He made many changes to the practice, becoming one of the first to have a health visitor who was employed by the local health authority, something which became common place later on. Another change he brought in was working with local district nursing services within the surgery itself. As he took on three partners a change to a larger surgery was necessary and they moved to Grove Health Centre. The surgery was opened in 1967 by Kenneth Robinson, the then Minister of Health, and it is said that the surgery was a great success and a 'model of its kind'. The RCGP awarded him MRCGP in 1958 and FRCGP in 1970. Also in 1970 he was appointed senior tutor in general practice at the Royal Postgraduate Medical School in Hammersmith Hospital.

With the RCGP Carne has undertaken many different roles. He was a member of College (and later RCGP) Council between 1961 and 1991 and has held the posts of honorary treasurer (1964–1981), chairman of North London Faculty (1972–1973), chairman of the North and West London Faculty (1974–1977), provost (1977–1980 and 1994–1997) and president (1988–1991). In 1981, he delivered the 29th James Mackenzie Lecture entitled 'A problem halved?' This lecture traced the history of the development of the referral system in the United Kingdom and commented on the role of the second opinion as it affects the three parties concerned: the patient, the specialist and the general practitioner. He had a huge influence on the RCGP and one of his many achievements was leading the team involved in acquiring the RCGP buildings at 15 Princes Gate in 1976. The acquisition of this site is said to have been made achievable through his 'financial flair as treasurer', ensuring the funds were available for the new buildings. He is said to have visited the RCGP daily, whilst juggling his role as a police surgeon and a general practitioner.

Carne's long-term commitment to general practice has enabled him to be a member of the Standing Medical Advisory Committee (SMAC). The SMAC was a statutory advisory non-departmental public body which advised the health minister and Central Health Services on matters relating to services provided under the NHS Act of 1946. He did this for 14 years and was chairman of it from 1982 to 1986.

Carne has had influence not just in the medical world but also in football. In 1959, he became the Honorary Medical Officer to Queens Park Rangers Football Club and he held this post for 30 years until 1989 when he retired and became vice-president of the club.

Carne has had the opportunity to travel to many different countries as part of many of his posts during his career, particularly through his links to WONCA. This organisation works to help people throughout the world by promoting high standards of care, including respect for human rights and gender equality. Before WONCA was established in 1972, however, there was an interim organisation. In 1970, he was appointed as chair of the Finance Committee, charged to produce for the 1972 council of this organisation a method whereby WONCA could be established and maintained. He later became the president of WONCA between 1976 and 1978.

Alongside these important positions Carne received other awards and did much research. He was awarded the Foundation Council Award in 1975 before being appointed both OBE (1977) and CBE (1986). He has written numerous articles in *The Lancet* and *BMJ* amongst others but paediatrics has been a special interest for him and he authored the book *Paediatric Care: Child Health in Family Practice* (1976). This book was the first of a kind, and discussed both the benefits and advantages of caring for children locally in the community. Other publications include the *Handbook of Contraceptive Practice* (1974), and numerous research papers surrounding the importance of general practice and basing health care in the community.

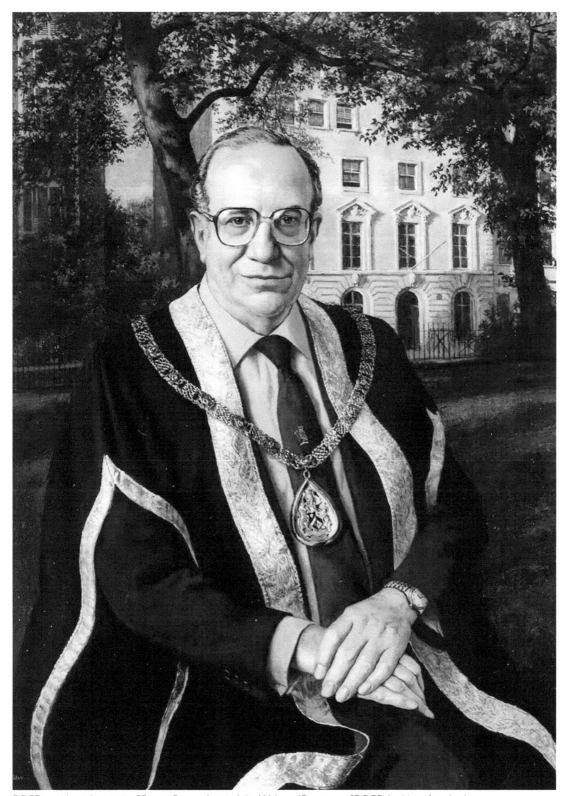

RCGP presidential portrait of Stuart Carne. Artist: John Walton. (Courtesy of RCGP Archives, London.)

Away from the medical world, Carne has interests in music, theatre, photography and stamp collecting. He particularly enjoys travelling to places such as Scotland so that he could obtain different editions of new stamp issues.

In terms of family life, he met his wife Yolande Cooper whilst at Middlesex Hospital Medical School, marrying in 1951. Yolande played a crucial role in his positions in office, not only by offering her constant support but also for her assistance in hosting many college functions, and her advice in the decoration and furnishing of the RCGP. They went on to have four children together.

Carne is loved by many, especially within the RCGP, and it was said on his retirement that 'his presence on Council will be missed as will his special sense of humour which has brightened so many conversations'. He has contributed a lot to general practice and his work within the RCGP has been a key contributor to its development.

Further Reading

Carne S. *Paediatric Care: Child Health in Family Practice*. Philadelphia, PA: Lippincott; 1976.

Carne S. General practitioner to a football club. *British Medical Journal* 1981;283:766–67.

Carne S. A problem halved? *The Journal of the Royal College of General Practitioners* 1982;32(234):10–31.

Donald A. Dr Stuart Carne. *Wonca News* 1992;18:iii–iv.

95 TERENCE JOHN KEMPLE (1952–)

Sohail A. Iftakhar

Terence (Terry) Kemple was born on 14 April 1952 in Cheltenham, Gloucestershire. He was the youngest of his parents' three children. He attended Whitefriars School (later renamed St. Edward's) in Cheltenham, and Belmont Abbey School in Hereford, for his early education. Initially, he had hoped to study science at university like his elder brother, Patrick. However, following his brother's advice, he opted to study medicine at Bristol Medical School.

During his time at medical school, Kemple developed a strong interest in general practice. He was particularly drawn towards its holistic approach and the personal nature of patient interactions. Upon graduating in 1975, he was, however, keen to explore other aspects of medicine before pursuing general practice. He gained additional qualifications in paediatrics and internal medicine in 1978 and 1980 respectively, before completing general practitioner training via the vocational training scheme. With regards to the RCGP, he was awarded MRCGP in 1981 and FRCGP in 1993. He was awarded FRCP in 2000.

Following locum appointments in Plymouth and Bristol, Kemple joined Horfield Health Centre in Bristol as a partner in 1982. Here he had a successful and fulfilling clinical career before retiring as senior partner in December 2015. Over this period, he accomplished many notable achievements: he helped in leading the Horfield Health Centre redevelopment programme, a multimillion-pound project to buy and redevelop the centre, as well as leading his practice to being given the RCGP Quality Practice Award three times. He commented that the key to attaining this prestigious level of recognition, of which only four practices nationally have achieved, was setting a shared goal with a realistic timeframe and sharing the burden of work fairly within the team. In addition to his role as a general practitioner, he has been involved in teaching medical students, training and appraising doctors and has led his practice's research interests through NHS funding.

During his career, Kemple travelled to many countries. This included Australia, New Zealand, the United States and Zambia. These had all been important formative experiences for his personal and professional development. During his time in the United States, he studied how to improve the performance of physicians, in particular the role of recertification. From this research, he concluded that recertification alone was not a sufficient means to assessing the provision of quality care; instead, emphasis should also be placed on assessing the process of recertification and its outcomes. He also contended that further research into the effectiveness of different forms of recertification was needed in order to establish a more meaningful and widely approved method for competency testing. Following this research, he was awarded the RCGP International Travel scholarship in 1995, which he used to travel to the WONCA world conference held in Hong Kong, where he led a workshop on recertification.

In 2012, following a friend's encouragement, Kemple decided to stand in the election for president of the RCGP. Having been unsuccessful in this attempt, he stood again for the role in 2015. He commented that, once upon a time, the RCGP was a visionary college which mapped an exciting future for general practice. However, he felt that it had become increasingly similar to that of a complacent corporation which mostly provided membership service. He believed that general practice was at a tipping point and that the RCGP reacted too little and too late to many of the contributors to this current crisis. During his campaign he stated that, if elected, he would prioritise a number of things which he felt needed improving: 'Reducing unnecessary workload for family doctors; increasing the general practitioner workforce by ensuring medical schools and the NHS are performance-managed to achieve the required number of general practitioners needed for the future; and finding the best ways to provide essential general practice efficiently and effectively and spread that best practice faster'. Another point that Kemple emphasised in his manifesto was to change the status of general practitioners from disease specialists, who have some knowledge of most diseases, to patient specialists, who understand the importance of everything that affects a patient. Through this proposed holistic awareness, the speciality would be able to deliver the high-quality, patient-centred, compassionate approach needed for excellent clinical care.

On 4 June 2015, the RCGP announced that Kemple was successful in his standing and was to be elected as its 24th President. Congratulating Kemple's appointment, RCGP Chief Executive and Returning Officer Neil Hunt (1954–) said: 'I am confident that the College will benefit greatly from his vast experience of general practice and providing excellent care to patients'.

Kemple announced that he would also use his presidency to promote the new Green Impact for Health project. The scheme started with a pilot in April 2015 and aims to help practices to improve their environmental, ethical and economic sustainability. He felt that this would in turn help practices to improve their efficiency, team morale and wellbeing. He continues to be the chair of this project after having completed his presidency of the RCGP in 2017. Away from

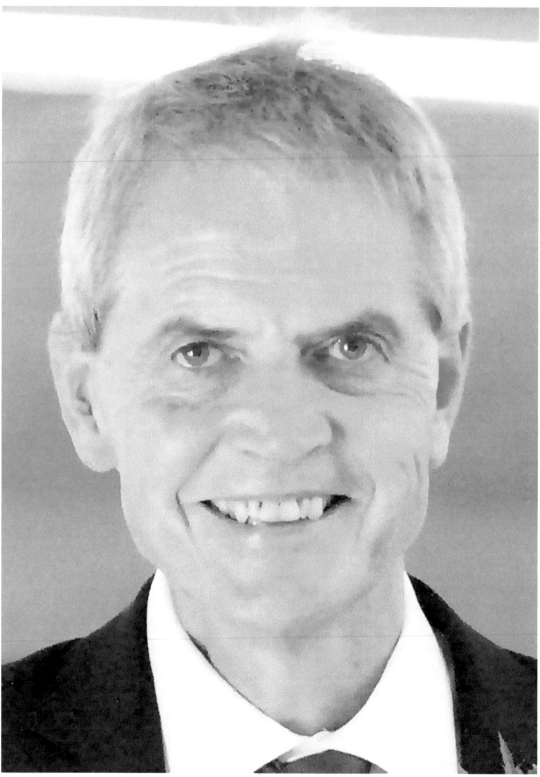

Terry Kemple. (Courtesy of Terry Kemple.)

the RCGP, he has roles as an appraiser and a general practice advisor for the National Institute for Health Research West of England Clinical Research Network.

In his spare time, Kemple has various hobbies and interests. He particularly enjoys running, often partaking in events including the London Marathon which he has completed three times. He also regularly updates his blog entitled *General Practice: Frequently Unasked Questions* (GPFUQ). Through this he encourages discussion on topics related to learning and quality improvement. He also enjoys spending time with his family. He lives with his wife, Rica Newbery (1951–), who has been awarded membership of the Royal College of Psychiatrists as well as MRCGP, whom he met during his time at medical school. Together, they have two children, Mariam and Maurice, both adopted as babies. Like their parents, they have chosen similar altruistic vocations: working towards humanitarian causes and entering the medical profession respectively.

Upon retiring from his work commitments altogether, Kemple intends to allow himself a 'gap year' with no particular plans other than discovering what emerges of interest. He remains open to the prospect of pursuing further opportunities which will allow him to advance his career.

Further Reading

Kemple T. Are UK revalidation proposals for GPs fit for purpose? *British Medical Journal* 2011;343(1):7906.

Kemple T. The Goldilocks problem in regulation. *British Medical Journal* 2016;354:3778.

96 LOTTE THERESE NEWMAN (1929–)
Fiona Watson

Lotte Therese Newman, second female president of the RCGP, was born in Germany in 1929 but like many Jewish families, the Neumanns left in 1938 to avoid the growing anti-Semitism and anti-Semitic legislation that had been accumulating since 1933. They settled in North London where Newman would go on to work in general practice from 1958 for more than 40 years. Both her mother, Tilly Meyet (1890–1966), and father, George Neumann (1900–1976), were general practitioners, although her mother stopped practising after she married, a factor that might have contributed to Newman's determined championship of women's place in medicine and general practice in particular. She not only worked tirelessly for equality for female practitioners but also for female patients. Her other major contribution to medicine was her international work. She became an important and well-known figure in the European medical community and was awarded the Baron Dr Ver Hayden de Lancey Memorial Award for advancing the status of general practice internationally in 1992. She was appointed OBE in 1991 and CBE in 1998 for her services to British general practice. Despite these astounding achievements she still found time to maintain a work–life balance with her husband, company director Norman Aronsohn and four children.

Never one to sit quietly on the sidelines, since she first became a member in 1967, Newman has been heavily involved with the work of the RCGP. Starting as an examiner in 1972, she then became secretary of the Board of Censors in 1981. Elected FRCGP in 1977 and a member of Council in 1980, she went on to do valuable work as provost of North East London Faculty (1982–1985) and vice-chair of the RCGP (1988–1989). Between 1994 and 1997 she was president of the RCGP. It was remarked that she was a very popular president and that her presidency was marked by both better attendances at RCGP meetings and involvement from younger members.

Further to her roles at the RCGP, Newman was also a member of the GMC in 1984 and medical director of St. John Ambulance for several years as well as being involved with the RAMC. She lectured on the RAMC course for the MRCGP, was invited to give the RAMC Sir David Bruce Lecture and was awarded the accompanying medal.

Newman originally entered the European medical scene in the mid-1980s as the British representative of the Societas Internationalis Medicinae Generalis (SIMG) of which she became the first female president. She was also later vice-president of the more recently founded European Society of General Practice (WONCA–Europe). The European medical environment had become increasingly crowded as WONCA's worldwide influence grew within Europe to match that of SIMG. There were also several other groups including the European Academy of Teachers in General Practice (EURACT), European General Practice Workshop (EGPRW) and European Working Party on Quality in Family Practice (EQuiP), whose activities were often in direct competition with WONCA. Amongst others Newman saw this duplication as a waste of effort and resources. Using her experience of SIMG and WONCA, she worked with Fons Sips (1940–2016), the subsequent president of SIMG, to bring them together.

Newman and Sips created and co-chaired the Group of Eight, a representative working party that laid the structural foundations for a new European organisation to be formed within WONCA but to include the work of SIMG and the other research groups. They first met in 1993, at the WONCA-SIMG congress in the Hague, and finally saw their goal accomplished at the first official council meeting of the WONCA–Europe and Family Medicine in 1995 on the morning of Friday 6 October in Strasbourg.

This pivotal role in the founding of the WONCA–Europe also meant Newman was heavily involved with the development of the *European Journal of General Practice*, its dedicated publication. In the first issue she expressed her joy saying:

> Now I have the privilege as president of the Royal College of General Practitioners, to welcome the existence of the new *European Journal of General Practice*, as a sister journal to our own *British Journal of General Practice*. I hope that the new journal will serve not only as an academic journal but also as a link between the growing family of general practice colleges and associations throughout Europe.

The involvement that Newman had in the international community continued for many years. She was awarded honorary fellowship of the Royal New Zealand College of General Practitioners for example. She often lectured internationally with visits including to countries such as Germany, Hungary, Switzerland and the United States. In 1996, she presented alongside Sips at the Baltic Conference on Family Medicine, talking about the successful alliance and future amalgamation of their organisations. Later still, at the WONCA conference in Vienna in 2000, she suggested and subsequently convened a special interest group on ethics in general practice.

In 1991, Newman was invited to give the 39th James MacKenzie Lecture and chose to focus on women's health and their place in the medical professions. The lecture was entitled 'Second among equals'. She spoke positively about the many crucial advances in medicine such as increased contraception, access to safe abortions, hormone

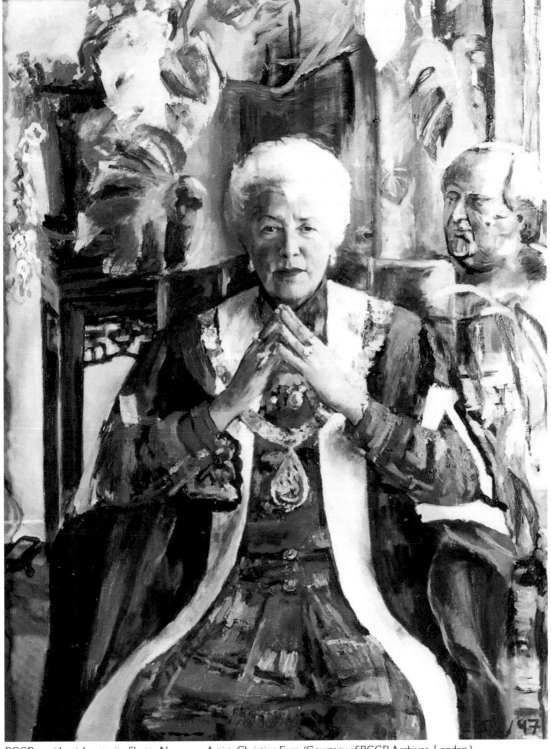

RCGP presidential portrait of Lotte Newman. Artist: Christian Furr. (Courtesy of RCGP Archives, London.)

replacement therapy and the Breast Screening Program that have combined to level opportunities career wise in general practice and emancipate women from the 'curses of our sex' and 'endless cycle of childbirth and child rearing'. However, she also emphasised that despite these advances inequality remained and women were, and are still, the greatest consumers of health care. Interestingly, her lecture 'Second among equals' was also given at a time when in almost half the practices in England, there was no female doctor. A far cry from today, when the RCGP have announced that 2009 was the first year in which over half of its membership were female.

Women's health remained one of Newman's key interests throughout her career. She was a member of the Department of Health and Social Security breast cancer screening advisory committee and spoke in favour of screening at a time when its future was still unsure. She also published many articles on breastfeeding and emotional problems in general practice. Her colleagues reported that she was also an excellent speaker and 'courageous in speaking at meetings, even on unpopular subjects'. She herself complained that as a woman there were only two options: 'if you speak out you're a shrieking harridan, if you keep quiet you're a shrinking violet'.

Similarly, Newman led discussions at the RCGP on 27 January 1995, along with members of the Royal College of Obstetricians and Gynaecologists, on 'The provision of emergency hormonal contraception'. Newman and the executive committee originally argued against the reclassification of emergency contraception from being a prescription-only medicine, to one offered over the counter at pharmacies. This was on the basis that women seeking emergency contraception often needed a more in-depth discussion of their options, which could be better provided in a general practitioner consultation than in public at the pharmacy. However, it was agreed that, on balance, wider availability was more important along with a need to maximise the drug's publicity and reclassification was approved.

Newman was vocal about the obstacles faced by female doctors and potential reforms to help the health services develop into a less biased system. She emphasised the 'glass ceiling' that prevented women rising in the most competitive specialities, including within obstetrics and gynaecology, as well as being elected to positions on the Royal Colleges' ruling councils and holding professorships at universities. Her explanation was simple: women are forced to choose between family life and their career. Reluctance to allow part-time work, insufficient and low paid maternity leave and lack of child care facilities all combined to make having children whilst pursuing a medical career as difficult as possible.

In 1987, Newman became president of the Medical Women's Federation and later chaired the 70th anniversary year conference on 'Women's Health and Work'. She later listed her involvement with the Federation as one of her proudest achievements. It is important to remember that whilst accomplishing all these things, she was still working 'at the coal face' in general practice, much of that at the Abbey Road Medical Centre in Kilburn, which she founded in 1968 along with Tony Antoniou (q. MBBS 1964). Under her presidency at the RCGP she pioneered the use of crèches at major RCGP events, a practice that, however insignificant it may seem, removed another barrier to particularly women's involvement with their profession and its governance. She worked to make the RCGP a more social and family orientated community and was herself an excellent hostess; organising many hugely successful events both for the RCGP and otherwise. In 2006 she was awarded the Foundation Council Award.

Outside of her work, Newman was a devout Jew and very devoted to her children and her husband, with whom she spent a great deal of time sailing around the Mediterranean. Despite her stunningly busy professional schedule she had no problem 'switching off' at the end of a day and had a great many hobbies. She learnt to horse ride in her 30s and to fly mostly small biplanes in her 40s. She was also a great art lover and collector; one of her children has gone on to become a successful artist and she gifted one of his bronzes to the RCGP. She attributed her remarkable success to 'luck, very good support from my family, being prepared to be unpopular at times – and always being at least as well prepared as the men at meetings!'

Further Reading

Hayden J. First among equals… Dr Lotte Newman OBE FRCGP. *British Journal of General Practice* 1998;48:938.

Newman L. James Mackenzie Lecture 1991: Second among equals. *British Journal of General Practice* 1992;42:71–74.

97 HAROLD SHIPMAN (1946–2004)
Daniel Ward

Harold Frederick Shipman was born on 14 January 1946 in Nottingham. The second of three children to working-class Methodist parents, he attended High Pavement Grammar School, where former teachers and fellow students remembered him as clever, confident, ambitious, strange and a loner. When 17 years old, his mother, Vera, died of lung cancer. He was very close to his mother and the young Shipman had helped nurse her through her illness, and saw first-hand the role of the general practitioner in providing care in a patient's final days, including the morphine injections he administered. In 1965, Shipman was accepted to study medicine at the University of Leeds. It was during his time at medical school that he, by his own admission, began abusing drugs, as well as meeting the woman that was to remain steadfastly by his side for the rest of his life, Primrose.

After graduating in 1970, Shipman's first employment as a doctor was at Pontefract Royal Infirmary. His first job as a general practitioner came in 1974, when he joined a practice in Todmorden, West Yorkshire. He soon developed a reputation as a caring and dedicated general practitioner, though he could be verbally sharp, even abusive, to junior members of staff. After concerns were raised by a local chemist about the number of prescriptions signed by Shipman for pethidine that came through his business, the doctor confessed to abusing the drug and to forging prescriptions to obtain a regular supply. He was dismissed from the practice but, having expressed remorse for his actions and a willingness to seek treatment, was fined £600 by magistrates for drug and forgery offences and allowed to maintain his place on the medical register. After a six-month period of rehabilitation, he took a position at a practice in Hyde, Greater Manchester. He remained there for 15 years until, in 1992, he fell out with fellow partners and left to start a single-handed practice close by. It is testament to his relationship with his patients that many followed him to his new premises.

In 1998, a general practitioner from another Hyde practice and the proprietors of a local funeral parlour reported concerns to the police about the disproportionately large number of cremation forms for elderly patients that Shipman had required to be countersigned. An investigation followed and, with no evidence found of wrongdoing on the doctor's part, largely due to the falsifying of records to create bogus medical histories, no further action was taken. On 24 June 1998, several hours after Shipman had visited her in her home, the lifeless body of 81-year-old Kathleen Grundy was found. Shipman was summoned and, reportedly not finding her death to be unexpected, signed the death certificate with 'old age' as the primary cause. To her friends and family, Mrs Grundy's passing came as a complete shock. Despite her advanced years, she was fit and active and, to those who saw her in her final days, in good spirits. When Grundy's will was opened it was discovered that she had left her entire fortune, a sum of around £386,000 to Shipman. Grundy's daughter, a solicitor, could not accept her mother would act in such a fashion and, finding the will and its accompanying letter to be poorly typewritten and in phraseology she did not recognise as that used by her mother, contacted the police. Mrs Grundy's body was exhumed and large amounts of diamorphine was found in her system. A search of Shipman's premises revealed the typewriter that had been used to forge the will and, on 7 September 1998, Shipman was arrested, interviewed and charged with the murder of Mrs Grundy and with other offences associated with the forgery.

A large-scale investigation followed, looking into a number of deaths of elderly patients that had occurred shortly after Shipman had conducted a home visit. Further exhumations took place and, when traces of diamorphine were found, more charges were brought. When the news broke, many of his patients refused to believe their dedicated general practitioner could be guilty of such horrific crimes. The news led to a number of people coming forward with suspicions regarding their own family member's deaths over the previous two decades.

In January 2000, Shipman was convicted on 15 counts of murder and was sentenced to life imprisonment. A subsequent inquiry by Dame Janet Smith found he had unlawfully killed 215 of his patients over a 23-year period from March 1975 to June 1998. At his most prolific, between 1995 and 1997, Shipman killed between 30 and 37 elderly patients a year. It is unlikely the true number of victims will ever be known but rational estimates range from 250 to 300.

'Each of your victims was your patient', commented Mr Justice Forbes upon sentencing Shipman, '[and] you murdered each and every one of your victims by a calculated and cold-blooded perversion of your medical skills'. The Judge went on to add: 'I have little doubt that each of your victims smiled and thanked you as [they] submitted to your deadly administrations'. Shipman showed no emotion when the verdict was announced. He made no further comment on the crimes and offered no explanation for them. His motives remain unknown.

On the morning of 13 January 2004, Shipman was discovered dead in his cell at Wakefield Prison. He had committed suicide by hanging himself with his bed sheets.

Shipman left a wife, Primrose, and four children. Primrose had met Shipman as a shy 16 year old during his first year at medical school and became pregnant within a few months. She was to remain loyally by his side throughout his career, trial and imprisonment. For a short time, Primrose had worked as his receptionist and even accompanied

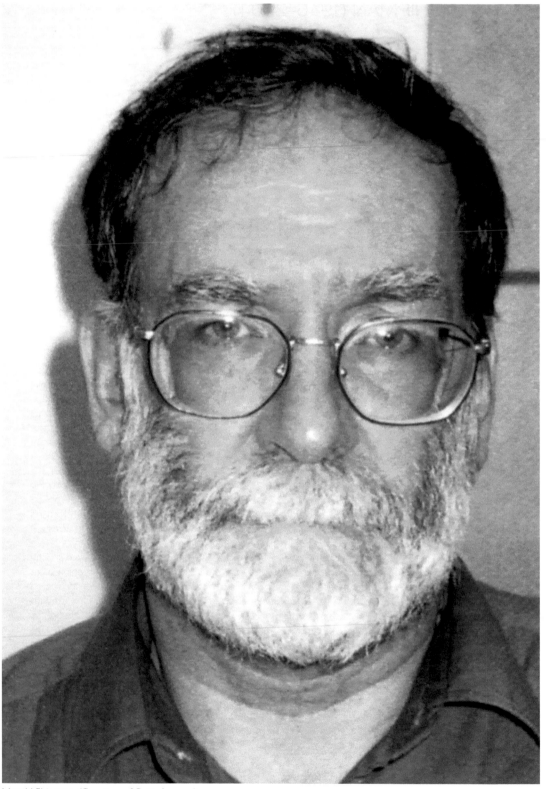

Harold Shipman. (Courtesy of Getty Images.)

him as he made house calls, waiting outside in the car as he murdered his victims. There is no suggestion that Primrose knew anything of her husband's crimes and she has not spoken publicly about them or offered any insight as to his motivations.

The case of Shipman had far-reaching implications for general practice and the wider medical landscape. Dame Janet Smith made clear in her report that the arrangements in place at that time for death registration, cremation certifications and coronial investigation in England and Wales were inadequate and had failed to either prevent Shipman's crimes nor detect them once they had taken place. New regulations for cremation certification, requiring a second practitioner to question the doctor who had originally completed the form, as well as speaking to any relatives and, if necessary, someone who had cared for the patient in their final illness, came into force in January 2009. These regulations also established the Medical Examiner's Office to provide better scrutiny of death certification, to collate and analyse data on causes of death and to provide advice to Coroners. Revalidation was introduced by the GMC in 2012 and, whilst not directly linked to the Shipman case, aims to highlight doctors for whom there are issues regarding fitness to practice. Whether revalidation would have prevented his crimes, or detected them earlier, remains a contentious issue.

Shipman murdered over 200 of his patients. He was not the first doctor to kill, and is unlikely to be the last, but it is heartening to remember that, in a number of surveys conducted since Shipman's horrific crimes, the trust people have in their doctors remains the highest across all professions.

Further Reading

Jackson T, Smith R. Obituary. *British Medical Journal* 2004:328:231.

Peters C. *Harold Shipman: Mind Set on Murder*. London: André Deutsch; 2006.

Smith J (Chmn.). *The Shipman Inquiry. (Reports 1 to 6)*. Norwich: Stationery Office; 2002–2005.

Whittle B, Ritchie J. *Harold Shipman: Prescription for Murder*. London: Little, Brown Book Group; 2000.

98 LIAM FOX (1961–)

Collette Isabel Stadler and Lukas Kurt Josef Stadler

The Right Honourable Liam Fox is a British MP for the Conservative Party as well as a member of the RCGP. Born in East Kilbride, Scotland, on 22 September 1961, he is of Irish Catholic descent and one of four siblings. At five years of age he stopped wanting to be a train driver and decided to become a doctor. He attended St. Bride's High School, East Kilbride, then Europe's largest school, before reading medicine at the University of Glasgow Medical School. It was during his time at university that his interest in politics grew. As such he held positions on the University Students' Representative Council, was a member of the Dialectic Society and became president of the University of Glasgow Conservative Association. Today, he is considered to be at the right edge of Conservatism and a foreshadowing of his political position came when he vocally supported the university union's opposition to letting the gay student's union join its ranks.

Following his graduation with MBChB in 1983, Fox undertook a number of junior doctor roles. During the infamous 'ice cream wars' in the 1980s in Glasgow, he was the casualty officer receiving victims of a ghastly arson attack. 'A family was effectively barricaded inside a house and it was set on fire', he recalled. 'I had never seen people horrendously burnt before. Something like that brings things into focus. I often think people in Westminster have an odd idea of a crisis. A crisis is not somebody saying something unpleasant about you in a newspaper'. He went into general practice training, and by the time he was 25 years old, he had become a general practice partner at Millbarn Surgery in Beaconsfield, Buckinghamshire.

However, Fox had spiritually and aspirationally begun to move towards Westminster. Firstly, he unsuccessfully contested a seat in his local council. A year later at the general election in 1987, he stood as a Conservative for the Roxburgh and Berwickshire seat but lost to the Liberals' Archy Kirkwood. A professional move away from hostile political territory to the Conservative-friendly South West, where he worked as a general practitioner and as a civilian army medical officer, finally brought success in the 1992 parliamentary elections, winning the seat of Woodspring, now North Somerset. Quickly gaining a reputation as an astute networker and for his sociable demeanour, he made friends easily. Outside of politics this included with the Australian singer Natalie Imbruglia, who thanked Fox on the inside cover of her debut album *Left of the Middle* (1997). He held a number of governmental positions in John Major's administration including being appointed a Senior Government Whip in November 1995 and between 1996 and 1997 as a Parliamentary Under Secretary of State at the Foreign and Commonwealth Office. During this role in 1996, he negotiated an agreement in the Civil War in Sri Lanka (1983–2009), called the Fox Peace Plan, which gained him recognition across party political boundaries.

Fox was Conservative Party Chairman from 2003 to 2005 but also during the Conservatives' time in opposition he served as Shadow Secretary of State for Health from 1999 to 2003. In this later role he drew on his experiences as a junior doctor and general practitioner to play an important role in shaping the 'Patient Passports' policy of his party. This scheme was designed to reduce waiting lists and give patients more freedom and control over where they would undergo an operation. Praised by its supporters for putting patients' interests first, it was criticised by its detractors for adding to the NHS's financial burden and promoting the private health care sector.

Following the Conservatives' third defeat to Tony Blair in 2005, Fox made apparent his ambitions for the very top of politics when he ran for the leadership of the Conservative Party, a contest he lost to David Cameron with David Davis coming second. Whilst politically defeated, he enjoyed more success in his private life, when in December that same year he married his long-term partner Jesme Baird (1968–), a fellow alumna of Glasgow Medical School.

During Cameron's time as leader of the opposition Fox was promoted to shadow Defence Secretary (2005–2010) and subsequently became Defence Secretary when the Conservatives entered the coalition government in 2010. His political success of this period was somewhat clouded by negative media attention as a result of his involvement in the expenses scandal and a clear case of nepotism during his tenure at the helm of the Ministry of Defence, which resulted in his eventual resignation as Defence Secretary. Those blemishes to his personal integrity notwithstanding, he remained a darling of the Conservative right by being a staunch supporter for the United Kingdom's exit from the European Union (EU) and having a vocal stance against abortion as well as same sex marriage, the latter at the time a central pillar of Cameron's social policy.

After his resignation as Defence Secretary and return to the backbenches, Fox dedicated time to furthering several charitable activities. A particular interest of his is the provision of mental health care to returning military personnel, a cause which fuses both his medical background as well as his experiences as Defence Secretary. He also wrote *Rising Tides: Facing the Challenges of a New Era* (2013) in which he argued that that world's institutions are not equipped for the economic and security challenges of the twenty-first century.

Following several years outside the public eye Fox made a return to the political limelight in 2016 as an ardent supporter of the campaign to leave the EU in that year's referendum on the matter. Buoyed by his campaign's success

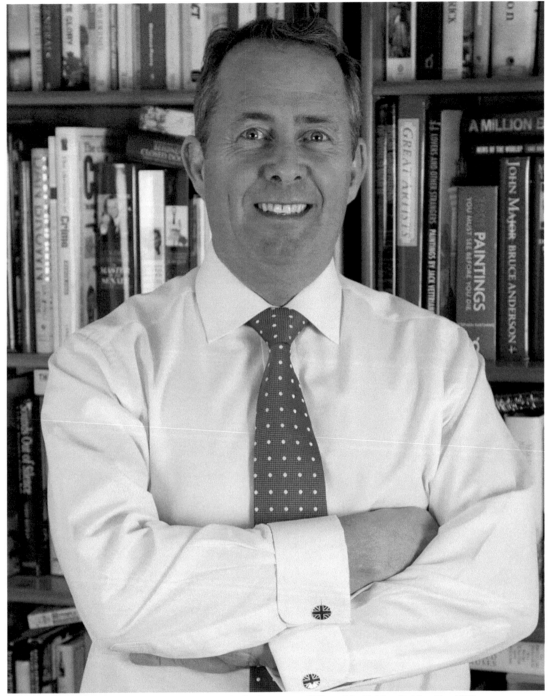

Liam Fox. (Courtesy of Ione Douglas, secretary at the Parliamentary Office of the Rt Hon Dr Liam Fox MP.)

and his resultant personal political boost, he again decided to stand in the Conservative leadership election, which was triggered by Cameron's resignation in the aftermath of the plebiscite. Whilst unsuccessful in his endeavour, he returned to the government's front benches under Theresa May's leadership, this time in the newly created post of Secretary of State for International Trade (2016–), thus tasked with forging new trade deals for the United Kingdom of Great Britain and Northern Ireland outside its membership of the EU. At the same time he is President of the Board of Trade (2016–).

Away from his earlier general practice career, Fox has had various interests including swimming, tennis and visiting the pub and the theatre to relax. He used to abseil, and once 'walked' on the wings of a plane for charity. He lives in Tickenham, North Somerset with his wife.

Thus, Fox, the general practitioner from a small Scottish town, has become a figure with significant power and influence over how the future of this country is shaped. Posterity will tell and historians will judge the value and benefit of his achievements as a committed public servant.

Further Reading

Craig O. Is this the Tories' First Lady-in-waiting? *The Telegraph* 2005; 2 October.

Grice E. A dose of Dr Fox's medicine. *The Telegraph* 2003; 29 September.

Harris D, Lister S. Who is Liam Fox? The right-wing Tory back in government just five years after resigning in disgrace. *Independent* 2016; 14 July.

Telegraph Reporters. Who is Liam Fox? Meet the new Secretary of State for International Trade. *The Telegraph* 2016; 14 July.

99 RICHARD BUDGETT (1959–)

Mason McGlynn and Neil Metcalfe

Richard Gordon McBride Budgett was born on 20 March 1959, in Glasgow. Having attended secondary school at Radley College, he entered Selwyn College, University of Cambridge, in 1977, to study medicine. Here, he was to add his name to the canon of great Selwyn oarsmen, competing as a member of the Hermes Club. Having completed his clinical years at Middlesex Hospital, University of London, he graduated in 1983, shortly before being selected for the British Olympic rowing crew.

Competing with Steven Redgrave, Martin Cross, Andy Holmes and Adrian Ellison in the Los Angeles 1984 Olympic Games, the British crew secured victory over the United States in the Coxed Fours event, in what proved an extremely close race. The British boat pulled ahead in the final 500 meters and emerged victorious by a margin of less than two seconds. At 25 years old, he had won Olympic gold, and in doing so helped to secure for Great Britain the highest rowing honour bestowed upon it since eventual general practitioner Ran Laurie (1915–1998) and Jack Wilson, Cambridge oarsmen themselves, had won gold at the London 1948 Olympic Games. Returning home following his victory, he began training as a general practitioner, with a view to entering the burgeoning field of sports medicine. In 1989, after completing three years of general practitioner training based at Northwick Park Hospital and the North West London vocational training scheme, he undertook a Master in Sports and Science Medicine at Queen Mary University of London, doing it part time at the same time as general practitioner partnership at Acton, West London. Continuing to coalesce his passions for medicine and sport, Budgett was appointed medical officer at the British Olympic Medical Centre in 1989 but continued as a general practitioner partner until 2004.

Following this, Budgett attended the 1992 and 1994 Winter Olympic Games in Albertville and Lillehammer respectively, as the doctor for the British bobsleigh team. In 1994, he was appointed the director of Medical Services at the British Olympic Association, and chairman of the Association's Medical Committee, posts he would hold until 2007. Remaining deeply involved in international sport, he has continued to faithfully attend both summer and winter games ever since. He served as Chief Medical Officer to the British team (Team GB) for the 1998, 2004 and 2006 Winter Olympic Games, held in Nagano, Salt Lake City and Turin respectively. In addition, he led the Team GB medical team at Atlanta 1996, Sydney 2000 and Athens 2004 Summer Games. In 2003, he was appointed lead sports physician for the southeast region of the English Institute of Sport, and in the same year he was appointed OBE for his services to sports.

In 2005, Budgett was appointed to the World Anti-Doping Agency list committee, which he chaired from 2010 to 2012. The same year, he returned to rowing in a professional capacity, becoming the doctor to the Team GB Rowing team, supporting the team through to their powerful performance in the Beijing 2008 Olympic Games. Team GB Rowing finished in Beijing with six medals, topping the leaderboard in an unprecedented victory. In 2007, he was elected to the council of the Faculty of Sports and Exercise Medicine, and in 2008 he was made chairman of the British Association of Sports and Exercise Medicine. Having published and lectured widely throughout his career, with a particular interest in athlete overtraining, he was awarded FRCP in 2011. The same year, he became a consultant physician in Sports and Exercise Medicine, based at the University College London Hospitals. In doing so, he registered to practise both as a general practitioner and a specialist.

In 2007, Budgett was appointed Chief Medical Officer of the London 2012 Olympic Games. This role meant overseeing all medical and anti-doping services. The London 2012 Olympic Games marked his 12th Olympic appearance, either as an olympian or doctor. Prior to his service at the London 2012 Olympic Games, he was tipped to succeed Patrick Schamasch (1947–) as the medical and scientific director of the International Olympic Committee, a post Schamasch had held for over 20 years. A strong anti-doping advocate, and indeed an expert consultant to the World Anti-doping Agency on prohibited substances, Budgett's remit in this new role extends to entail wider medical and anti-doping responsibilities within the Olympic Federation.

In 2015, Budgett was awarded HRH Prince Philip, Duke of Edinburgh himself, on behalf of the Institute of Sports and Exercise Medicine, in recognition of his outstanding contribution to Sports and Exercise Medicine. He received the accolade in the presence of his wife, Sue, and children. This endowment, only the third since the inception of the Institute in 1958, afforded him the opportunity to remark upon his plans for the future. In his address, he outlined his work with the International Olympic Committee, and his ongoing support for the Active Cities program, an initiative dedicated to addressing growing public health concerns over inactivity in industrialised nations. Budgett, through the vehicle of the International Olympic Committee, remains dedicated to enshrining the benefits of sporting activity, for all.

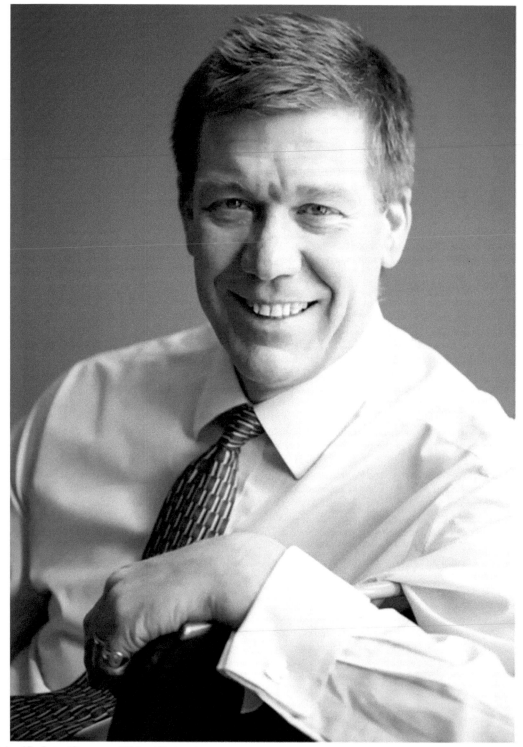

Richard Budgett. (Courtesy of Richard Budgett.)

Further Reading

Budgett R. The road to success in international rowing. *British Journal of Sports Medicine* 1989;23(1):49–50.

Budgett R. Overtraining syndrome. *British Journal of Sports Medicine* 1990;24(4):231–36.

Budgett R. The role of the British Olympic Association. *British Journal of Sports Medicine* 1996;30(2):80–81.

00 STEPHANIE COOK (1972–)
Neil Metcalfe

Stephanie Jayne Cook was born to Paul and Valerie Cook on 7 February 1972 at Irvine, North Ayrshire, in Scotland. She attended Bedford High School and then The Perse School for Girls, Cambridge. During her schooling she was a keen sportswoman particularly excelling in hockey and cross-country. She read medicine at Peterhouse, University of Cambridge (1991–1994) before completing her degree at Lincoln College, University of Oxford (1994–1997).

During her time at the university, Cook continued her sporting interests. During her time at Peterhouse she rowed for the university lightweight crew before a stress fracture of a rib affected her winter training regimen whilst president of the club. It was after reading a poster on a college bulletin board in 1995 that she first became aware of, and eventually joined, the Oxford University Modern Pentathlon Association (OUMPA). Based on the exploits of an heroic army officer evading capture, the sport at the time incorporated the five diverse events of pistol shooting, epee fencing, 200 metres freestyle swimming, show jumping on an unfamiliar horse and a 3000 metres cross-country run. Having been involved in her local pony club as a child and been a runner at the University of Cambridge she was already skilled in two of the events and as a capable swimmer had experience in the third. Although she was a novice at shooting and fencing, she quickly became adept at both. She became president of the Oxford University Modern Pentathlon Association for the 1995 to 1996 academic year and then won the women's individual title in the varsity match against the University of Cambridge in 1997. In addition to her training with OUMPA, she also represented University of Oxford at cross-country, athletics and fencing, and went on to win the National Modern Triathlon Championships in 1996, the National Modern Tetrathlon Championships in 1999 and the National Modern Biathlon Championships in 2000.

After university and national sporting honours, international honours soon followed for Cook. She was selected to represent Great Britain at the modern pentathlon European Championships in Moscow but the dates clashed with her medical finals and so she was unable to participate in the event. Her house officer jobs were completed in Poole and then Oxford and during these roles she won a silver medal in the Women's Team event at the 1998 World Championships in Mexico City as well as a bronze medal in the Women's Team Relay. She was also the highest placed British competitor gaining eighth place in the individual event. This overall performance helped her become eligible to receive Lottery funding in the run up to the Sydney 2000 Olympic Games. Her training for this went full-time after conducting vascular surgery research with Mark Whiteley (1962–) from August 1998 to November 1999 at Guildford. This training occurred at the University of Bath, which was the home of the new National Training Centre for Modern Pentathlon. On looking back at this stage of her career she mentioned 'It was a huge risk to put my medical career on hold as I had no guarantees that my sporting career would be successful, but the fear of failure has never stopped me from trying, and I believe that if you are determined enough then you will find a way to achieve your dreams'. In 1999, she won team relay gold and team silver at the World Championships in Budapest as well as team silver at the European Championships in Tampere, Finland. The following year at the World Championships in Pesaro, Italy, there were team relay and team silvers and at the European Championships in Székesfehérvár, Hungary, she won individual silver, team relay gold and team silver. In the World Cup series she came first in the individual event in Mexico, which meant that she had qualified for the Sydney 2000 Olympic Games later that year.

The modern pentathlon competition at the Sydney 2000 Olympic Games was on the last day of the Games. All five of the events occurred within a 10-hour period on 1 October 2000. Out of the competitors, her teammate and training partner Kate Allenby and United States' Emily de Reil, who was a fellow OUMPA member, were well known to her. Going into the final round de Reil had not been out of a medal position and Cook, despite recording a personal best in the swimming, was trailing in eighth place but was still in touch with the leaders. The 3000 m cross-country run was the final event. Modern pentathlon uses a staggered start, with starting positions to reflect the points differential after four events. Cook was to start 49 seconds behind de Reil. However, running was known not to be de Reil's strong point, whereas Cook had regularly finished a minute faster than any other international competitor in previous competitions. In an exciting race which brought the stadium to its feet, she passed the leader, de Riel, with just 250 m to go, crossing the line in 10 minutes 3 seconds, which was an event time 51 seconds faster than de Riel and meant she clinched the gold by eight points, winning with a total of 5318 points. De Reil and Allenby won silver and bronze respectively. As she crossed the line Cook made history in being the first woman to win Olympic gold in modern pentathlon and her life would never be quite the same again.

Following her Olympic gold medal, Cook received many awards and had further golden sporting success. She was awarded *The Sunday Times* Sportswoman of the year 2000 and then won additional gold medals at both the 2001 World and European Championships in Millfield, England and Sofia, Bulgaria respectively. This included World golds in the individual, team relay and team events as well as European golds in the individual and team events, together with a team relay bronze. That year she received the Great Britain Sports Writers Association Sportswoman of The Year,

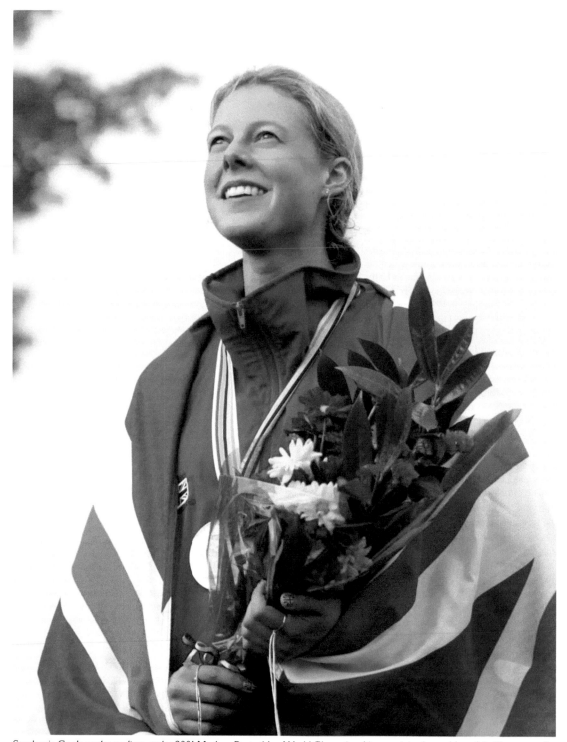

Stephanie Cook on the podium at the 2001 Modern Pentathlon World Championships receiving her gold medal. (Courtesy of Matchtight.)

the *Sunday Times* Helen Rollason Award for inspiration and these, in combination with simultaneously holding the European, World and Olympic titles, a rarity in British sportsmen and women, was why it was a surprise to many when she retired from the sport at 29 years of age. On the timing of her retirement, she mentioned 'it was never a question of if I would return to medicine, just a matter of finding the right time, and what better time to bow out than at the top of your game – I had nothing more that I could achieve'. In the same year she was appointed MBE for services to sport.

The resumption of Cook's medical career occurred very quickly after her last event. A week after her retirement from pentathlon she travelled as an ambassador of the medical charity Merlin which helped treat the victims of the Gujuarat earthquake in India. On returning to the United Kingdom, she undertook a surgical training rotation in Bath and was awarded MRCS in 2003. Time as an Ear Nose Throat (ENT) registrar followed in the South West of England and she was awarded an honorary fellowship from Lincoln College, University of Oxford, in 2005. During a period of maternity leave, in which in 2008 she was awarded MD from the University of Bath, she felt it was right to move to general practice. A place on the Brighton and mid-Sussex general practitioner Training Programme was commenced in August 2008. She completed her general practice training and awarded her MRCGP in 2012. Posts as a general practitioner with a specialist interest in ENT and as a general practitioner locum followed before a partnership at Ship Street surgery in East Grinstead, Sussex was commenced in 2014.

Away from medicine Cook is married to Dan Carroll, an equine vet, and has two sons, Oliver and William. She is, or has been, Patron to Merlin, Helen Rollason Cancer Charity, SportsAid, Access Sport, Against Malaria Foundation, Crimestoppers Trust and Bedfordshire Rural Communities Charity. She has not ceased her sporting involvement completely, however, for she was an ambassador for the London 2012 Olympic Games bid and then a member of the athletes committee for the London Organising Committee of the Olympic and Paralympic Games. She was a foundation member of the Faculty of Sport and Exercise medicine established in July 2007, and in 2008 took part in the 'Excellence in Health – The Olympic Ideal' conference organised by the BMA. She commentated for the BBC at the Athens 2004, London 2012 and Rio de Janeiro 2016 Olympics Games. In November 2016, she was amongst the first 10 athletes to be inducted into the prestigious Union Internationale de Pentathlon Moderne Hall of Fame. She continues to enjoy running and riding over the Ashdown Forest near to her home.

Further Reading

Union Internationale de Pentathlon Moderne. *Annual Yearbook*. Monte Carlo, Monaco: Union Internationale de Pentathlon Moderne; 2014–16.

INDEX